MEDICAL ETHICS

Edited by

Robert M. Veatch

Kennedy Institute of Ethics
Georgetown University

Jones and Bartlett Publishers
Boston • London

Editorial, Sales and Customer Services Offices

Jones and Bartlett Publishers
One Exeter Plaza
Boston, MA 02116

Jones and Bartlett Publishers Int'l
P.O. Box 1498
London W6 7RS
England

Library of Congress Cataloging-in-Publication Data
Medical ethics.
   Includes bibliographies.
   1. Medical ethics. I. Veatch, Robert M.
R724.M2927 1989 174'.2 88-28462
ISBN 0-86720-074-X

Printed in the United States of America
10 9 8 7 6 5 4

Production   Michael Bass & Associates
Cover and text design   Rafael Millán

ISBN 0-86720-074-X

Publisher's   Note:

A book of readings, entitled *Cross Cultural
Perspectives in Medical Ethics: Readings*
(ISBN: 0-86720-075-8), edited by Robert
M. Veatch is available from Jones and Bartlett
Publishers to accompany *Medical Ethics*.

PREFACE

Ethical problems in medicine and the biological sciences have, in the past few years, exploded into the public consciousness at an exponential rate. Partly this is a result of new, increasingly complex technologies: ventilators, artificial kidney machines, new life-saving medications, and transplant technologies. Partly it is a result of increasing access to existing medical services brought on by better insurance. Partly it comes from increased public awareness of medical decisions that have always been made in the privacy of the health professional's conscience.

Underlying all of these developments is an increasingly complex set of ethical and other value choices that must be made by patients and their agents, by public officials such as judges and legislators, as well as by health professionals. We now recognize that someone must decide whether to stop a ventilator on a patient who has suffered a stroke and will never again regain consciousness. A choice must be made whether it is morally appropriate to abort a pregnancy when a genetic test reveals a disease incompatible with life. A decision must be made about who will get a scarce piece of biomedical equipment like a bed in an intensive care unit when there are more persons in need than there are beds.

It was once thought that these were "medical" choices in the sense that they should be made by people with medical expertise, perhaps on the assumption that we should, as a society, do everything we can to prolong life as long as possible and that people with medical expertise were the ones best equipped to determine how life could be prolonged. The prolongation life of the permanently unconscious octogenarian and the controversy over the justification of abortion make clear, however, that not everyone believes that it is automatically morally correct to prolong life in all circumstances.

Moreover, many continuing ethical problems in health care have nothing to do with prolonging life. They involve problems of privacy and confidentiality, consent, disclosure of critical illness or contagious disease, or problems in psychiatry. It is becoming increasingly clear that different ethical positions will lead to different conclusions about what is morally appropriate in these circumstances. Someone committed to an ethic emphasizing liberty may well come to a different conclusion than someone committed to maximizing patient welfare or someone committed to the priority of equality in allocating resources. There is no reason to assume that being skilled in medical science will make one an expert in choosing among these basic philosophical and ethical positions.

Medical ethics is now, as never before, for everyone: for patients, parents and other family members, public officials, and educators as well as for health professionals. Among health professionals it is for nurses, pharmacists, dentists, social workers, and chaplains as well as for physicians.

As these ethical issues and responsibilities emerged in the 1970s, articles on specific issues began appearing with increasing frequency. Some adventuresome critics began writing whole volumes on the issues of medical ethics. Others, recognizing the enormousness of the field, began collecting together essays by others or excerpts of such essays to publish as anthologies and readers.

Medical ethics in a way has paralleled the development of medicine more generally. Now only the most ambitious, some would say immodest, author would attempt to write a textbook of medicine, surgery, or the other clinical sciences. The most authoritative volumes are now produced by large teams of authors, each a specialist in some aspect of medicine. Even books in the basic medical sciences are now routinely authored by large groups with each author writing on an area in which he or she has specialized.

It is time for the field of medical ethics to be approached in the same way as medical science if we are to have authoritative, critical examinations of the issues inherent in its various subspecialties. This volume brings together for the first time the leading authorities in medical ethics wherein each has developed a survey of the most critical issues in major subareas of the field. For each chapter a leading scholar has developed a discussion of the critical concepts, arguments, and positions of an aspect of medical ethics and its state-of-the-art. The combined result is a level of discussion that represents the current state of the debate in medical ethics within a format accessible to the undergraduate or graduate student. Each chapter begins with a summary and concludes with a set of questions for further exploration of the issues. A glossary of terms is included at the back of the book.

This volume is a cooperative project with many of the authors not only writing their own chapters but reading and commenting upon other chapters. A number of reviewers and colleagues also have read and provided helpful comments on single chapters or the entire volume. Several people deserve special mention for their help in the preparation of the manuscript. Joseph Burns, the editor at Jones and Bartlett, has been very supportive and patient throughout. Carol Mason and Karen Roberts have provided research and editing assistance and Denise Brooks, Michelle Lewis, and Nancy Martin have helped in manuscript preparation. To them I and the other authors owe our gratitude.

Every reader, whether a health professional or a responsible decisionmaker about his or her own health, is encouraged to explore the importance of different ethical positions in deciding what counts as responsible medical choices.

CONTRIBUTORS' LIST

CHAPTER 1
Robert M. Veatch is Professor of Medical Ethics at Georgetown University's Kennedy Institute of Ethics; Professor of Philosophy at Georgetown University; Adjunct Professor, Departments of Community and Family Medicine, and Obstetrics and Gynecology at the Georgetown University School of Medicine.

CHAPTER 2
James F. Childress is Professor of Religious Studies at the University of Virginia.

CHAPTER 3
Arthur L. Caplan is Director of the Center for Bioethics at the University of Minnesota.

CHAPTER 4
Howard Brody is a member of the Department of Human Development, at the Michigan State University College of Human Medicine, East Lansing.

CHAPTER 5
Judith Areen is Professor of Law at the Georgetown University Law Center; and Professor of Community and Family Medicine at the Georgetown University School of Medicine.

CHAPTER 6
A. M. Capron is Norman Topping Professor of Law, Medicine and Public Policy at the University of Southern California. He gratefully acknowledges the support of the USC Law Center faculty summer research fund, and the assistance of Tami Byram, Class of 1989.

CHAPTER 7
Tom L. Beauchamp is Professor of Philosophy at Georgetown University, and Senior Research Scholar at the Georgetown University Kennedy Institute of Ethics.

CHAPTER 8

LeRoy Walters is Director of the Center for Bioethics at Georgetown University's Kennedy Institute of Ethics.

CHAPTER 9

Albert R. Jonsen is Professor of Ethics in Medicine and Chairman of Biomedical History at the University of Washington School of Medicine.

CHAPTER 10

Loretta M. Kopelman is Professor of Humanities and Chair of the Department of Medical Humanities at the East Carolina University School of Medicine.

CHAPTER 11

Allen Buchanan is Professor of Philosophy at the University of Arizona.

CHAPTER 12

Dan Brock is a member of the Department of Philosophy at Brown University.

CONTENTS

1

Medical Ethics: An Introduction

Robert M. Veatch

SUMMARY

Ethics is the enterprise of disciplined reflection on the moral intuitions and moral choices that people make. Medical ethics is the analysis of choices in medicine. As used in this volume, medicine refers to the entire range of choices made in the medical sphere. Medical ethics covers not only choices made by physicians, but also by other health professionals—nurses, pharmacists, hospital chaplains, and so forth. More importantly, it covers choices made by medical lay people—patients, parents, legislators, public officials, and judges.

Chapter one provides an introduction to the more or less well-thought-out views about the ethics of medical choices, what could be called basic theories or systems in medical ethics. The chapter also surveys the history of medical ethical systems and the traditions of medical professionals that have gained prominence in the West. The most well-known of these is the Hippocratic Oath; the medical tradition based on the Hippocratic Oath has given rise to several professional ethical codes in modern times and they are discussed in the chapter. Also, the origin and development of Percival's eighteenth century medical ethics, the ethical codes of the American Medical Association, and the codes of other health professionals are traced, and the chapter explores the influences they have had on medicine and health care.

The second section of this chapter shifts emphasis away from professional codes and examines the development and impact of ethical positions developed in the Western religious and political traditions outside of organized professional groups. These include the Jewish, Roman Catholic, and Protestant traditions and secular philosophical thought. Each of these schools of ethics has a distinct history and a special impact upon health care. Ethical systems also exist beyond those of the Anglo-American West. The chapter explores the medical ethical positions prevalent in Eastern Europe, Islam, China, India, and Japan.

In studying medical ethical traditions it is important to examine the role codes of ethics should play in ethical decision making. The chapter considers the debate over whether ethical codes should be treated as rules, guidelines, covenants, or contracts, and the implications for each. Finally, the chapter explores the different bases for adopting an articulation of an ethical code as one's own.

Ethical problems increasingly command the attention of medical decisionmakers, health professionals and lay persons alike. They arise not only in the ethically obvious decisions: abortion, euthanasia, heart transplants, treatment of AIDS patients, and research on human subjects, but also in everyday medical decisions: what physicians should tell patients about their diseases, what treatments patients should consent to (or refuse), how much of a society's funds should be spent on health care, and how will it be divided among patients. In fact it is the very nature of medical decisions that value choices must be made constantly. To decide to pursue a particular course is to decide that it is better or more right than available alternatives, and deciding that something is better or more right means making value judgments. Many of those value judgments involve ethical choices. Thus for people to make choices about their health is at its core an exercise in ethics. For patients interacting with health-care professionals to propose, accept or reject a treatment plan is necessarily a value choice.

Many ethical and other value choices can be made instinctively, drawing on one's long-standing beliefs, commitments, and habits. Not every ethical or value choice in life requires conscious reflection. Medical choices are no different. In some cases, however, our intuitions fail us. They do not give us a clear answer. In other cases they may deceive us, giving clear signals that may nevertheless, upon reflection, be erroneous. We may be confronted by others who have equally clear intuitions that conflict with our own. A person who has just experienced the long, painful death of a loved one may be convinced that merciful hastening of death is the only thing that makes sense. He may be confronted by someone else who, believing that life is sacred, is equally certain that great wrong would come from policies permitting "euthanasia." Consider the following case involving an AIDS patient, a medical problem that is ethically controversial in part because it raises so many different problems about which intuitions differ.

Case 1. Twenty-seven-year-old Billy Harnack had been admitted to the intensive care unit for the fourth time in the past nine months. He had experienced severe difficulty breathing through the night. Dr. Karen Gladnow, the chief of the intensive care unit, was convinced even without the lab work that it was another episode of *pneumocystis carinii* pneumonia, one of the most common AIDS-related infections. Each occurrence of the disease was more difficult to treat. Mr. Harnack also had Kaposi's sarcoma, a tumor of the blood vessel cells, and his prognosis was very bleak: he was virtually certain to be dead in a matter of months. In fact, his quality of life had deteriorated to the point where Dr. Gladnow was convinced that were she the patient, she would refuse further treatment. She thought the time had come where death should no longer be opposed.

Her first problem was whether to write an order not to resuscitate the patient in case of a cardio-pulmonary arrest. She believed that such an action was realistically in the patient's interest and her traditional Hippocratic duty would be to serve her patient by doing what she thought was in his interest. She was fairly certain, however, that Mr. Harnack was not ready to end his struggle against his disease. If the pneumonia was arrested, he could survive several more months. Some of that time might be miserable, but parts of it might be good. He hoped to return to his work as a part-time clerk in a liquor store. Is the physician to do what she thinks is best or respect the patient's autonomous choice even though she perceives it wrong?

Since Mr. Harnack was too sick and too feeble to discuss the matter at the time, she could consult his family for their opinion. There were several problems with that, however. First, she was not sure whether the family's opinion should count any more than hers if it differed from the patient's views. Second, she was fairly sure that the family really did not understand Mr. Harnack's diagnosis. They knew he had been sick for sometime and had been told he had pneumonia and a type of cancer, but apparently they did not know he had AIDS. Could she really discuss the case with them without breaking the confidence of her patient?

Another dimension to the case that troubled Dr. Gladnow was that she had learned from Mr. Harnack during a previous admission that he had never really adjusted to his illness. He had become angry that he had been struck down, almost irrational in striking out at others for the hand that fate had dealt him. She strongly suspected that he had remained sexually active, running the risk of exposing his sexual partners to the AIDS virus. In fact, he had apparently decided that since he had been treated so unkindly by fate, he would take as many others with him as he could. Dr. Gladnow realized that were she to treat this episode, he would likely purposely expose others to a fatal illness. Could she purposely let her patient die in order to protect others or should she remain true to her traditional ethical obligation to serve only the welfare of the patient while excluding the welfare of others from moral consideration? Does the irresponsible behavior on the part of her patient justify sacrificing his interests in order to protect others? If she treated her patient's pneumonia, should she at least report Mr. Harnack's behavior to authorities or would that also be a violation of confidentiality?

Even if Dr. Gladnow ought morally to avoid sacrificing her patient's medical interests in order to protect others in the society, Dr. Gladnow faced still another problem. The ICU is a very busy place and beds are scarce. Treating Mr. Harnack aggressively in the ICU this time would only mean he would live to return again for further treatment. Other patients currently could be served by the unit. One was recovering from a heart attack and probably would do all right if moved to the step-down unit. Another was clearly terminal with muscular dystrophy and probably was not going to live through the night in any case. Other patients were competing for these beds. Dr. Gladnow had to make a choice about how Mr. Harnack's needs compared with the needs of these other patients.

One moral approach in allocating scarce medical resources like ICU beds is to ask how the beds can do the most good. That can include assessment not only of the medical benefits, but the social benefits as well. Dr. Gladnow had real doubts about the benefits that would accrue from aggressive treatment of Mr. Harnack. He was not going to do well medically in the long run, but more than that, his temporary improvement was not going to do anyone much good. In fact, to be realistic about it, she thought his treatment would probably result in substantial net harm to others. Is that a relevant consideration in deciding whether he should be treated?

Another complicating dimension in Dr. Gladnow's decision about treatment in the ICU was that Dr. Gladnow believed that Mr. Harnack got his exposure to AIDS through behaviors he voluntarily chose. He was both an active homosexual and an intravenous drug abuser. Dr. Gladnow believed that even if she should not generally take into account social factors in deciding which patients get treated, here was a case where the patient had, in a certain way, brought on his own illness. Can it be, she asked herself, that medicine must treat the problems that people bring on themselves with the same priority care required of the patient with muscular dystrophy, for instance, or some other genetic disease clearly unrelated to personal choice?

Here in one case we have a wide range of serious and controversial medical ethical issues: autonomy and paternalism, confidentiality, conflict between the individual patient's interests and those of society, the ethics of the allocation of resources and the role voluntary behavior ought to play, if any, in allocating resources. In other settings AIDS also introduces questions of compulsory testing, reporting and treatment. Public health has traditionally been seen as a justification for overriding both the right to refuse treatment and the privacy of the confidential relation. AIDS, however, is a public health problem of a special sort. Its mode of transmission is different from many of the traditional infectious diseases. Public health ethics is being challenged by the AIDS epidemic, as is the ethics of medical research. Researchers are being asked to give special priority to a disease that many of them would just as soon not become involved with. Both researchers and clinicians are asking whether they have the right to refuse to participate in the care of AIDS patients because of the risks the disease might pose to them, no matter how small.

In short, AIDS presents to us an amazing mix of extremely complicated ethical issues. While no one issue is terribly new, the urgency with which they are presented and the combination of them in one complex disease phenomenon is new. What is needed is a discipline for teasing out the issues and reflecting on our moral intuitions about them.

Ethics is the enterprise of disciplined reflection on moral intuitions and moral choices. It often begins with intuitions and long-held convictions. It attempts to compare them for consistency, to formulate rules of conduct accounting for our considered judgments, and, to articulate general principles that might underlie these judgments and rules. It confronts questions such as how these more general rules and principles relate to each other and to our judgments. Finally, it deals with basic questions of what we mean when we say something is ethical or unethical and how we can know what is right or wrong.

Ethics is a branch of the disciplines that deal with basic questions of meaning and value: of philosophy and theology. Some philosophers and theologians can spend entire lifetimes dealing with these issues on a rather abstract or theoretical level. Increasingly, however, ethics is becoming a discipline that is applied to real world problems such as medicine. Applied ethics takes various rules and principles and integrates them with detailed knowledge of the relevant facts and customs of a particular sphere of life such as politics or race relations or the work place. This volume explores the application of ethics to the sphere of medicine.

Medicine is a more ambiguous term than many people realize. Sometimes medical ethics is assumed to be the ethics of decisions made by physicians. Medicine is taken to be the work of doctors. Many other health professionals are engaged in the medical enterprise, however. Nurses, pharmacists, dentists, hospital chaplains, and health-care administrators are all part of what is sometimes called the health-care team. They are an integral part of the decisionmaking process. Sometimes they face unique problems, such as what a nurse should do when she is given an "order" from a physician *not* to resuscitate a patient in the event of a cardiac arrest when the nurse feels (perhaps because she thinks she knows the patient's wishes) that failing to resuscitate would be unethical. These decisions faced by other members of the health-care team are also part of the ethics of medicine.

More importantly, many of the choices made by lay people are also decisions in the medical sphere. The woman who decides to be sterilized, the parent who decides not to seek psychiatric counsel for a disturbed child, the legislator who votes for a "natural death act," or the judge who decides that a patient's consent was not adequately informed are all making decisions that naturally fall within the scope of medical ethics. Medicine, then, is a term that applies to all decisions having to do with health and disease. Most such decisions are made by lay people. Medical ethics, as considered in this volume, will cover all such choices, not just those made by health-care professionals.

Sometimes the term "bioethics" is used in place of medical ethics. The terms are now used almost interchangeably. Sometimes bioethics has a slightly broader meaning, including ethical problems of the biological sciences outside of medicine: research on animals, efforts to manipulate the genetic makeup of nonhuman species, and so forth. We shall not make a sharp distinction between the two terms.

This volume will examine systematically the major ethical issues arising in medicine and, to some extent, the biological sciences.

THE HISTORY OF MEDICAL ETHICAL SYSTEMS

While individual health-care professionals and lay persons may have collections of more or less well thought out views about the ethics of medical choices, a number of major positions have gained enough prominence that they can be considered "systems" or "traditions" in medical ethics. The most well known, at least in the West, is the Hippocratic tradition.

Professional Codes in the West

THE HIPPOCRATIC TRADITION

The Hippocratic Oath is often acknowledged by both physicians and lay people to be the foundation of medical ethics for physicians in the West. Although the ethics of physician behavior is only one part of medical ethics, it has been historically the part to receive the greatest attention. Until very recently, medical choices were thought to be the province of trained professionals. Sometimes choices were thought to be too complex for uneducated or untrained lay persons. Sometimes they were thought to rest directly on esoteric, scientific knowledge that was only accessible to those socialized into the profession of medicine. Sometimes physicians were seen as a "profession" in the sense that in addition to having a body of specialized knowledge, they were committed to a special ethic that bound the members of the profession to special norms, duties, and virtues. For whatever reason, physicians have had a special ethical tradition and that tradition is best summarized in the Hippocratic Oath.

The Hippocratic Oath is of uncertain origin. It is traced to a group of physicians in ancient Greece. At the time there was no single school of medical orthodoxy. Different "schools" of physicians reflected different medical and philosophical beliefs. One of these schools had its center on the island of Cos. It emerged in the fifth century BC and produced a large body of scientific and ethical writings. Its acknowledged head was Hippocrates, but not all of the writings were, in fact, authored by him. These writings were later gathered together into various collections and referred to as the Hippocratic corpus. Since as early as the time of Galen (circa 130–200 AD), there are well-documented disputes over the authorship of many of these writings (Carrick 1985; Edelstein 1967; Smith 1979).

While some of the writings describe human anatomy or deal with scientific problems, others are decidedly ethical in tone. These include *Precepts, Aphorisms, Law,* and *On Decorum.* Of these the *Oath* is the shortest and, by far, the most important historically. It is of the Hippocratic Oath that Western physicians in the Hippocratic tradition trace the foundations of their ethics.

The date of the *Oath* is uncertain, although there is substantial evidence that it dates from the late fourth century BC (Edelstein 1967, 55–61). This is based in part on linguistic considerations and in part on its content. The doctrines it contains are not consistent with much Greek thought, but are characteristic of the Pythagorean school of that time.

The *Oath* is divided into two parts. The first, an oath of allegiance, pledges the Hippocratic physician to consider his teacher as equal to his parents and to regard his teacher's offspring as equal to his brothers. It is as if the student is being initiated into a Greek cult. He pledges to share the precepts or instruction only with those who have "signed the covenant," a notion strangely at odds with modern commitments to share medical knowledge, but understandable in the context of Greek society's famous secret groups. The arrangement whereby the student honors his teacher as a father by adoption is distinctively a pattern of fourth century Pythagoreans. The new initiate even pledges to help his teacher financially in time of need.

The opening covenant is separated from the second part, often referred to as the code of ethics. The requirements of the code are also quite unique for Greek ethics (or any other ethical system for that matter). Medicine is divided into three parts: dietetics, pharmacology, and surgery. The Hippocratic physician pledges in the section on dietetics to apply measures "for the benefit of the sick according to my ability and judgment." This is probably the most important line in the *Oath*. It is the thought that many modern physicians carry with them as the essence of the Hippocratic ethic. They expand it beyond its original literal applications to dietetics to apply to all medical treatment, in fact, to all behavior affecting the patient.

In the section on pharmacology, the physician pledges not to administer a deadly drug or to give a woman an abortive remedy, both distinctively Pythagorean ethical positions. Also, the virtues of "purity and holiness," both characteristically religious terms, are extolled.

In the section on surgery a strange prohibition is included. The Hippocratic physician will not use the knife (perform surgery) "even on sufferers from stone [presumably kidney stones], but will withdraw in favor of such men as are engaged in this work." There is thus a division of labor with Hippocratic physicians eschewing surgery. It is not that they consider surgery immoral per se but rather that it should be left for others. One explanation is that Pythagoreans viewed surgery as defiling their divine purity (Edelstein 1967, 32). They could, thus, leave surgery for those who did not need to worry about ritual contamination.

The remaining sentences of the *Oath* proscribe sexual relations with patients and enjoin confidentiality (by ambiguously prohibiting disclosure of "those things that ought not to be spread abroad"). Finally, the *Oath* closes by having the physician ask that if he keeps the oath he be granted enjoyment of life and fame for all time to come, but that if he break it, the opposite should be his lot.

The *Oath* is thus a mixture of apparently uncontroversial maxims (such as benefitting the patient and confidentiality) and injunctions that are hard for the modern mind to understand (such as the prohibition on surgery and a pledge of secrecy). In fact, even the apparently uncontroversial maxims have generated debate recently. Sometimes the maxim that the physician should benefit the patient according to his ability and judgment has been cited as an authorization for treating patients against their wishes or for deceiving patients by withholding a diagnosis of terminal illness. Critics have accused the Hippocratic Oath of condoning paternalism. They have also questioned the confidentiality clause, pointing out that prohibiting disclosure of that which should not be "spread abroad" appears to condone disclosures of those things that should be "spread abroad," thus opening the door for toleration of disclosures for either paternalistic or social reasons. In any case, at least since the time of Galen, the Hippocratic Oath has been elevated to premier status among physicians as the summary of their sense of ethical obligation. What was once a code of a minority medical group became the dominant ethical document for all professional medicine in the West.

The Hippocratic Oath Insofar as a Christian May Swear It

Some people have suggested that the reason the Hippocratic Oath survived was that, after Constantine and the Christianization of Europe, other Greek ethical systems lost favor while the Hippocratic ethic was elevated because of its similarities to Christian ethics. There are, in fact, points of similarity. A new version of the Oath, called "The Oath According to Hippocrates in so far as a Christian May Swear It" (Jones 1926), emerged for Christian physicians. Some obvious changes were made such as the removal of references to the Greek gods and goddesses. There were also more subtle changes. The entire covenant including the pledge of secrecy and the ritualistic adoption of the teacher as father were dropped. The abortion prohibition was strengthened and the prohibition against surgery was dropped.

From the title of the Christian version it is clear that even in the middle ages there was a sense among Christians of tension between Hippocratic and Christian ethics. In fact there is virtually no evidence that early Christian writers were aware of the Hippocratic Oath, much less endorsed it or adopted it as their own. It was not until about the tenth century, when many Greek writings including the Hippocratic writings were recovered from Arabic sources, that interest in the Hippocratic ethic began to increase.

Percival and Eighteenth-Century Medical Ethics

In modern times the first major interest in medical ethics in the Anglo-Saxon world appeared in the eighteenth century. The most important example of a comprehensive medical ethics is John Gregory's (1724–1773) *Lectures on the Duties and Qualifications of a Physician*. It is not so much dependent on the Hippocratic tradition as on the broader philosophical thought of the day, including the Scottish moralists such as David Hume and Frances Hutcheson.

The most influential development of the time, however, turned out to be the by-product of a local dispute at the Manchester Infirmary. In 1789 an epidemic struck taxing the infirmary staff and creating a feud among the physicians, surgeons, and apothecaries. The trustees approached a distinguished physician, Thomas Percival, who had been on the staff before a physical disability forced him to resign. They asked him to draw up a "scheme of professional conduct" to prevent such disputes in the future. The result was Percival's *Medical Ethics,* which became the foundation of modern Anglo-American professional physician ethics. It has many features in common with the Hippocratic Oath, but there are some differences as well. It focuses much more on the institutional ethics of health care. It deals with physician's relations with hospitals and with other health professionals. It is a document with a greater social perspective than the Hippocratic Oath.

To the extent that Percival's *Medical Ethics* communicates with ethics beyond the medical profession, it states the ethic of the British gentleman more than anything else. The religious virtues of purity and holiness of the Hippocratic Oath are replaced with the virtues of the gentleman: physicians should "unite *tenderness* with *steadiness,* and *condescension* with *authority*" (Percival 1927, 71). In the introduction Percival commends the study of professional ethics as a practice that will "soften your manners, expand your affections, and form you to that propriety and dignity of conduct, which are essential to the character of a GENTLEMAN" (Percival 1927, 63).

THE ETHICAL CODES OF THE AMERICAN MEDICAL ASSOCIATION

Some half century later, American medicine was involved in a dispute among several schools of medicine. What eventually became known as the orthodox practitioners formed the American Medical Association in 1847. It is clear from the founding documents that "self-constituted doctors and doctresses" and other so-called quack practitioners were a great concern.

One of the documents growing out of the founding convention in Philadelphia was the *Code of Medical Ethics.* It followed the pattern of Percival's *Medical Ethics.* It contained three sections beginning with "Of the duties of physicians to their patients, and the obligations of patients to their physicians." This was followed by "Of the duties of physicians to each other, and to the profession at large." The influence of Percival is unmistakable. Whole paragraphs are used verbatim, including the explicit references to tenderness, firmness, condescension, and authority.

Revisions occurred in 1903, 1912, and 1947, and then in 1957 an entirely new format was adopted ("Principles of Medical Ethics"). In place of the lengthy document, ten succinct principles were adopted. These were supplemented by more lengthy opinions of the AMA's Judicial Council, the body responsible for interpreting the AMA's principles. The principles were general and sometimes platitudinous. They committed the AMA physician to "render service to humanity." The language condemning other practitioners as unscientific was toned down and, in contrast to the Hippocratic Oath, there was a clearly acknowledged responsibility to the society as well as to the individual. Nevertheless, there still remained an unmistakable paternalistic quality. In the opinion of the AMA, for instance, confidences could be broken when it became necessary to protect the welfare of the individual as well as the community.

In 1980 the most recent revision was adopted (American Medical Association 1981). It probably represented the most substantive ethical change in the history of codes of ethics for physicians written within the profession. The result was a set of seven general principles, but with a tone quite different from anything previously written by a professional organization of physicians. AMA physicians now are to be dedicated to service with compassion and respect for human dignity. They are to respect the law and to deal honestly with patients, a radical change from the previously widely held view that physicians had the right (if not the duty) to deceive patients whenever they thought it was in the interest of the patient to do so (when the truth about a cancer diagnosis would disturb the patient, for instance). For the first time in any codification written by physicians, there is an explicit commitment to the rights of patients. While in previous codes the welfare of patients had received attention, never had patients' rights been acknowledged. In place of the confidentiality principle that permitted exceptions in the interest of the welfare of the patient or the community, the new provision commits the AMA physician to safeguard patient confidences within the constraints of the law.

As in all of the editions of the AMA Principles since 1957, the 1980 version is supplemented with the current opinions of the Judicial Council. Sometimes those opinions reveal traditional thinking and Hippocratic influences. For example, with regard to confidentiality, at one point the opinion of the Judicial Council repeats the position in the Principles: "The physician should not reveal confidential communications or information without the express consent of the patient, unless required to do so by law" (American Medical Association 1984, 19). However, later in the text the older, more paternalistic formulation is revived with exceptions permitted for the welfare of the individual or community (American Medical Association 1984, 26). At another point after making a strong commitment to the notion of informed consent (a notion totally absent from the Hippocratic tradition), the Judicial Council states its opinion that consent need not be obtained "when risk-disclosure poses such a serious psychological threat of detriment to the patient as to be medically contraindicated" (American Medical Association 1984, 30). The older Hippocratic notion that information can be "medically contraindicated" when it would upset the patient, takes precedence once again over the more liberal philosophical notion of respect for the individual autonomy of the patient.

OTHER CONTEMPORARY PHYSICIAN CODES

To make matters more confusing there are many other professionally written codes of ethics purporting to specify proper ethical conduct for physicians. Many other national medical associations have their own codes. Moreover, the World Medical Association, a federation of national medical associations, has adopted two codes of ethics, The Declaration of Geneva in 1948 and the International Code of Medical Ethics in 1949. The Declaration of Geneva is consciously patterned after the Hippocratic Oath. It is meant to be an updating. It retains a pledge to give teachers "respect and gratitude" (but no money). Reminiscent of the Hippocratic pledge that

TABLE 1–1.   Professional Associations with Codes of Ethics

1. American Academy of Allergy
2. American Association of Nurse Anesthetists
3. American Chiropractic Association
4. American Dental Assistants Association
5. American Dental Hygienists' Association
6. American Dental Association
7. The American Dietetic Association
8. American Geriatrics Society
9. American Board of Health Physics
10. American College of Hospital Administrators
11. Society for Clinical and Experimental Hypnosis
12. American Medical Technologists
13. American Society of Medical Technology
14. International Society of Clinical Laboratory Technologists
15. American Medical Record Association
16. American Nurses' Association
17. National Association for Practical Nurse Education and Service
18. American College of Nursing Home Administrators
19. American Occupational Therapy Association
20. Association of Operating Room Technicians
21. American Association of Opthamology
22. Guild of Prescription Opticians of America
23. American Optometric Association
24. American Pharmaceutical Association
25. American Physical Therapy Association
26. American Osteopathic Association
27. American Podiatry Association
28. American Proctologic Society
29. National Association of Human Service Technologies
30. American Psychiatric Association
31. American Psychoanalytic Association
32. American Board of Professional Psychology
33. American Psychological Association
34. American Registry of Clinical Radiography Technologists
35. American Registry of Radiologic Technologists
36. American Corrective Therapy Association
37. National Rehabilitation Counseling Association
38. American Association for Respiratory Therapy
39. American Speech and Hearing Association
40. American Association of Neurological Surgeons
41. American Academy of Physician Assistants

From Clapp, Jane. *Professional Ethics and Insignia.* Metuchen, N.J.: The Scarecrow Press, 1974; and other sources.

physicians will work for the benefit of the patient according to their ability and judgment, the Declaration of Geneva has the new physician pledge "The health of my patient will be my first consideration." In contrast to the ambiguous provision in the Hippocratic Oath, it contains an apparently exceptionless confidentiality clause: "I will respect the secrets confided in me." It has the physician treat colleagues as brothers and "maintain . . . the honor and the noble traditions of the medical profession."

THE CODES OF THE OTHER HEALTH PROFESSIONS

Just as the physician is not the only member of the health professional team, so physicians are not the only group with professionally articulated codes of ethics. Table 1-1 lists several other professional codes. These professional association codes vary considerably with regard to the themes outlined above. Some are still very much in accord with the Hippocratic model; the health professional is expected to be the decisionmaker acting in what he or she believes to be the patient's interest. Others have moved away from that paternalistic mode. The American Nurses' Association *Code for Nurses* states, for example, that respect for persons is the most fundamental principle and that self-determination is basic to respect for persons. It is committed to having clients "as fully involved as possible in the planning and implementation of their own health care" and to clients having the "moral right to determine what will be done with their own person; to be given accurate information, and all the information necessary for making informed judgments . . . ; [and] to accept, refuse, or terminate treatment without coercion." By contrast the American Pharmaceutical Association Code claims, in a manner similar to the Declaration of Geneva, "a pharmacist should hold the health and safety of patients to be of first consideration."

Other Codifications in Western Thought

There are many different formulations of the health professional's duty written by professional groups at different times and places. They do not always agree with one another. The matter becomes even more complicated when one realizes that professional groups are not the only ones writing codes of ethics governing medical practice. Ethics has long been a matter of importance to religious groups, and most religious groups have codified positions on the ethics of medical decisionmaking.

RELIGIOUS GROUPS

Judaism. Jewish scholars have long recognized that Judaism includes a set of laws that provide uniquely Jewish views on such matters as autopsy, circumcision, and abortion. Orthodox scholars of the Talmud hold that life is sacred and to be preserved until the time when the patient is *gesisah,* or moribund (Bleich 1979, 33–35).

A Hebrew physician's oath is preserved from the seventh century. Referred to as the Oath of Asaf, it was administered by a teacher to his students (Etziony 1973, 24–26). It contains prohibitions on causing death, on performing an abortion (for the adulterous wife), and revealing confidences. In contrast with the almost complete lack of concern about the needy in the Hippocratic tradition, there is also a specific injunction to show mercy to the poor and the needy, a provision one would expect in Jewish ethics. There is also a warning to avoid sorcery, magic, and witchcraft.

Another Jewish text is the prayer of Yehuda Halevi, an eleventh to twelfth century Judeo-Spanish philosopher and physician. It, like the Oath of Asaf, emphasizes that it is God who heals, not the physician. The most well known Jewish document is a prayer attributed to the twelfth century Jewish physician, Moses Maimonides although it probably dates from eighteenth century Germany. It condemns "thirst for profit" and "ambition for renown and admiration." These, together with more recent writings on Jewish medical ethics (Franck 1980; Rosner and Bleich 1979; Tendler 1975), provide a framework for medical ethics quite different from the professionally articulated codes.

Roman Catholicism.   Roman Catholic scholars since the middle ages have written on medical ethical problems from the perspective of Christian theological ethics. Papal statements on abortion, contraception and sexual ethics are well known. Of equal importance, however, are well-developed positions on many other medical issues including the care of the critically and terminally-ill patient. The opposition to active killing of terminally-ill patients on grounds of mercy is counterbalanced with a nuanced doctrine of the justifiability of withholding treatments that are considered "extraordinary" in the sense that they involve disproportionate burden (Congregation for the Doctrine of the Faith 1980; Pope Pius XII 1958). Catholic thought also has developed what is referred to as the doctrine of double effect, whereby indirect evil effects of an action can be tolerated under certain conditions provided they are not intended. The doctrine is applied in medical ethics to justify the unavoidable killing of a fetus while removing a cancerous uterus or the unintended killing of a cancer patient with a narcotic given to relieve pain.

The document of greatest importance to medical ethics in the American context is the *Ethical and Religious Directives for Catholic Health Facilities* of the United States Catholic Conference. It is a succinct compendium of the positions of Catholic thought on the full range of medical ethical issues.

Protestant Thought.   Virtually every major Protestant denomination has endorsed official positions on the full range of medical ethical issues. The variety of their positions is considerable, but certain patterns can be recognized. Although many conservative Protestant groups still have serious reservations, since 1930 there has been a widening of Protestant thought regarding contraception, sterilization, and abortion. There has generally been an openness toward refusal of life-prolonging treatments, although only occasionally does that encompass an acceptance of the ethics of active killing. Here the Protestants have followed Catholic thinkers closely.

Perhaps the most important contribution of Protestant thinkers to medical ethics has not been over specific substantive issues, but more in their approach to medical ethical problems. Protestants are, by tradition, committed to giving the lay person an increased role in ethical and theological matters. Protestants believe that the text ought to be in the hands of the lay person. This has manifest itself in medical ethics with a heavy emphasis on the role of the lay person having access to medical information and in making medical decisions about his or her own care. The patients' rights movement has had great affinity with Protestant thought. In fact, many of the persons working in the current generation of medical ethics are trained in Protestant theology. Their anti-paternalism can be accounted for, in part, from their Protestant heritage.

SECULAR PHILOSOPHICAL THOUGHT

Although the patients' rights movement has considerable support from religious ethics, especially Protestant, it also resonates well with many secular philosophical trends, especially those grounded in liberal political philosophy. The concept of rights, totally alien to the Hippocratic ethical tradition, has its roots in liberal political philosophy. Many secular ethical thinkers standing in this tradition have developed medical ethical positions that can be thought of as a "school of medical ethics." They draw on the historical concepts and documents of the liberal tradition including Locke, Jefferson, and the Bill of Rights. That tradition, far more than the tradition of Hippocratic medicine, has been manifested in the legal decisions that have become such a prominent part of the American medical ethics scene since about 1960.

The first important expression of this began with the Nuremburg trials of the late 1940s. In those trials, in which those who conducted horrifying research on prisoners were condemned, a Nuremburg Code was produced. It became the first major publicly produced code of ethics for a branch of medical practice. It has a legal and moral status quite different from earlier codes generated by the professional groups themselves. The Nuremburg Code abandons the older notion that subjects of research should be protected solely by the commitment of the professional to the subject, and replaces it with a notion of self-determination for potential subjects that gives rise to a requirement for informed consent.

At the national level a similar emergence of a legal commitment to patient self-determination was emerging in case law. A doctrine of informed consent rooted in a right to self-determination that is quite different from anything in the Hippocratic tradition has emerged in the courts and jurisprudential scholarship.

Similar trends were manifest in two national governmental commissions. In 1973 the National Commission for the Protection of Human Subjects of Biomedical and Behavioral Research was established. Stimulated by a then recent exposure of research that had withheld treatment from patients with syphilis for decades, its mandate was to provide a public review of the ethical and legal problems of human subjects research. In the process it developed the first formal governmental analysis of the ethical principles that underlie medical ethical decisions from the point of view of a secular, nonprofessional body. That commission was the first secular body working in medical ethics that, by law, had a majority of members from outside the health professions (National Commission for the Protection of Human Subjects of Biomedical and Behavioral Research 1978).

The successor to this commission devoted to medical research was the President's Commission on the Study of Ethical Problems in Medicine and Biomedical and Behavioral Research (1983). Its mandate was broader; it dealt with the full range of medical ethical issues including the care of the dying, genetics, issues of health-care decisions such as informed consent, and allocation of health resources. Its reports, produced in a number of volumes, have become definitive treatises on medical ethics in a secular, public context.

While they represent the consensus mainstream thought of the American secular public on these topics, it is important to realize that subcultural groups, religious and secular, also have special more or less well-developed positions on important medical ethical issues. These are not limited to groups such as Jehovah's Witnesses and Christian Scientists, who have special views on blood transfusions or medical interventions more generally. They also include groups with special ethnic, cultural and ideological perspectives. There has yet to be written a medical ethics of Black culture or Hispanic culture or feminist culture, but they exist, at least in the thinking of members of these groups. They sometimes provide a radical contrast to more orthodox thinking whether it be from health professionals or lay people. Patients coming from any of these groups, whether from the mainstream of liberal thought or minority groups, can provide a real challenge to the ethical thinking of health professionals who encounter them in hospital emergency rooms, clinics, and physicians' offices.

Medical Ethics in Other Cultures

The diversity of medical ethical positions is great even within Anglo-American Western culture. It is even greater if the net is cast more broadly. Patients or health-care workers coming from cultures outside the Anglo-American West may bring with them belief systems with medical ethical implications difficult for Westerners to comprehend. People concerned about problems in medical ethics are wise to examine these positions as well as those from more familiar traditions if they want to grasp the full range of possible positions on a medical ethical issue.

EASTERN EUROPE

One might expect that Eastern European countries would have a medical ethic that differs in some respects from the traditions described thus far. The Eastern European countries all express their own nuance. The Oath of Soviet Physicians is fundamentally different from the Hippocratic Oath and the codes of the Western professional associations in that it was produced by the Presidium of the Supreme Soviet, not by a professional organization. All graduating Soviet medical students are required to take this oath. There is a stronger emphasis on preventive medicine than in the Western codes. There is also a much stronger commitment to the interests of society. The Soviet physician pledges "to work conscientiously wherever the interests of the society will require it;" "to conduct all my actions according to the principles of the Communist [morality];" and "to always keep in mind the . . . high responsibility I have to my people and to the Soviet government." At the same time, many of the traditional themes of Western professional oaths are included: a pledge to keep professional secrets, to improve knowledge, to consult colleagues, and to never refuse to give advice or help.

ISLAM

The people of the Islamic tradition also have a history of views on medical ethics. As might be anticipated, the ethics are based on Quranic teaching. The Oath of the Islamic Medical Association of the USA and Canada (Rahman, Amine, and Elkadi 1981) contains a strong prohibition on killing similar to that seen in Jewish thought. Islamic physicians are committed to the virtues of "strength," "fortitude," "wisdom," and "understanding." They are to be honest, modest, merciful, and objective. There is a strong commitment to serving mankind "poor or rich, wise or illiterate, Muslim or non-Muslim, black or white."

Sometimes Muslims express an almost fatalistic reliance on the will of Allah. This has been expressed in reluctance to authorize nontreatment decisions for comatose patients and opposition to birth control, although Muslim scholars offer no formal opposition to the practice of contraception.

CHINA

The cultures of the East also have long historical traditions of interest in medical ethics. In China records exist of medical ethical writings as early as Sun Szu-miao's in the seventh century (Unschuld 1979, 24–33). These writings, in contrast to many key documents in Hippocratic medical ethics, are closely dependent upon the major philosophical/ethical systems of the broader culture. Sun Szu-miao was identified with Taoism, but also reflected significant Buddhist influences. Confucian thought provides the background of many other early Chinese medical ethical texts.

Several themes that are alien to Western professional medical ethics repeatedly occur in these Chinese writings. The Confucian writings have long shown an acceptance of the limits of the human capacity to struggle against death. There is a constant concern for the care given to the poor. Injunctions are repeated over and over to treat the poor and the rich without regard for financial status.

The three classical virtues are humaneness, compassion, and filial piety. The last is linked to a notion completely foreign to Hippocratic ethics. Loyalty to one's family has always been important in Chinese culture. Originally in Confucian society, someone in the family was responsible for medical knowledge. Loyalty to one's brother became the moral basis for rendering health care. As knowledge became more complex, professionalization emerged. When people could not get care from the designated family member, they would have to be satisfied with a mere professional physician—one acting on a professional basis rather than out of a sense of familial loyalty. This is a far cry from the exalted status of the professional in Western medicine where it is considered unethical, or at least irresponsible, for the physician to treat a family member.

INDIA

Indian medical ethics is also closely dependent upon the ethical traditions of the broader culture. The most important texts in ancient Indian medical ethics are the Caraka Samhita, which is a part of a Vedic religious writing on medicine, and the Susruta Samhita. The Caraka Samhita, written in about the first century AD, contains maxims appropriate for the elite of Indian culture. The physician should lead the life of a celibate, grow his hair and beard, speak only the truth, eat no meat, eat only pure particles of food, be free from envy, and carry no arms. The physician should endeavor to relieve patients, should not desert or injure them, and should never cause another's death. The physician is committed to being helpful to the patient which leads, as in Hippocratic ethics, to benevolent decisions not to tell patients of their terminal illnesses. "Even knowing that the patient's span of life has come to its close, it shall not be mentioned by thee there, where if so done, it would cause shock to the patient or to others."

The most provocative paragraph is one that can only be understood in the context of the Indian doctrine of karma, the doctrine that links one's present status in life with the way one has led previous incarnations. One of the earliest codes to address the problem of allocating health resources, the Caraka states, "No persons, who are hated by the king or who are haters of the king or who are hated by the public or who are haters of the public, shall receive treatment. Similarly, those who are extremely abnormal, wicked, and of miserable character and conduct, those who have not vindicated their honor, those who are on the point of death, and similarly women who are unattended by their husbands or guardians shall not receive treatment." Contrast that text with the strong commitment to the needy in Judeo-Christian and Chinese medical ethics and the silence on these matters in the Hippocratic tradition.

JAPAN

Like the other Eastern cultures, Japan's medical ethics has also been influenced by the broader cultural traditions, in this case indigenous Shinto as well as Buddhist and Confucian thought both brought from China. Also as a modern culture, in Japan as well as in all the other cultures mentioned, many Western themes from both the Hippocratic and liberal traditions have been influential. One example of a traditional Japanese code of medical ethics comes from the Ri-shu school of medical practice dating from about the sixteenth century. The code, the Seventeen Rules of Enjuin, has many similarities with the Hippocratic Oath including secrecy and a strong commitment to serving the patient. The physician is to protect against disclosing any secrets he learns during his medical education. He is even given instructions to make sure that his books are returned to the school upon his death.

OTHER CULTURES

Other cultures also have their own medical ethical systems. Most national medical groups have a code of ethics that reflects the unique character of the culture as well as the physicians in that culture. Much remains to be learned about some cultures. The medical ethics of African cultures, for example, are virtually unknown in the West. In studying medical ethics it is important to keep in mind that the number of medical ethical codes (and the systems they reflect) is great, and that cultural traditions vary tremendously in the ethical practices they expect of health professionals and lay people.

THE ROLE OF CODES

The existence of this wide variety of codes of ethics in medicine raises some interesting questions about the way codes ought to be used. Presumably they represent the collective wisdom of the group that authored and endorsed them. As such, they at times may sound platitudinous. Still they manage to express some very controversial notions, ideas that are at least controversial to those outside the group endorsing the code.

Rules versus Guidelines

Even among those who endorse codes there is some question about roles. Some people attempt to interpret ethical codes as a set of rules spelling out exactly what conduct is appropriate for medical decisionmakers. In extreme cases they are viewed essentially as law where violation is cause for legal or quasi-legal action. Some disciplinary proceedings of medical professional organizations come complete with legal counsel, due process, and juries. Sometimes codes are introduced into public judicial proceedings as if they were legally binding on members of professional groups.

On the other hand, some people view codes as mere guidelines; general principles of appropriate conduct that should guide the individual as he or she makes moral choices. That seems to be the view in the minds of the drafters of the 1980 revision of the American Medical Association's Principles of Medical Ethics. The Preface says the principles "are not laws, but standards of conduct which define the essentials of honorable behavior for the physician." They are "intended as guides to responsible professional behavior, but they are not presented as the sole or only route to medical morality." At the same time, failure to conform can result in disciplinary proceedings within the association. There is an ambivalence that probably reflects a gradual historical evolution in the concept of a code of ethics.

While professional codes are viewed even by their authors as guidelines from which the individual clinician must make responsible moral decisions, there is another view of a code that is much more stringent. As we have seen, some of the codes of medical ethics have a status far different from expressions of professional consensus. The Nuremburg Code, for example, has the status of international law. The positions of the President's Commission on the Study of Ethical Problems in Medicine and Biomedical and Behavioral Research (1983) are not legally binding, but they are increasingly taken to represent the collective wisdom of the American population. In both cases it is hard to discount the positions expressed as "mere opinion" without legitimate authority. The status of the Nuremburg Code is least ambiguous. Presumably anyone violating it is guilty not only of unethical conduct but of violation of international law as well. On the other hand someone who went against the wisdom of the President's Commission would not necessarily be violating a law, but would at least have a moral burden of proof. In legal cases where the "reasonable person" standard is used, such as in informed consent cases, the views of the Commission could be (in fact have been) introduced as evidence of national policy.

A similar tension between codes as guidelines and as rigid rules may occur within various religious traditions. Some traditions, for example, Protestantism, may tend to view church pronouncements as matters for guidance of members and anyone else in the general public who cares to listen. In other cases, pronouncements have a more binding quality, at least to the extent that violation can lead to expulsion from membership in the group.

Thus codes sometimes have legal standing and function to determine what the law requires while in other cases they are more moral documents articulating the moral positions of members of various groups. Among those codes that are viewed as moral codes, some groups expect their members to treat them as guides for individual moral judgment while others assume that members will follow them as moral rules of conduct.

Codes, Covenants, and Contracts

The dispute over whether ethical codes are rules of conduct or guidelines is not the only disagreement. Not all medical ethics writings are, by any means, in the form of codes. Some are essays, written by individuals attempting to defend a particular moral point of view or offer an analysis of several points of view. Others are what could be termed "covenants" or "contracts."

William May, currently a professor at Southern Methodist University, has written a provocative analysis entitled "Code, Covenant, Contract, or Philanthropy?"

(1985). In it he examines the general form of the code as an ethical document. A code, he suggests, is a compilation of patterns of behavior for particular groups of people. It is particularly relevant to "inner circles within certain societies," among friends or professionals within a guild. They tend to make conduct matters of aesthetics. Morality becomes a matter of conforming elegantly to an ideal of character envisioned in the code.

More important, a code does not encourage or necessitate personal involvement with other persons. A code is created unilaterally. May cites the Hemingway hero—the bull-fighter or the soldier—as examples. They live by a code that eschews involvement. The ideal is created entirely by the group itself without participation by others.

May contrasts the code as a mode of articulating an ethic with a covenant. A covenant has its roots in specific historical events. "It always has reference to specific historical exchange between partners leading to a promissory event." The pledge that the young physician makes to his teacher in the Hippocratic Oath is a covenant. The obligations he takes on vis-a-vis patients constitute a code. Patients play no role in the articulation of the moral duties of either party. The same thing has happened in the creation of other professional codes: Percival, the AMA, and the World Medical Association. The American Medical Association meeting in 1847 articulated the obligations of patients to physicians as well as physicians to patients, but patients played no part in the specification of these obligations. The covenant, whether in its prototypical religious form or in the form establishing mutual promises among professionals and lay people, involves a mutuality, a promise that shapes both partners and binds them in the future. The code on the other hand has philanthropy as its ideal. The commitment is unilateral; the commitment is bestowed gratuitously on the other party rather than being responsive and reciprocal.

May and others also have questioned the relationship between a covenant model and one referred to as a contract. Both involve mutual participation of the parties. But May defines contract quite specifically to involve agreements in which "two parties calculate their own best interests and agree upon some joint project in which both derive roughly equivalent benefits for goods contributed by each." He seems to have in mind the contemporary idea of a legal or business contract, with the overtones of legalism, self-interest, and individual "deal making."

While the above is one use of the term contract, there are others that do not have these overtones. In particular, modern liberal thought is based on what philosophers refer to as a "social contract." In some cases, the concept of the social contract is a highly qualified, metaphorical image in which members of the society agree on what the basic principles of the society should be. Sometimes they are even seen as agreeing on what a set of pre-existing principles are. In this broader usage, contract is a general term that implies mutuality; promising (but not necessarily limited to) arrangements between individuals and having no legal implications. The term, marriage contract, is only one example of this broader usage in which the parties may not have in mind exclusively self-interest and legal obligations. Some people use the term contract to include what May calls covenants as well as other types of mutual promises. May, in response, considers the term, contract, too infiltrated with negative connotation and prefers to stay with the term, covenant. Regardless of the term used, the idea that ethical obligations between professionals and lay people may be based on mutual promises provides an alternative to the ethics of codes.

Codes raise a particularly interesting problem when the other party does not acknowledge or even desire the commitment made by the philanthropic gesture. For example, physicians pledge to act so as to benefit their patients according to their ability and judgment. This has given rise to well-meaning disclosures of confidential information even in cases where the patient might not want it disclosed. It has given rise to medical treatments believed by the physician to be for the benefit of the patient even in cases where patients may not want the treatments. There is the possibility with a unilaterally generated code that a group of persons may promise to engage in what they take to be benevolent actions toward outsiders when, in reality, some of those outsiders do not want the purported benefits. May and others prefer that the mode of mutual participation be the basis for articulating sets of duties in professional relationships such as between health professionals and patients. This would have the impact of viewing the patient as well as the professional as an active participant with the potential for obligations as well as claims against the other party.

The American Medical Association is apparently aware of this tension between unilaterally articulated codes and mutually agreed upon sets of moral obligations. In the report of the committee of the AMA that revised the Principles of Medical Ethics, it states that "The profession does not exist for itself; it exists for a purpose, and increasingly that purpose will be defined by society." Nevertheless the 1980 revision was a project written by and approved by members of the AMA only.

CHOOSING AMONG PROFESSIONAL AND OTHER CODIFICATIONS

Once one recognizes that there are many different codifications of the duties of health professionals and lay people for decisions in a medical context, the question of choosing among them becomes critical. We must ask why persons would feel obligated to follow one particular codification or another.

One basis for adopting an articulation of an ethical code as one's own is that one has voluntarily become a member of a group and, in doing so, has subscribed to its moral formulation. Thus the Hippocratic medical student on the Isle of Cos could be viewed as voluntarily committing himself to the obligations to teachers, colleagues, and patients called for by the Hippocratic guild.

This is a peculiarly modern notion of the origin of moral obligation, however. It rests on the idea that moral duties arise only when people voluntarily commit themselves to them. That may work for the twentieth century physician who seeks to join the AMA, but it hardly applies to the ancient physician. It probably does not work very well in other cultures even in the modern period. For example, are Soviet physicians thought to be bound to the Soviet Oath because they voluntarily decided to join the guild of Soviet physicians?

It presents even bigger problems for those physicians and other health professionals who are not members of their professional organization. Approximately half the physicians licensed to practice medicine in the United States are not members of the AMA. Does that mean they are exempt from the professional duties articulated by the AMA? If so, are they bound by some other ethic? Which one?

An even more complicated problem arises for persons who voluntarily join (or accept themselves as members of) two groups each of which has a set of medical ethical standards that it considers authoritative. This might arise if a physician specializing in some branch of medicine such as obstetrics or neurology is simultaneously a member of a specialty association and the state or national medical organization. It could arise if a physician considers himself or herself bound by both a national association and the World Medical Association codes when the two may conflict. Most commonly it can arise when a person is simultaneously a member of a medical professional organization and some other group purporting to speak on matters of medical ethics. A Jewish physician, for example, may feel simultaneously bound by the Talmudic obligation to preserve life as well as the AMA's commitment to accept treatment refusal decisions from competent patients even though the result will be a quicker death.

This Jewish physician is forced to decide which group he considers to be authoritative morally (or how he will combine the moral insights of each with his own moral judgments). Eventually he must face the question of the nature of the claims of each of these groups to be morally authoritative. Religious groups have traditionally claimed to be legitimate sources of moral insight for their members. They may claim to have knowledge of revelation or be capable of using reason to discern moral laws. Some of these groups have established patterns of moral authority—persons identified as authoritative teachers. Others may give substantial latitude for individual members to discern moral requirements based on their individual interpretation of Scripture and doctrine.

Those who approach ethics secularly also must make decisions about how moral knowledge is acquired. Some might yield to the state as the authority to establish ethical requirements. Others will turn to reason and intuition or the authority of individuals or groups. The question critical for those who make use of professionally articulated codes is to what extent these professional groups are legitimately recognized as authoritative in identifying moral obligations for members of their profession.

While professional groups have long written codes of ethics and assumed they were binding on their members, the exact nature of their claim to authority has never been fully analyzed. Some groups have claimed that the group is authoritative because the group literally creates the ethic. One official of a major professional organization once referred to his organization's code of ethics as one that the members have "imposed upon themselves." This would easily explain why members ought to feel bound, but it gives the agreement no weight for nonmembers, professional or lay. It also seems to fly in the face of what most people believe to be the nature of ethics. Ethical obligations are not merely self-imposed duties. Rather they are perceived as coming from outside the individual.

In other cases, somewhat more sophisticated professional organizations claim that they do not literally create the obligations, but rather they articulate them. They argue that only by being socialized into the profession and understanding the complex and esoteric nature of the professional role can one possibly understand the moral duties that the member of the profession must bear. The professional group, it is claimed, is responsible for articulating the professional duty although it is not something the group invents.

Different views of ethics have been held by certain groups in certain periods of history. The predominant view was that only people with special skills or knowledge or training can know ethical truths. In fact, that seems to be the position of the Hippocratic group. It is a controversial position in modern society, however, one that many people have rejected in favor of a position acknowledging that all may have moral insight. This is usually based on the belief that morality is universal in the sense that some common set of principles, some common system of ethics, applies universally and can be known without special esoteric skills.

This is no way implies that all persons have exactly the same duties. Surely, parents or police or physicians have duties that are unique to their roles. But holders of this latter view maintain that in principle anyone can recognize and understand the special duties of the parent or policeman or physician. By the same token anyone can, according to this view, understand the duties of the lay person. It is this framework that appears to underlie the position of those who are striving to make medical ethics more a matter of mutuality in which professionals and lay persons have a shared understanding of each other's rights and duties.

REFERENCES

American Medical Association. *Code of Medical Ethics: Adopted by the American Medical Association at Philadelphia, May, 1847, and by the New York Academy of Medicine in October, 1847.* New York: H. Ludwig, 1848.

American Medical Association. *Current Opinions of the Judicial Council of the American Medical Association.* Chicago: American Medical Association, 1981.

American Medical Association. *Current Opinions of the Judicial Council of the American Medical Association—1984: Including the Principles of Medical Ethics and Rules of the Judicial Council.* Chicago: American Medical Association, 1984.

Bleich, J. David. "The Obligation to Heal in the Judaic Tradition: A Comparative Analysis." In *Jewish Bioethics*, edited by Fred Rosner and J. David Bleich, 1–44. New York: Sanhedrin Press, 1979.

British Medical Association. *The Handbook of Medical Ethics.* Luton and London: Leagrave Press, 1984.

Carrick, Paul. *Medical Ethics in Antiquity: Philosophical Perspectives on Abortion and Euthanasia.* Dordrecht, Holland: D. Reidel, 1985.

Congregation for the Doctrine of the Faith. *Declaration On Euthanasia*. Rome: The Sacred Congregation for the Doctrine of the Faith, May 5, 1980.

Edelstein, Ludwig. "The Hippocratic Oath: Text, Translation and Interpretation." In *Ancient Medicine: Selected Papers of Ludwig Edelstein*, edited by Owsei Temkin and C. Lilian Temkin, 3–64. Baltimore: Johns Hopkins Press, 1967.

Etziony, M. B. *The Physician's Creed: An Anthology of Medical Prayers, Oaths and Codes of Ethics Written and Recited by Medical Practitioners Through the Ages*. Springfield, Ill.: Thomas, 1973.

Franck, Isaac, ed. *Biomedical Ethics in Perspective of Jewish Teaching and Tradition: Proceedings of an Academic Conference*. Washington, D.C.: College of Jewish Studies of Greater Washington, D.C., 1980.

Gregory, John. *Lectures on the Duties and Qualifications of a Physician*. Philadelphia: M. Carey & Son, 1817.

Jones, W. H. S. *The Doctor's Oath: An Essay in the History of Medicine*. Cambridge, Mass.: Cambridge University Press, 1926.

Judicial Council, American Medical Association. *Current Opinions of the Judicial Council of the American Medical Association—1984: Including the Principles of Medical Ethics and Rules of the Judicial Council*. Chicago: American Medical Association, 1984.

May, William F. "Code, Covenant, Contract, or Philanthropy?" *Hastings Cent Rep* 5 (Dec. 1975): 29–38.

National Commission for the Protection of Human Subjects of Biomedical and Behavioral Research. *The Belmont Report: Ethical Principles and Guidelines for the Protection of Human Subjects of Research*. Washington, D.C.: Government Printing Office, 1978.

"Oath of Initiation (Caraka Samhita)." In *Encylopedia of Bioethics*, Vol. 4, edited by Warren T. Reich, 1732–1733. New York: The Free Press, 1978.

Percival, Thomas. *Percival's Medical Ethics, 1803*. Reprint. Edited by Chauncey D. Leake. Baltimore: Williams & Wilkins, 1927.

Pope Pius XII. "The Prolongation of Life: An Address of Pope Pius XII to an International Congress of Anesthesiologists." *The Pope Speaks* 4 (1958): 393–398.

President's Commission for the Study of Ethical Problems in Medicine and Biomedical and Behavioral Research. *Summing Up: Final Report on Studies of the Ethical and Legal Problems in Medicine and Biomedical and Behavioral Research*. Washington, D.C.: Government Printing Office, 1983.

"Principles of Medical Ethics of the American Medical Association." *JAMA* 164 (1957): 11119–11120.

Rahman, Abdul, C. Amine, and Ahmed Elkadi. "Islamic Code of Medical Professional Ethics." Papers Presented to the First International Conference on Islamic Medicine Celebrating the Advent of the Fifteenth Century Hijri. Kuwait: Kuwait Ministry of Health, 1981.

Rosner, Fred, and David J. Bleich, eds. *Jewish Bioethics*. New York: Sanhedrin Press, 1979.

Smith, Wesley D. *The Hippocratic Tradition*. Ithaca, N.Y.: Cornell University Press, 1979.

Tendler, M. D., ed. *Medical Ethics: A Compendium of Jewish Moral, Ethical and Religious Principles in Medical Practice*, 5th ed. New York: Committee of Religious Affairs, Federation of Jewish Philanthropies of New York, 1975.

The Oath of Soviet Physicians. Translated by Zenonas Danilevicius. *JAMA* 217 (1971): 834.

United States Catholic Conference, Department of Health Affairs. *Ethical and Religious Directives for Catholic Health Facilities*. Washington, D.C.: United States Catholic Conference, 1971.

Unschuld, Paul U. *Medical Ethics in Imperial China: A Study in Historical Anthropology*, Berkeley, Calif.: University of California Press, 1979.

World Medical Association. "International Code of Medical Ethics." *World Med J* 3 (1956), supplement, p. 12.

World Medical Association. "Declaration of Geneva." *World Med J* 3, suppl. (1956): 12.

DISCUSSION QUESTIONS

1. How has the Hippocratic system of medical ethics changed over the years? Is it possible for an ethical code or oath produced for a particular group of physicians in the culture of ancient Greece to be meaningful today for physicians in a different culture?

2. What are the key differences between the ethics of the Hippocratic tradition and the ethics of the nursing profession? Ought nursing be governed by the ethics articulated by physicians? If not, how ought ethical conflicts between physicians and nurses be resolved?

3. Is it reasonable for patients, legislators, judges, and other medical lay people to assume that the ethics for professional-lay relationships should be governed by professionally articulated ethical positions?

4. If a physician is a member of a professional group and also of a religious group that in some way differs from the professional group on some key ethical issue, by which ethical tradition ought the physician be guided?

5. Should physicians who come from non-Western ethical traditions be guided by their own ethical traditions or by that of Western medicine? What should a physician do who encounters a patient standing in an ethical tradition that is in conflict with the ethics of the physician? Should people from other parts of the world or from different ethical traditions in the West be exempt from the ethics of Western medicine?

2

The Normative
Principles of
Medical Ethics

James F. Childress

SUMMARY

Moral dilemmas are often generated by conflicts among moral principles. Normative principles are action guides specifying which type of actions are morally required, prohibited, or permitted. They are very general, describing the characteristics of actions that make them morally right or wrong: for example, beneficence (doing good), nonmaleficence (avoiding evil), autonomy, and justice. This chapter analyzes the debate about normative principles in biomedical ethics, indicating the major issues and lines of argument. The first section of the chapter addresses the issues of moral justification, moral theories, and dilemmas which derive from conflicts among moral principles.

Although principles in biomedical ethics represent similar sorts of moral considerations they are often denominated differently by various groups. Sometimes, moral obligations are expressed as principles, other times, as rules. Principles are more general and frequently serve as sources of foundations of rules, which specify in more detail the type of prohibited, required, or permitted action.

It is possible to justify an action from many different perspectives including those of the agent, the act itself, the end, and the consequences. The role of ethical principles and rules in these assessments are explored. Even among proponents of the same principles and rules, there is often wide disagreement about what those principles and rules imply for particular cases largely due to disputes about their meaning and weight. Several major views are presented of the weight or stringency of moral principles and rules and of how they may be applied to justify moral judgment.

As there are different viewpoints about the meaning and nature of moral principles and rules, as well as many moral principles and rules, there are also several types of dilemmas to which they can give rise. The first type involves a conflict between moral principles and self-interest. The second involves an apparent conflict among moral principles, some indicating that an act is right, others that it is wrong. In the third type of dilemma, the conflict between moral principles persists even after careful and imaginative reflection.

The final section surveys various criticisms of ethical rules and principles. Throughout this chapter, the author suggests that the difficult question is not whether to invoke or apply principles and rules but rather which rules and principles should be adopted, how they should be interpreted, how much weight and strength they should be accorded, which have priority in a conflict, and in what relations and situations they apply.

MORAL JUSTIFICATION AND MORAL THEORIES

Many disputes in biomedical ethics are largely disputes about normative principles—which principles, if any, are applicable, how much weight they have, especially if they are in conflict, and what they imply for particular cases. This chapter will analyze the debate about normative principles in biomedical ethics, indicating the major issues and lines of argument. Case 1 focuses on some major issues of moral justification and ethical reflection.

Case 1. For the last three years a five-year-old girl has suffered from progressive renal failure as a result of glomerulonephritis. She was not doing well on chronic renal dialysis, and the staff proposed transplantation after determining that there was "a clear possibility" that a transplanted kidney would not undergo the same disease process. The parents accepted this proposal. It was clear from tissue typing that the patient would be difficult to match. Her two siblings, ages two and four, were too young to be organ donors, and her mother was not histocompatible, but her father was quite compatible. When the nephrologist met with the father and informed him of the test results, as well as the uncertain prognosis for his daughter even with a kidney transplant, the father decided not to donate one of his kidneys to his daughter. He gave several reasons for his decision: In addition to the uncertain prognosis for his daughter, there was a possibility of a cadaver kidney, his daughter had already undergone a great deal of suffering, and he lacked the courage to make the donation. However, the father was afraid that if the family knew the truth, they would blame him for allowing his daughter to die and then the family itself would be wrecked. Therefore, he asked the physician to tell the members of the family that he was not histocompatible, when in fact he was. The physician did not feel comfortable about carrying out this request, but he finally agreed to tell the man's

> wife that the father could not donate a kidney "for medical reasons" (Levine, Scott, and Curran 1977, 205).

The physician felt uncomfortable in carrying out the father's request because of what he experienced as a moral conflict, quandary, or dilemma. Moral dilemmas are generated by conflicts between moral principles. As a character in Tom Stoppard's play *Professional Foul* (1978, 99) notes, "there would be no moral dilemmas if moral principles worked in straight lines and never crossed each other." However, in science, medicine, and health care, as well as elsewhere, agents experience such conflicts. Because these conflicts are set by principles, they can only be resolved by probing those principles, their meaning and their weight, to see what ought to be done in the situation, all things considered. In this case the physician balanced such moral considerations as truthfulness, not lying, acting in the daughter's interest, confidentiality, protecting the father, and preserving the family.

Some of these moral considerations may be viewed as principles, others as rules. Both principles and rules are "general action guides specifying that some type of action is prohibited, required, or permitted in certain circumstances" (Solomon 1978, 1, 408). Even though the term "principles" often encompasses rules, it is useful to distinguish principles from rules for this discussion. Principles are more general and frequently serve as sources or foundations of rules, which specify in more detail the type of prohibited, required, or permitted action. With this distinction, it is possible to think about the process of moral justification in an appellate fashion, with the justification of particular moral judgments often involving more general moral appeals. This process can be sketched in terms of tiers or three levels of moral justification (Beauchamp and Childress 1983, Chapter 1):

1. Principles (These might be stated as either duties/obligations or rights)
2. Rules
3. Particular Judgments

Apparently the physician believed that it was wrong to lie and thus refrained from saying directly that the father was not histocompatible. If asked why he thought it was wrong to lie to the mother he might have appealed to a moral rule that prohibits lying, and he might have justified this moral rule by appealing to various principles such as respect for persons and utility (maximizing welfare)— for example, a rule against lying is important to maintain trust between professionals and patients. If the moral rule against lying had been the only moral consideration in this case, the physician would not have experienced a dilemma. However, there were other moral considerations, including confidentiality (the physician had gained information about the father in the course of an examination and the rule of confidentiality limits the disclosure of such information to other parties without the examinee's consent) and not wrecking the family (which reflects the principle of utility). The physician found what he deemed a satisfactory moral compromise. He did not directly lie because "medical reasons" may include psychological reasons, but he also did not disclose the full truth in order to protect the confidentiality of the information he had gained, and in order to avoid wrecking the family.

The physician's action could be assessed from several different standpoints.

Aspects of Human Action:

(1) Agent (2) Acts (3) Ends and (4) Consequences.

Ethical theories differ in part according to which aspect of human action they emphasize. *Virtue* theories emphasize aspect (1), holding that actions are right or wrong depending on what they express about the agent. Actions are right if they express virtue, wrong if they express vice. Although it may be difficult to come to a conclusive judgment in this case, the actions could be assessed according to what they express about the agents. For example, both the father's cowardice in not wanting to donate or to face blame from the family and his concern for his daughter and his family are relevant. (Virtue theories will be considered again at the end of this chapter.)

Deontological theories emphasize aspect (2), acts in and of themselves, holding that some inherent or intrinsic features of actions make them right or wrong, not simply their ends and their consequences. For example, it might be argued that the father violated an implicit commitment to his daughter when he refused to accept the risk of organ donation for her, or that the physician's actions did not violate the rule against lying. As a deontologist, the physician might have argued that the rule of confidentiality outweighed the rule of truthfulness.

Teleological theories emphasize aspect (3), the ends of action, while *consequentialist* theories emphasize aspect (4), the consequences or effects of action. Both of these theories downplay or even deny the importance of intrinsic or inherent features of actions, such as whether actions are in accord with a moral rule against lying, in order to concentrate on what actions are intended to produce or actually produce. For example, the physician's actions might be assessed as means to his goal of not wrecking the family. Then it would be necessary to determine whether the means would probably be effective (e.g., the family might not be salvageable or the mother might press questions about "medical reasons") and also whether if effective the actions would produce other bad consequences that might outweigh the good ones (e.g., the father might later experience guilt that would destroy the family).

This chapter concentrates on the debate about the adequacy of teleological-consequentialist theories, which affirm principles regarding the production of good and avoidance of bad consequences, and deontological theories, which affirm principles regarding the inherent or intrinsic rightness or wrongness of actions. Many theories of biomedical ethics attempt to provide room for both rules and consequences and thus determine the rightness or wrongness of actions according to whether they conform to principles and rules and maximize good consequences. Exactly how they attempt to do this will be considered later.

MORAL PRINCIPLES AND RULES

The literature in biomedical ethics in the last fifteen or twenty years has identified several moral principles, often but not always the same ones. For example, the National Commission for the Protection of Human Subjects of Biomedical and Behavioral Research (1978) justified its recommendations for policies by appealing to three major principles: respect for persons, beneficence (which includes what some have called nonmaleficence), and justice. Whatever the principles in biomedical ethics are called, they represent the following sorts of moral considerations: obligations to respect the wishes of competent persons (respect for persons or autonomy); obligations not to harm others, including not killing them or treating them cruelly (nonmaleficence); obligations to benefit others (beneficence); obligations to produce a net balance of benefits over harms (utility); obligations to distribute benefits and harms fairly (justice); obligations to keep promises and contracts (fidelity); obligations of truthfulness; obligations to disclose information; and obligations to respect privacy and to protect confidential information (confidentiality). Sometimes these obligations are stated as principles; sometimes as rules. Some obligations are viewed as primary and fundamental; others as secondary and derivative. For example, Beauchamp and Childress (1983) recognize primary principles of autonomy, nonmaleficence, beneficence (including utility), justice, and derivative principles or rules of veracity, fidelity, privacy and confidentiality. Veatch's (1981) list of primary principles overlaps in important respects but differs in others: beneficence; contract-keeping; autonomy; honesty; avoiding killing; and justice. He also recognizes several moral rules or intermediate moral formulations, such as informed consent. In a much shorter list, Tristram Engelhardt (1986) accepts only the principles of autonomy and beneficence, reducing justice to these two considerations, but he then recognizes several derivative obligations. Thus, one major difference among ethical theories is how they sort out different obligations. Some theories may encompass several obligations under a few general headings, while others may view them as distinct and even separable obligations.

Other principles and rules have been proposed in addition to those already identified. For example, universalizability is widely accepted as a principle of morality. It is often viewed as a formal principle of morality, that is, as a necessary condition for any moral judgment. It is also widely viewed as a formal principle of justice within morality: treat similar cases in a similar way. This principle has affinities with the Golden Rule—do unto others as you would have them do unto you. Sometimes the Golden Rule is invoked in biomedical ethics as though it is all that agents need to make their decisions. It is easy to dismiss the Golden Rule if it is viewed as a sufficient principle but much harder to dismiss if it is viewed only as a necessary principle. It is probably best viewed as a test of reasons for action, especially to determine if one is making an unjustified exception of oneself. It thus functions best, as Marcus Singer (1963) indicates, when it is conceived in terms of general rather than specific desires or general rules rather than particular actions. If the Golden Rule (perhaps more properly construed as a principle than as a rule) is applied to specific desires or particular actions it may be plausibly viewed as "morally dangerous" (Veatch 1981, 313). For example, physicians may decide whether to tell the patient the truth about a diagnosis of cancer and a prognosis of death by asking whether the bad news would upset them if they were in the patient's situation. However, the principle of universalizability or the Golden Rule is more properly applied in the following way. The physician should ask by what rule he/she would want to be treated in such circumstances. As a necessary condition of moral judgments, whether general or particular, the principle itself is not dangerous, though unsophisticated applications may be dangerous.

Ethical theories differ not only according to which aspects of human action they emphasize and which moral principles and rules they propose, but also according to the grounds or foundations they offer for those principles and rules. Sometimes the debate between utilitarians and deontologists has been misplaced because some utilitarians suppose that deontologists have a more difficult time than they in laying foundations for their ethical principles and rules. This misplaced debate may stem from the tendency to view deontological theories as reflecting common morality. However, the problems faced by deontologists in justifying several distinct principles and rules of obligation are not different from those faced by the utilitarian in justifying the ultimate principle of utility. Deontologists and utilitarians then may appeal to the same foundations: revelation (e.g., the divine will); intuition; reason (e.g., the nature of practical reason); human nature (e.g., natural law); a hypothetical contract; tradition; etc. The debates about the acceptability or superiority of any ethical theory will hinge on such obvious formal criteria as consistency, coherence, simplicity, and comprehensiveness, and, more controversially, on such substantive criteria as the theory's capacity to account for and to direct moral experience.

THE MEANING AND WEIGHT OF PRINCIPLES AND RULES

Even among proponents of the same principles and rules, there is wide disagreement about what those principles and rules imply for particular cases because of disputes about their meaning and weight. It is important to consider meaning and weight together. For example, in Case 1, the physician might have held that the rule of confidentiality outweighed the rule of truthfulness or that the avoidance of bad consequences (wrecking the family) outweighed the rule of truthfulness. However, there are different interpretations of the meaning of the rules of confidentiality and truthfulness, as well as of their weight and stringency. Consider two possibilities. First, if lying is defined as an intentionally deceptive statement, it might be held that the physician told a lie when he said that for "medical reasons" the father should not donate a kidney. In view of this definition, the moral debate would focus on whether the rule against lying could be overridden in this case by another rule (the rule of confidentiality) or by the consequences (avoiding the destruction of the family). Whatever is held about this particular case, few if any ethical theories consistently hold that lying so defined is absolutely wrong. Second, if lying is defined as intentionally withholding information from or deceiving someone who has a right to the truth, the moral debate about this case would focus on whether the physician actually lied and ultimately on whether the wife had a right to the information that had emerged in the relationship between her husband and the nephrologist. If this second definition of lying is accepted, it would be possible to hold that the rule against lying is absolute, for all of the difficult moral questions would be answered by determining who has a right to the truth. As this example suggests, it is essential to examine both the meaning and the weight of any principle or rule.

The following categories suggest several major views of the weight or stringency of moral principles and rules:

Legalism   Antinomianism

Absolute/ Prima Facie/Relative

Joseph Fletcher (1966) offered his method of "situation ethics" as a view between the extremes of legalism and antinomianism. He insisted that there is only one absolute principle—that of neighbor-love, or utility—and all other principles and rules are mere maxims or rules of thumb, such as "don't bunt on third strike." These other principles and rules suggest actions that people have found to produce or subvert good consequences. They only illuminate courses of action, they do not prescribe what ought to be done. By reducing all principles and rules to mere maxims regarding utility, Fletcher came perilously close to antinomianism. His position failed to recognize that principles and rules can be prescriptive, without being absolute. They can be prima facie binding, i.e., binding other things being equal. As prima facie, they direct courses of action but they can be overridden or outweighed by other prima facie principles and rules when they conflict.

Beauchamp and Childress (1983) argue that the principles they identify—autonomy, nonmaleficence, beneficence (including utility or proportionality), and justice, along with such derivative principles or rules as veracity, fidelity, privacy, and confidentiality—are only prima facie binding. None can be considered as absolute. And these principles and rules have to be weighed and balanced in situations of decision. This perspective might appear to be very close to Fletcher's maxims or rules of thumb, but there is an important difference. For Beauchamp and Childress, the principles and rules are prima facie binding and thus prescriptive, whereas for Fletcher they only illuminate the application of the one ultimate principle of neighbor-love (or utility). For Beauchamp and Childress, the moral agent has to justify departures from moral principles and rules by showing that in the situation some other principles and rules have more weight. However, the assignment of weight or priority depends on the situation rather than on an abstract, *a priori* ranking. Their approach suffers from the limitations of any pluralistic approach that does not assign weights or priorities to various principles in advance. A great deal rests on what has been variously called prudence, practical moral reasoning, or discernment in the situation.

A rule-utilitarian may find the pluralistic approach to moral principles and rules less troubling than a rule-deontologist, because the former at least has the ultimate principle of utility which justifies various other principles and rules and also adjudicates conflicts among them. Some deontologists have explored priority rules, for example, contending that the principle of autonomy always trumps or overrides the principle of beneficence, when the only beneficiary is the competent person whose wishes, choices or actions are overridden. A major effort to find a lexical or serial ordering of principles appears in Robert Veatch's *A Theory of Medical Ethics* (1981), wherein all deontological or nonconsequentialist principles "are given lexical priority over the principle of beneficence." However, in cases of conflict, the deontological or nonconsequentialist principles are themselves balanced against each other in what Veatch labels a "balancing strategy." Veatch thus finds "a solution to the inevitable unacceptable tension between Hippocratic individualism and the utilitarian drive toward aggregate net benefit." This solution "comes from the articulation of other nonconsequentialist principles that will necessarily have a bearing on medical ethical decisions: contract keeping, autonomy, honesty, avoiding killing, and justice" and from assigning them collective priority over the production of good consequences for individuals (Hippocratic individualism) or society (utilitarianism). Nonconsequentialist principles are thus given "coequal ranking" in relation to each other and "lexical ranking" over the principle of beneficence. Similarly, Engelhardt (1986) gives the principle of autonomy priority over the principle of beneficence. The problems of ranking and ordering principles in the context of moral conflicts, and the application of principles to cases, are further explored below.

MORAL CONFLICTS AND THE APPLICATION OF PRINCIPLES

Earlier I suggested that moral dilemmas are generated by conflicts among moral principles. Adapting a proposal by John Lemmon (1962), it is possible to distinguish several types of dilemmas. The first type involves a conflict between moral principles and self-interest. For example, the father in Case 1 may have experienced a dilemma in this sense. He felt a moral obligation to donate a kidney in order to try to save his daughter's life, but he lacked the courage to risk his health and survival. Whether such a conflict should even be construed as a *moral* dilemma is debatable. Some deny that it is a moral dilemma because morality is on one side and self-interest on the other, but others would define morality so as to include self-interest.

The second type of dilemma involves an apparent conflict between moral principles, some of which indicate that an act is wrong, others that it is right. The physician in the first case may have experienced such a dilemma as he considered the principles of confidentiality, truthfulness, and utility. Sometimes a dilemma of this second type is only a matter of uncertainty that can be resolved when the relevant principles are properly balanced or interpreted. Some ethicists deny that this second type of conflict is genuinely dilemmatic if the perplexity dissolves upon closer examination.

In the third type of dilemma, however, the conflict between moral principles persists even after careful and imaginative reflection; there is clear evidence that an act is right and clear evidence that it is wrong. There is general agreement that this third type of situation—where the moral conflict is not in principle resolvable if limitations of knowledge could be overcome—is a genuine dilemma, but there is disagreement about whether such dilemmas exist. It is not clear that the physician in the first case experienced this kind of dilemma. At least he found what was for him an acceptable moral compromise by saying that for "medical reasons" the father should not donate a kidney. For purposes of this discussion both the second and the third types of conflicts are called "dilemmas." The following are three situations of conflict that illuminate debates about the application of principles.

The first situation is research involving human subjects. A straightforward consequentialist approach to research, particularly one based on utilitarian calculation and unfettered by deontological restraints (or rule-utilitarian restraints), might justify research that is deceptive or coercive in order to produce significant benefits for a large number of people. Such an approach, further tainted by a racist ideology, was adopted by Nazi Germany. However, utilitarianism may avoid such a conclusion by being truly universalistic (rather than denying the relevance of harms to some human beings) and by considering a broad range of goods over time (rather than simply immediate scientific progress). By contrast, a rule-deontologist, such as Ramsey (1970), would hold that the ends justify only the means that pass an independent moral audit or inspection. For the deontologist, actions have features other than their effectiveness and efficiency as means; they should also be assessed in relation to such independent principles as autonomy and justice.

Most ethical assessments of research involving human subjects appeal to both consequentialist and deontological considerations and to a wide range of moral principles and rules, as is evident in the following conditions or criteria of ethically justified research (see Childress 1981; Walters 1977). (1) The end of the research—the knowledge sought—should be important. (2) There should be a reasonable prospect that the research will generate the knowledge that is sought. (3) The use of human subjects in a research project should be a matter of last resort. Their use should be preceded by other studies, including animal experimentation, and should be necessary. The Nuremberg Code (Beauchamp and Childress 1983, 338) holds that "the experiment should be such as to yield fruitful results for the good of society, unprocurable by other methods or means of study." (4) The risks to the subjects should be minimized. (5) The research should meet the principle of utility or proportionality in the balance of probable benefits to the society, including the subjects, and the risks, burdens, and costs to subjects.

The first five conditions focus on the probable consequences of the research for the society and the subjects, as viewed in relation to the principles of beneficence, nonmaleficence and utility. While these conditions are necessary, they are not sufficient from most ethical perspectives. Even though it can be argued that these conditions should be considered first, some other conditions are also necessary and may morally invalidate research that satisfies the first five conditions. (6) The selection of research subjects should be fair and equitable (the principle of justice), and (7) the research must have the subjects' (or the proxy's where appropriate) voluntary and informed consent to participate (the principle of respect for persons). In addition, (8) the principles or rules of privacy, confidentiality, and promise-keeping set limits on the conduct of the research. There is no moral right to seek research subjects unless the first five conditions have been met (as often determined by an Institutional Review Board), there is no moral right to proceed with these research subjects unless conditions six and seven have been met, and the research is wrongly conducted unless the eighth condition is met. If all of these conditions are necessary for ethically justified research with human subjects, then research that meets the principles of beneficence, nonmaleficence, and utility, but not the principles of justice, autonomy, privacy, confidentiality, and promise-keeping, is unjustified. The conflict between producing good for the society through research and not wronging research subjects is not a dilemma in the third sense above; it should be resolved through assigning priority to the nonconsequentialist principles in cases of conflict.

From this perspective, it is necessary to view as morally unacceptable the 1979 randomized clinical trial of intestinal bypass in comparison to medication in the treatment of gross obesity. Patients who were referred to participating institutions were informed about the benefits, risks, side-effects, and uncertainties of the surgical procedure before being randomly assigned to the surgical and medical groups. However, the investigators wrote: "We did not ask for informed consent for randomisation. Patients allocated to medical treatment were told that the surgery had to be postponed for an undetermined period primarily because liver-biopsy findings showed fatty infiltration" (Danish Obesity Project 1979). The investigators not only failed to disclose the use of randomization but also deliberately deceived those assigned to the medical group. Their actions were not warranted even to increase the number of participants in order to conduct more valid research.

A conflict between utility and justice (or equity) can be seen in the debate about policies to control hypertension in the American population. Some ethical problems are obvious. While such a policy to control hypertension as a concern of public health may be justified on grounds of its cost-effectiveness, it may be problematic from the standpoint of distributive justice or equity. Many poor people and blacks would not know of their hypertension because they are not under medical care. For example, blacks, who comprise 18 percent of hypertensives but only 9 percent of the total US population, have not had equal access to good medical care. In addition, if hypertension as a disease of modern industrial society is exacerbated by the unequal distribution of power there may be other claims of injustice (Guttmacher 1981). Finally, it might be argued that the society has a stronger moral obligation to inform everyone of his/her hypertension through public screening than "to cajole people to take care of themselves when others might be denied the basic information about their condition that would even allow them to make a choice" (Weinstein and Stason 1977).

Case 2. In the mid-1970s it was estimated that 17 percent of adults (approximately 24 million persons) had hypertension, which can lead to major health problems. According to Milton Weinstein and William B. Stason (1977), minimally adequate treatment for all of these people would cost over $5 billion annually. Treatment is difficult because almost half of the people with hypertension are not aware of their problem and only one-sixth of those who know about their problem are receiving proper treatment. Weinstein and Stason tried to determine the most cost-effective way to control hypertension. As an expression of the principle of utility, cost-effectiveness analysis is an attempt to determine which policy would produce the greatest aggregate benefits, such as quality-adjusted life years for the money. (Cost-effectiveness analysis differs from cost-benefit analysis in that it does not convert the benefits along with the costs into a common denominator of money.) Several factors were important in the analysis, including the difficulty of convincing people identified as hypertensives through mass screening and education programs to seek medical treatment and to comply with the recommended treatment. Their analysis led Weinstein and Stason (1977, 28) to conclude that a "community with limited resources would probably do better to concentrate its efforts on improving adherence of known hypertensives, even at a sacrifice in terms of the numbers screened. This conclusion holds even if such proadherence interventions are rather expensive and only moderately effective, and even if screening is very inexpensive." Furthermore, they concluded, screening patients already under the care of a physician is more cost-effective than public screening.

A final example of a dilemma (at least in the second sense) involves the deceptive use of a placebo and an apparent conflict between the principle of beneficence and the principles of autonomy and truthfulness.

Case 3. Mr. X, a 65-year-old retired army officer who had been very successful in the military and in teaching and research, had had several abdominal operations for gallstones, postoperative adhesions, and bowel obstructions. Because of chronic pain, he was somewhat depressed, had lost weight, had poor hygiene, and had withdrawn socially because he had to assume awkward or embarrassing postures in order to control his pain. He had used Talwin six times a day for more than two years to control the pain, but now he had so much tissue and muscle damage that he had trouble finding injection sites. And Talwin itself may be addictive. Stating his goal as "to get more out of life in spite of my pain," Mr. X voluntarily entered a psychiatric ward, which included individual behavior therapy programs, daily group therapy, etc. Although Mr. X reduced his Talwin usage to four times a day, he insisted that this level was necessary to control his pain. After considerable discussion with their colleagues, the therapists decided to withdraw the Talwin over time without the patient's knowledge by diluting it with increasing proportions of normal saline. Although Mr. X experienced nausea, diarrhea, and cramps, he thought that these withdrawal symptoms were actually the result of Elavil (Amitriptyline), which the therapists had introduced to relieve the withdrawal symptoms. Self-control techniques were continued, and the intervals between injections were increased. Although the patient was aware of the changes in intervals, he was not aware that he was receiving only saline. After three weeks, his therapists disclosed that he was receiving a placebo, not Talwin. After initial anger, he asked that the saline be discontinued and the self-control techniques continued. When he was discharged three weeks later, he reported that he could control his abdominal pain more effectively with the self-control techniques than he could earlier with Talwin. A follow-up six months later showed that he was still using the relaxation techniques and had resumed social activities and part-time teaching. The therapists justified this deceptive use of a placebo on grounds of its effectiveness: "We felt ethically obliged to use a treatment that had a high probability of success. To withhold the procedure may have protected some standard of openness but may not have been in his [the patient's] best interests. We saw no option without ethical problems. Although it is precarious to justify the means by the end, we felt most obliged to use a procedure designed to help the patient achieve a personally and medically desirable goal" (Levendusky and Pankratz 1975, 165–168).

On one level this case appears to involve a straightforward conflict between the principle of beneficence and the principles of autonomy and veracity. The therapists saw "no option without ethical problems," and concluded that the ends justified the means in this case. Thus, ranking consequentialist principles over nonconsequentialist ones, at least in this sort of case, they justified paternalistic actions in apparent violation of the principles of autonomy and veracity. There is considerable debate about whether paternalistic actions—refusals to acquiesce in a person's wishes, choices, and actions for that person's own benefit—can be justified. Both a conceptual point and a normative point are involved.

Normatively, some consequentialists argue that beneficence (as well as nonmaleficence and utility) toward a patient can justify overriding that patient's autonomy. By contrast, some nonconsequentialists contend that the principle of autonomy always trumps the principle of beneficence, when only the patient's welfare is involved (i.e., there is no harm to other parties). In this case nonconsequentialists could argue that the therapists unjustifiably violated the patient's autonomy when they deceptively used a placebo. Clearly this debate in ethical theory has considerable significance for resolving this case.

The conceptual point concerns the definition of paternalism. Some philosophers insist that paternalism has both strong (or extended) and weak (or limited) forms. Strong paternalism overrides an *autonomous* person's wishes, choices or actions, while weak paternalism overrides a *nonautonomous* person's wishes, choices or actions (or temporarily intervenes in order to determine if a person is acting autonomously). It is clear that strong paternalism raises the most serious moral questions, and some philosophers insist that weak paternalism is not even paternalism, at least in any morally interesting sense, because it does not involve a conflict between beneficence and autonomy (because the target of beneficence is not autonomous). In this case, there could be debate about whether Mr. X's autonomy has been sufficiently compromised both by his pain and by his use of Talwin, an addictive drug, so as to justify overriding his choices as nonautonomous—whether or not this intervention is called weak paternalism. In any event, despite their differences about whether a person's diminished autonomy is a necessary condition to justify paternalism, both weak and strong paternalists have to meet some consequentialist conditions that focus on the probability of harm or loss of benefit without intervention and the probability of a net balance of benefit over harm with the intervention. In addition, some ethicists argue, even if the principle of respect for persons is overridden, it still requires that the least insulting, humiliating, disrespectful, and restrictive intervention be chosen (see Childress 1982).

Another possible response to this case also focuses on the meaning of the principle of autonomy. According to this interpretation the therapists did not violate Mr. X's autonomous choices but rather acted in accord with them. It could be claimed that the patient implicitly consented to the modification in medication, even though he continued explicitly to refuse it, because he voluntarily admitted himself to a psychiatric ward where adjustment in medication was a clear expectation and because he accepted the goals of therapy—"to get more out of life in spite of . . . pain." Or it might be argued that Mr. X's current refusal to further modify his Talwin usage should be put in the context of his *past consent* and his *probable future consent*. The issue of past consent usually surfaces when a person has previously accepted a course of action that he or she now repudiates; as in the case of implicit consent, the question is exactly what Mr. X consented to when he voluntarily entered the psychiatric ward. While the appeal to implicit or past consent might succeed if we had no other information about Mr. X's wishes, we do have other information: he now expressly refuses to allow further reduction in the Talwin dosage level. Thus, many would argue, we cannot appeal to implied consent or to past consent to override current express refusals unless we can show that the patient now has diminished autonomy (i.e., some defect, encumbrance, or limitation in decisionmaking).

Is it possible for the therapists to appeal to Mr. X's probable future consent and thus invoke the principle of autonomy to justify their actions? The therapists apparently believed that Mr. X retrospectively ratified their decision to use the placebo when he decided to continue the self-control techniques. However, it is difficult to hold that either actual or predicted future consent satisfies the condition of respect for persons. There is a danger that the intervention itself will create the consent, but, even where this danger is not present, the prediction of future consent can only provide some evidence that the criteria for justifying paternalism have been met. That prediction does not itself make the intervention a matter of respect for autonomy.

Finally, the therapists noted that they saw "no option without ethical problems." In order to be justified, deception must be necessary to meet the goal that is sought. If the goal can be obtained by some other morally appropriate means, deception is unjustified. This claim may be based on the recognition of the principle of veracity as having at least prima facie moral weight so that any violation requires justification. The therapists believed that they had a duty to "use a treatment that had a high probability of success" even if they had to violate "some standard of openness." They had to choose between openness and effectiveness in seeking a goal which the patient also desired. It is not clear, however, that all moral options had been exhausted. One possibility would have been to obtain the patient's consent to several drugs, including placebos. Such consent might have been obtained at the outset. Indeed, when the placebo was given, Mr. X was informed that a modification of his medication regimen would be undertaken, but he did not receive any specific details. However, since he still insisted on maintaining the same Talwin dosage level (though not the same frequency), he could not be said to have consented to the placebo. Another possibility may have been excluded as an option because of the staff's therapeutic perspective. The staff defined the "problem" in terms of specific behaviors, and perhaps they paid inadequate attention to the "person responsible for those behaviors" (Kelman 1975). If the therapists had conceived the problem in a different way, they might have considered alternative procedures with high probabilities of success and without ethical problems.

These cases and problem areas suggest some complexities in the appeal to principles in ethical deliberation and justification. Not only are there difficult questions about which principles are relevant, there are also difficult questions about their meaning and their weight. Even the appeal to shared principles does not ensure agreement about their application to particular cases, because there may be disagreements about the meaning and weight of the relevant moral principles and rules as well as about the facts of the case. The metaphor of "application" itself may distort the process, especially if it suggests a mechanical or legalistic use of principles and rules. The metaphor of "discernment" may be more helpful as long as it is not combined with efforts to replace principles and rules altogether. Perhaps it would also be appropriate to view the relation between principles and particular judgments about cases as circular or dialectical. Agents move back and forth between them, using principles to make judgments about particular cases but sometimes modifying their interpretation of the meaning and stringency of principles in the light of particular cases. Sometimes it will be unclear whether the principles or the particular judgments require modification.

CRITICISMS OF PRINCIPLES

In recent years several criticisms have been levelled against principles and rules in biomedical ethics. One such criticism emerged in our discussion of situation ethics.

As the major contemporary form of consequentialism, utilitarianism may, as we have seen, appeal to utility to derive other principles and rules, which then determine the rightness or wrongness of particular acts (rule utilitarianism), or to assess acts directly (act utilitarianism). Act utilitarians hold that principles and rules other than utility are indefensible unless they function only as maxims or rules of thumb without prescriptive, binding power. Thus, from the standpoint of act utilitarians, both rule utilitarians and rule deontologists are more alike than different; both make too much of principles and rules and too little of the consequences of particular acts. Principles and rules, act consequentialists contend, create victims of morality—people suffer bad consequences because of adherence to principles and rules.

A closely related version of this criticism of principles and rules—which does not necessarily entail act utilitarianism—focuses on casuistry and holds that moral agents can make discerning judgments about particular cases even though they disagree about the principles and rules that justify those judgments. For example, in reflecting on the work of the National Commission for the Protection of Human Subjects, Stephen Toulmin, who was a staff philosopher for the Commission, argues that the appeal to principles by the commissioners was unnecessary and misleading. For, he insists, the commissioners "were, quite evidently, surer about these shared particular judgments (e.g., about the kind of consent procedures required in biomedical research using five-year-old children) than they were about the discordant general principles on which, in theory, their practical judgments were based" (Toulmin 1981, 31). So, Toulmin contends, appeals to principles do not provide "a more solid foundation" for particular ethical judgments, but rather connect ethical conclusions with nonethical commitments. "Such principles serve less as foundations, adding intellectual strength or force to particular moral opinions, than they do as corridors or curtain walls linking the moral perceptions of all reflective human beings, with other, more general positions—theological, philosophical, ideological, or Weltanschaulich." Toulmin's target is not clear, for he shoots indiscriminately at "the tyranny of principles," the "absoluteness of moral principles," "tyrannical absolutism," "the cult of absolute principles," "unchallengeable principles," "a single principle held as absolute," "a morality based entirely on general rules and principles," etc. It may be possible and desirable to escape the tyranny of absolute, single, unchallengeable principles, but it may not be possible or desirable to escape all principles.

In response to such criticisms, rule utilitarians and rule deontologists contend that principles and rules are necessary to solve problems of coordination, cooperation, and trust in human interaction. For example, G. J. Warnock (1971, 33) asks us to consider the expectations that would be appropriate in an encounter between an act-utilitarian physician and an act-utilitarian patient. Warnock notes that the patient could only expect the physician to try to cure him of his afflictions, "*unless* his (the physician's) assessment of the 'general happiness' leads him to do otherwise." Asking the act-utilitarian physician to declare his intentions truthfully or to promise to consider only the patient's welfare, in accord with the Hippocratic tradition, would not help, because all of the physician's promises and declarations would themselves be subject to utilitarian calculation. Trust that the physician will act for the patient's own advantage disappears because of the physician's lack of commitment to moral principles other than utility. (Similar and more serious problems arise from the standpoint of act deontology's critique of principles and rules. At least act utilitarianism requires that agents attempt to calculate the greatest good for the greater number; by contrast act deontologists appeal to intuition, conscience, the divine command, etc., and their predictability becomes even less secure than the act utilitarians'.)

Another criticism of principles and rules in biomedical ethics holds that they are appropriate in interactions among strangers but not among friends and intimates. While attacking principles, Toulmin (1981) concedes that they are important in relations among strangers in contrast to relations among intimates. Hence, a fundamental question is whether in our society patients and physicians or other health care professionals interact as friends or as strangers. Major changes in health care have rendered problematic a conception of medicine in terms of friendship—pluralism in values, the decline of close, intimate contact over time between professionals and patients, the rise of specialists who treat only part of the whole person, and the growth of large, impersonal, and bureaucratic institutions of health care have all contributed to the loss of intimacy and community. Trust among strangers cannot presuppose knowledge of their traits of character or their values. In the absence of community, principles, rules, and procedures become increasingly important. As reconceived in a pluralistic setting, trust may be confidence in and reliance upon health care professionals to adhere to principles such as autonomy and truthfulness which do not presuppose knowledge of the professionals' interpretation of benefits and burdens or harms. Thus, rights within health care, as distinct from rights to health care, may limit and constrain the professional's actions even when they are putatively directed at the patient's welfare. Trust may be expressed as confidence in and reliance upon others to adhere to moral limits that derive from respect for persons, justice, etc., rather than from beneficence. In short, principles and rules may provide the basis for interaction among "friendly strangers." They are not friends, but they are not estranged and hostile. Even though they do not have (or at least do not know if they have) shared conceptions of the good life, including balances of benefits and harms, they can trust each other to respect common principles and rules. As MacIntyre (1977) has noted,

> When a community of moral and metaphysical beliefs is lacking, trust between strangers becomes much more questionable than when we can safely assume such a community. Nobody can rely on anyone else's judgments on his or her behalf until he or she knows what the other person believes. It follows that nobody can accept the moral authority of another in virtue simply of his professional position. We are thrust back into a form of moral autonomy.

Our social situation thus supports claims not only about the importance of moral principles and rules for interaction among strangers but also about the importance of some moral principles and rules over others. Expounding a theory of bioethics for secular, pluralistic societies, Engelhardt (1986) has argued that physicians "must come to terms with the moral commitments and views of individuals from various moral communities while preserving the moral fabric of a peaceable, secular, pluralist society."

In addition to their arguments for the significance of principles and rules for human interaction, rule utilitarians and rule deontologists contend that particular judgments imply rules because of the principle of universalizability: To hold that act X is wrong is to imply that all relevantly similar X's are wrong. Defenders of principles and rules also note that their critics frequently employ principles and rules, even when they fail to acknowledge them. For example, Fletcher, who expressly recognizes only the ultimate principle of utility and reduces other principles and rules to the status of suggestive maxims, appears to affirm at least one other strong rule when he holds that no "unwanted and unintended baby should ever be born" (Fletcher 1966, 39).

Also defending the primacy of casuistry against principles and rules, Albert Jonsen, Mark Siegler, and William Winslade in *Clinical Ethics* (1986) identify four main moral considerations for the cases they examine: medical indications; patient preferences; quality of life; and external factors. These four factors correlate closely with what others call moral principles—e.g., medical indications and quality of life both involve principles of beneficence and nonmaleficence; patient preferences involve respect for persons and their autonomy; and the external factors, which focus on the impact of actions on others, including family and society, involve considerations of utility and justice. In fact these ethical factors or considerations function in their argument about clinical ethics in roughly the way that similar principles and rules function for some other theories of biomedical ethics. They are prima facie or presumptive rather than absolute, but they are more than maxims. It is not clear that fear of the tyranny of principles that are absolute, simplistic, etc., is sufficient reason to discard the language of principles altogether, especially when these ethical considerations function as principles.

Another major criticism of principles and rules comes from virtue theories. In a virtue theory of morality, actions are assessed according to what they express about the agent. Such a theory holds that deontologists and utilitarians, in both their act and their rule forms, neglect the primary role of the virtues in the moral life when they emphasize principles and rules. Deontologists and utilitarians address a common question "What ought I do?" rather than "What ought I to be?", and they tend to emphasize moral dilemmas, quandaries, and problems that are set by conflicts of principles and have to be resolved by interpreting and balancing those principles. By contrast virtue theorists—though by no means a uniform group—emphasize (1) that a virtuous professional can *discern* the right course of action in the situation without reliance on principles and rules, and/or (2) that a virtuous person will *desire* to do what is right and avoid what is wrong. The first approach is often combined with situation ethics, and it downplays rules and often principles in moral decisionmaking. Leon Kass articulates this viewpoint: "I increasingly believe that the attempt to replace the often inarticulate yet prudent judgments of discerning physicians with explicit rules or procedures will not lead to better decisions" (1980, 1811). However, if we try to determine which approach will lead to "better decisions," it is necessary to appeal to principles and rules to identify courses of action that are right, obligatory, wrong, or permitted. And when agents, such as the physician in Case 1, have to justify their conduct, it is not sufficient for them to appeal to their discernment or prudence or conscience without reference to principles and rules. There is simply no assurance that good people will discern what is right.

The second approach to virtues concentrates on the agent's motivation to do what is right, assuming that what is right is clear in most situations and that the major problem is the lack of motivation to do what is right. In my interpretation of Case 1, I noted that the father's dilemma could be construed as a conflict between morality and self-interest. In such a conflict, the problem is not one of knowledge but of motivation, and virtues dispose people to act in certain ways. For example, according to Gregory Pence (1980, 177), "the ultimate argument" why biomedical ethics should be discussed "in the framework of the virtues" is that researchers, physicians, and other professionals can subvert such rules as informed consent if they desire. Thus, it is important to create a climate in which professionals have the right kind of desires. Pence is certainly correct to emphasize the role of virtues in disposing people to right actions, but it is necessary to have an independent assessment of acts in light of moral principles. Virtues include dispositions to right actions, but are not themselves sufficient to determine right actions. In Case 1 it is not clear what a virtuous physician would have done; perhaps at least he/she would have refused to be an instrument for the father's wishes, but, as we have seen, the case is complicated. And, for the most part, the determination of which virtues should be developed depends on principles of action. Many virtues are correlated with principles and rules (e.g., benevolence with beneficence, truthfulness with veracity) and other virtues (e.g., conscientiousness and courage) are important for morality as a whole.

A final criticism of principles and rules in biomedical ethics could be built on the arguments offered by Carol Gilligan (1982) about male and female moralities. Noting that Piaget and Kohlberg both omitted girls and women from their studies of moral development, Gilligan contends that women are not morally retarded, as some tests suggest, but rather speak in a different moral voice, which is not adequately recorded by the tests developed on male models. In particular, Gilligan notes that women tend to concentrate on narrative, context, and relationships rather than on tiers of moral principles and rules with a logic of hierarchical justification, as in male perspectives on morality. She argues that women see and resolve moral problems differently. This is a very important argument, but it needs further clarification and elaboration. Gilligan emphasizes that what is involved is not gender but socialization, and she insists that what is needed is a recognition of the complementarity of the two moralities of care and justice, including rights. While this complementarity is possible within an individual's life over time, it is not yet clear what it would imply for some social roles, such as medicine. Would female and male physicians have viewed the problem differently in Case 1? Would they come to different conclusions? It is hard to predict with confidence that they would have, not only because the socialization process in medicine may inculcate male morality, but because the major question is the *moral significance* of the nephrologist's relationships with the father and with the other members of the family. Hence, the physician in that case would have to determine, at least in part through principles and rules, how much weight each relationship should have. It is plausible to hold that some moral principles and rules as well as modes of moral reasoning will be more important in some settings than in others, whether females or males occupy the social roles. Within research, medicine, and health care, which, as we have seen, often involve relations among strangers, the appeal to principles and rules may be important and even indispensable, whether the strangers are male or female.

In conclusion, the difficult questions of biomedical ethics do not concern whether to invoke and to apply principles and rules. Rather the difficult questions are which principles and rules should be adopted, how should they be interpreted, how much weight and strength should they have, which should have priority in cases of conflict, and in what relations and situations do they apply? Answers to these questions are not easy, but seeking the answers in the context of science, medicine, and health care is the fundamental task of biomedical ethics.

REFERENCES

Beauchamp, Tom L., and Childress, James F. *Principles of Biomedical Ethics*, 2d ed. New York: Oxford University Press, 1983.

Childress, James F. *Priorities in Biomedical Ethics*. Philadelphia: Westminster Press, 1981.

———. *Who Should Decide? Paternalism in Health Care*. New York: Oxford University Press, 1982.

The Danish Obesity Project. "Randomised Trial of Jejunoileal Bypass Versus Medical Treatment in Morbid Obesity." *The Lancet* (15 Dec. 1979): 1255–1257.

Engelhardt, H. Tristram, Jr. *The Foundations of Bioethics*. New York: Oxford University Press, 1986.

Fletcher, Joseph. *Situation Ethics: The New Morality*. Philadelphia: Westminster Press, 1966.

Gilligan, Carol. *In a Different Voice*. Cambridge, Mass.: Harvard University Press, 1982.

Guttmacher, Sally, et al. "Ethics and Preventive Medicine: The Case of Borderline Hypertension." *The Hastings Cent Rep* 11 (Feb. 1981): 12–20.

Jonsen, Albert R., Mark Siegler, and William J. Winslade. *Clinical Ethics: A Practical Approach to Ethical Decisions in Clinical Medicine*, 2d ed. New York: Macmillan, 1986.

Kass, Leon R. "Ethical Dilemmas in the Care of the Ill." *JAMA* 244 (17 Oct. 1980): 1811–1816.

Kelman, Herbert C. "Was Deception Justified—And Was It Necessary? Comments on Self-Control Techniques as an Alternative to Pain Medication." *J Abnorm Psychol* 84 (1975): 172–174.

Lemmon, John. "Moral Dilemmas." *Philosophical Review* 71 (1962): 139–158.

Levendusky, Philip, and Pankratz, Loren. "Self-Control Techniques as an Alternative to Pain Medication." *J Abnorm Psychol* 84 (1975): 165–168.

Levine, Melvin D., Lee Scott, and William J. Curran. "Ethics Rounds in a Children's Medical Center: Evaluation of a Hospital-Based Program for Continuing Education in Medical Ethics." *Pediatrics* 60 (Aug. 1977).

MacIntyre, Alasdair. "Patients as Agents." In *Philosophical Medical Ethics: Its Nature and Significance*, edited by Stuart F. Spicker and H. Tristram Engelhardt, Jr. Boston: D. Reidel, 1977.

THE NORMATIVE PRINCIPLES OF MEDICAL ETHICS

National Commission for the Protection of Human Subjects of Biomedical and Behavioral Research. *The Belmont Report: Ethical Guidelines for the Protection of Human Subjects of Research.* DHEW Publication No. (OS) 78–0012, 1978.

Pence, Gregory E. *Ethical Options in Medicine.* Oradell, N.J.: Medical Economics, Book Division, 1980.

Ramsey, Paul. *The Patient as Person.* New Haven: Yale University Press, 1970.

Singer, Marcus G. "The Golden Rule." *Philosophy* 38, no. 146 (Oct. 1963): 293–314.

Solomon, William David. "Rules and Principles." *Encyclopedia of Bioethics*, edited by Warren T. Reich, 407–413. New York: Macmillan and Free Press, 1978.

Stoppard, Tom. *Every Good Boy Deserves Favor and Professional Foul.* New York: Grove Press, 1978.

Toulmin, Stephen. "The Tyranny of Principles." *Hastings Cent Rep* 11 (Dec. 1981): 31–39.

Veatch, Robert M. *A Theory of Medical Ethics.* New York: Basic Books, 1981.

Walters, LeRoy. "Some Ethical Issues in Research Involving Human Subjects." *Perspect Biol Med* 20, no. 2 (Winter 1977): 193–211.

Warnock, G. J. *The Object of Morality.* London: Methuen, 1971.

Weinstein, Milton C., and William B. Stason. "Allocating Resources for Hypertension." *Hastings Cent Rep* 7, no. 5 (Oct. 1977): pp. 24–29.

DISCUSSION QUESTIONS

1. Are beneficence and nonmaleficence merely the positive and negative aspects of the same moral principle or is the moral duty to avoid evil morally prior or more stringent? Does the ethical slogan in medicine, first of all do no harm, imply that avoiding harm is a more rigorous or prior duty for physicians? Would this imply that when a physician must choose between a conservative course (one that can do little harm, but little good) and a more aggressive course (one that can do much harm but also much good), the physician ought to choose the one that at least does little harm?

2. Do the consequences of actions—the benefits and harms expected—always tell us what is morally required or are there other characteristics that can determine whether an action is right or wrong (such as whether the action involves violating another's autonomy, lying, breaking a promise, or taking a life)?

3. What should happen when two principles come into conflict? For example, if a physician believes that respecting the patient's autonomy by getting consent from the patient for giving a toxic cancer treatment will do more harm than good for the patient, should the physician be guided by beneficence and omit the request for consent or should he or she still be guided by autonomy and try to get the consent nevertheless?

4. What is the relationship between the principle of justice and producing the greatest amount of good possible? What should a health planner do when a scarce resource could be allocated in different ways—one of which would produce the greatest amount of good and another of which would distribute the resources more evenly or fairly?

5. Are moral rules (such as the rule to always obtain consent before surgery) always morally binding or are they only guidelines to be assessed in each case by ascertaining whether the outcome of following the rule is in accord with the basic moral principles?

3

The Concepts of Health and Disease

Arthur L. Caplan

SUMMARY

The concepts of health and disease play a pivotal role in defining the boundaries of medical concern, professional control, and social obligation. Defining what does or does not constitute a disease determines both the authority and power of those charged with alleviating its consequences as well as the scope of the social obligations of those beset by medical problems. Thus, in order to delineate the proper scope and domain of medicine and the related healing arts, it is necessary to develop a clear and concise understanding of these concepts.

First, the nature of the relationship between health and disease must be established. This relationship, when looked at uncritically, seems to be that health is nothing more than the absence of disease and disease is any impairment in a person's sense of well-being or fitness. However, some philosophers and health-care professionals have pointed out that matters are not so simple as this.

In understanding health or disease, two facts are important. First, disease does not always impair or threaten health. Consider the case of persons who carry the sickle cell trait. Those with sickle cell disease are prone to certain blood disorders. Sickle cell carriers are better protected against malaria than someone lacking this genetic endowment.

Second, some health-care professionals see their jobs as being more than just the alleviation of pain or eradication of disease. They see their role as improving or optimizing functions. While the view that health and disease are conceptual opposites may be valid, establishing this requires a sustained argument.

The remainder of the chapter considers three major views concerning the analysis of health and disease. The first view suggests that because all organisms are the product of a long course of biological evolution, health is the functioning of any organism in conformity with its natural design. Another view holds that disease is anything that is statistically abnormal. Health is what has been most commonly detected by statistical measurement, as normal, i.e., blood pressure, cholesterol level, IQ, etc.

A third view suggests that health and disease are concepts that cannot be defined without reference to values. Holders of this position are sometimes referred to as normativists. In this view, health and disease are inherently value-laden, and to fully understand these concepts, one must realize that decisions about states of the mind or body involve considerations of what is good, bad, desirable, or undesirable.

THE SPECIAL SIGNIFICANCE OF HEALTH AND DISEASE IN AMERICAN SOCIETY

Health and disease are concepts of extraordinary importance in the daily life of Americans. We spend more than any other nation on the planet for health care and health-related services. In 1987, well over five hundred billion dollars (more than eleven percent of the entire gross national product) was spent on doctor fees, hospital costs, medical insurance and government programs as varied as the Public Health Service, Medicare, the Indian Health Service and the Veterans Administration hospital system.

As Talcott Parsons has noted (1958), as well as many other social scientists, Americans seem peculiarly fascinated and preoccupied by matters pertaining to health and disease. While the exercise and diet boom make it seem as if health is an obsession unique to our own time, Americans have long been interested in health and health promotion. The nineteenth century counterparts of today's beansprouts and yogurt were the Graham cracker and W. K. Kellogg's cornflake (Whorton 1982). Many nineteenth century Americans were convinced of the importance of diet and exercise in the pursuit of mental health, purity of character and longevity.

The current fascination with the concept of health in our society may be a function of the historical attention paid in some Christian theological writings between health and moral character. Disease and disability were sometimes seen by the devout as reflections of God's displeasure with sinners and the impure in mind if not in deed. Certainly our interest in health reflects a perennial Western obsession with longevity and immortality, but more is involved in the explanation of the prominence of the value placed upon health in our society than the concern for one's character or lifespan.

Techonology has come to play an increasingly important role in our health-care system. Americans have long exhibited a fondness for technology and technological innovation. This is reflected in our health-care-delivery system's emphasis on the treatment of acute medical problems in hospital settings (Rosner 1981). The proliferation of neonatal units, CAT scanners and organ transplants is a reflection of our collective faith in the power of technology and our desire to use it to try and control the evils of disease and disability.

The fact is that prior to World War II there was relatively little that physicians or anyone else could do to combat the effects of disease and disability. The introduction of antibiotics, vaccines, powerful diagnostic technologies and technologically-based therapies in the decades following the War transformed medicine from a profession focused on caring to one with at least a serious interest in curing. The expectations of physicians and patients have grown considerably and, as a result, the desire to be returned to a state of health after the onset of disease or injury seems more a matter of finding a competent professional than it does a matter for hopes, wishes, and prayers.

While it is relatively easy to understand why health and disease have attained sociological and technological prominence in our society, it is perhaps less clear that there are also important political and social values characteristic of American society that result in our placing a special premium on health and the avoidance of disease. Health and the alleviation of disease and disability play key roles in a highly competitive society that places great weight on equality of opportunities (Stone 1980).

Ours is a highly individualistic society deeply committed to freedom and autonomy as the core values of both our law and our morality. Sickness and disease are more threatening to our sense of selfhood and self-assurance than they might be in societies less committed to individualism and less worried about using personal achievement as the measure of a person's worth.

Sickness and disease often signify disability and dependence—states that are abhorred by a nation with a can-do ethic and the belief that life finds its greatest value in the expression of individual choice and action. If, as some commentators suggest, Americans define themselves by their work or occupations as much as by any other criteria, then health is crucial to our self-perception since it is a necessary means to the achievement of productive work and, thus, self-respect.

Americans are also firm believers in equality, but only with respect to opportunity, not outcome. We tolerate differences in wealth, property, ownership, and the distribution of material goods that those in many other nations find difficult to fathom. But we are firm believers that these differences are tolerable only in so far as they are the product of individual initiative, merit and industriousness, or, their absence.

The moral assessment of the inequalities of power, possessions and property that exist all around us is contingent upon our view of the opportunities and individual efforts that have created such inequities relative to the distribution of social goods. If some people are rich because they work hard and others are poor because they are lazy then so be it. As long as a relative equality of opportunity exists for all, then any differences that result are morally acceptable to most Americans (Engelhardt 1986).

If equality of opportunity is a critical moral component of the legal, political, and societal norms of a capitalistic society, then health and disease must be accorded special status. Those who are born with congenital deformities and those who suffer from disabling or chronic diseases, especially infants and children, cannot be said to have an equal opportunity to compete with their peers for the goods and benefits that a competitive society makes available. The alleviation of disease and disability and the promotion of health are important political and cultural goals for our society for the same reasons special priority is given in our social policies to the provision of education, shelter, and food. All of these factors influence the extent to which equality can legitimately be said to exist with respect to opportunities and, therefore, to the extent to which the inequalities which necessarily result from a free-market approach to the distribution of social resources can be viewed as morally palatable (Daniels 1985; President's Commission 1983).

As Norman Daniels has recently argued (1985), disease is disvalued in our society because it is seen as a threat to equal opportunity. The reductions in abilities and capacities that usually accompany diseases are threatening not only because they cause intrinsic harms to those beset by them but also because they undermine our social commitment to the equity of competition and the fairness of the market as efficient methods for distributing social resources. Despite the fact that it may be expensive to redress the effects of disease or to prevent its occurrence, if fundamental inequities exist among people because of serious but remediable differences in their health and well-being, this would seem to be a state of affairs that is simply incompatible with a socioeconomic orientation that seeks to reward striving, performance, and individual achievement.

Health, Disease, and the Scope of Medicine

If it is true that health and disease play powerful and instrumental roles in legitimizing key presuppositions of our socio-economic arrangements, it is obvious why so much attention has been placed in recent years on their meaning and definition (Caplan, Engelhardt, and McCartney 1981). The definitions accorded these concepts play a pivotal role in establishing the boundaries of not only medical concern and professional control but also social obligation.

Prima facie obligations will arise for government and legislators to correct the inequalities wrought by disease and illness. Thus, the definition of these terms is more than a philosophical exercise. The answer to the question of what does or does not constitute a disease will determine both the scope of social obligations and the authority and power assigned to those responsible for alleviating the consequences of disease—physicians, nurses, public health officials, social workers, and other health-care professionals.

There has been much concern on the part of a variety of social commentators and ethicists from both ends of the political spectrum (Kass 1975; Susser 1974) about the growing power and influence of medicine and other health-care professions in our society. Conservatives worry that physicians, nurses, and psychologists will introduce public high school students to liberal attitudes toward sexual conduct in the guise of health education. Liberals fear that the classification of homosexuality as a disease rather than a matter of personal behavioral preference will result in discriminatory treatment of gays and the promotion of the kinds of negative stereotypes associated with most forms of mental illness (Bayer 1981; Engelhardt and Caplan 1987).

Physicians are now able to control access to a wide variety of social and economic resources by the use of their authority as gate-keepers of eligibility for a wide spectrum of public and private programs (Stone 1980). Getting a job, receiving life insurance, admission to school, entry into and out of the armed services, and the ability to marry and raise a family are all controlled to some extent by physicians. Similarly, decisions about who will or will not be forced to receive medical care in hospital or institutional settings and what is or is not an acceptable form of medical treatment are controlled by physicians and other health-care personnel (Starr 1983).

Physicians and other health-care providers not only have the authority to en-franchise some members of society with social benefits or privileges, they also have the authority to excuse behavior that, without medical exculpation, might be the object of educational or judicial attention (Flew 1973). Many groups have fought long and hard to have particular behavioral dispositions labelled as diseases. Alco-holics, gamblers, and the mentally ill are but a few of the groups who have lobbied persistently to have their conditions labelled as diseases. The disease label excuses certain behavior that might otherwise be viewed as criminal, sinful, or both.

Conversely, many groups such as homosexuals have struggled to free them-selves from being categorized as ill or diseased (Bayer 1981). Disease labels, while often exculpatory in terms of liability or responsibility, carry other burdens such as the stigma attached to illness and the assumption that those who are ill or diseased require treatment and cure from legitimate experts.

If the proper scope and domain of medicine and the related healing arts are to be delineated, this will require a clear understanding of the concepts of health and disease. Since both the health professions and society in general view the proper role of health care as the struggle against disease and the endeavor to maintain, restore or promote health, the definitions that are given to these concepts are critical both for understanding the possibilities and limits of health care as well as for under-standing the moral obligations, rights, and responsibilities that ought prevail be-tween patients and providers in health care contexts.

The Relationship Between the Concepts of Health and Disease

What is the nature of the relationship between health and disease? Many health care-professionals and a large percentage of the general public appear to view health and disease as logical opposites. When asked if they are healthy or feel well, most will answer affirmatively if they are not suffering from any particular disease or disorder at the time the question is asked. Looked at uncritically, health would seem to be no more than the absence of disease, and disease any impairment in a person's sense of well-being or fitness.

But some philosophers and physicians have pointed out that there are powerful reasons for questioning the appropriateness of viewing health and disease merely as conceptual opposites (Whitbeck 1981). Even if someone is not afflicted with a particular disease it is still possible to say of such a person that they appear healthier or are healthier at certain times than at others. The average marathon runner or professional athlete is probably healthier, with respect to overall physical well-being, than the average philosophy professor even if no members of any of these classes happens to be afflicted with a specific disease.

Some health-care professionals see their job as more than simply the alleviation of disease. Psychoanalysts, cosmetic surgeons, nutritionists, and sports physiologists are interested not only in the prevention or alleviation of disease, but also, and perhaps sometimes only, the promotion of health. If health and disease were logically related to one another as contradictory concepts, it would be impossible to make any sense of the ideas expressed by such terms as "health promotion" or "positive mental health." Yet, these ideas, as well as the notion of relative degrees of health in the absence of disease, do appear to be meaningful and coherent.

Diseases do not always impair or threaten health. Some diseases are unpleasant and disabling but do not compromise the health of the individual who has them. For example, enduring a short bout of the measles or mumps during childhood, either through infection or innoculation, may actually be conducive to health. A person can be riddled with cancer or suffering from hypertension and yet remain entirely unaware of any physical dysfunctions. And a person who is the carrier of the sickle cell trait, while prone to certain blood disorders under some highly unusual circumstances, is better protected against malaria than someone lacking this genetic endowment.

Some behaviors that are viewed as diseases in at least some circles, such as gambling, homosexuality, or drug-addiction, have tenuous logical connections to the concept of health. Certainly it is much less difficult to obtain agreement across social classes and different cultures about those states of the mind and body that constitute diseases than it is to secure agreement about which states are to be viewed as healthy. The use of addictive drugs is viewed quite differently in Jamaica and Burma than it is in the United States or the Soviet Union (Murray 1984).

While the view of health and disease as conceptual opposites may be valid, it makes more sense to view the conceptual contradiction of health as being unhealthy and the logical contradictory of being diseased as being non-diseased rather than to see health and disease as defined only in terms of one another.

Normativism Versus Nonnormativism in the Definition of Disease

Perhaps the major point of contention among philosophers, physicians, and other health-care experts who have examined the meaning of health and disease is the extent to which value judgments are requisite for or are implicit in the definitions of these concepts. Many physicians and not a few philosophers believe that there is no need to resort to considerations of value in general or morality in particular to identify, understand, or analyze the concepts of health and disease (Boorse 1975; King 1980; Murphy 1976; Scadding 1967). They believe that determinations of health and disease are matters of empirical fact and nothing more.

The clearest expression of the view that health and disease can be defined without explicit reference to any moral values or ethical norms has been offered by the philosopher Christopher Boorse (1975, 1977). He argues that while it is true that different social, ethnic, and economic groups do not agree on the reference class of the terms health and disease, and while it is also true that professionals often disagree about the disease status of a particular condition or behavior, it would be wrong to conclude from such facts that an objective definition of health or disease that does not rely on values is impossible.

Boorse contends that while it is possible for different people or groups to disagree about the specific application of a definition to a particular case, this does nothing to disprove the possibility of locating an objective, value-free definition of disease or any other concept. Since, Boorse argues, all organisms including human beings are the product of a long course of biological evolution which is a process that has been driven by a wide variety of environmental demands, it makes sense to say that health consists in the functioning of any organism in conformity with its natural design as determined by natural selection.

In other words, if it is the case that kidneys evolved in response to the forces of natural selection to remove impurities from the body, and hearts to pump blood to organs and tissues, then in any organism possessing a kidney or a heart, health consists, in part, in having a kidney that removes impurities from the blood and a heart that pumps blood to organs and tissues. These organs were designed by evolution to perform such functions and when they do so the organism that possesses them can be said to be healthy or to have a healthy pair of kidneys or a healthy heart.

In general, Boorse notes, evolution has placed a premium on survival and reproduction. These goals have required all organisms to be adaptable to increase their probability of survival. Organisms that lacked the genotypes and phenotypes requisite for survival and reproduction simply died-out; those with the necessary adaptive traits survived and reproduced.

As a result of the interaction of genes, phenotypes and environments over time, organisms evolved certain advantageous traits in the struggle for existence. Disease develops whenever there is any impairment of the functions typical of a particular biological species; functions required to achieve the natural goals set by the twin demands of survival and reproduction. Boorse's analysis may seem, at first glance, to smuggle in premises or assumptions about values into the analysis of the meanings of health and disease. Perhaps concepts such as survival and reproduction are themselves value-laden? But neither of these terms are used in his analysis in any moralistic or evaluative sense.

Boorse need only borrow from the findings of empirical science—evolutionary biology to be exact—to make his case. If one accepts the view that the goals of survival and reproduction have guided the evolution of every living organism on this planet, then health and disease can be understood solely in terms of the causal contributions various states, conditions, and behaviors make to the achievement of these ends. No resort to ethics or any other sort of value-judgment is necessary. All that must be done is to determine whether the causal contribution of a particular trait or behavior is positive or negative in terms of the overall capacity of a particular organism to achieve its biologically designed ends. The extent to which this is so will be determinative of whether or not the trait or behavior is to be classified as healthy or diseased.

Indeed, as Boorse himself notes, the best evidence that values play no role or at least need play no role in the definitions of health and disease is that the analysis he proposes works as well for assessing the health status of plants and animals as it does for humans. Veterinarians know what it means for a cat or a pig to be sick. Few would want to argue that before they could say that an animal was sick or dying they would need to resort to a complex moral theory or set of moral norms based upon the animal's own values!

Boorse's view, that disease can be defined without reference to anything other than the empirical assessment of functions based solely upon the understanding of the purposes the functions were meant to achieve in the light of evolution, is closely related to one of the most frequently utilized definitions of health and disease in medicine today. Many physicians, if pressed to define health and disease, will respond that disease is anything that is abnormal and health is what is normal (Murphy 1976). The sense of normal and abnormal used here is intended to impart some sense of statistical normalcy, not to reflect any sort of value judgment about a particular state or behavior. The unusual and the extreme become candidates for classification as disease within this view. Those states and behaviors that cluster around the mean or for which there is relatively small variance become the reference class of health (Weinstein and Stason 1977).

The statistical conception of health and disease has prevailed for many decades in many different areas of medicine. Physicians often do equate abnormal measures of blood pressure, blood chemistry, or body weight with disease—regardless of whether dysfunction or pain are present. But the primary problem with the attempt to establish a value-free definition of both health and disease is that anything "unusual" is considered a disease state even when it is not at all clear why it is unhealthy to be unusually tall, intelligent, strong, fast or agile.

Despite the problem raised by the advantages conferred by some forms of statistical deviancy, the statistical approach to the definition of health and disease would seem to be useful only as a rough approximation of health and disease. If a value-free conception of these concepts is to be found it would seem that Boorse's attempt to root disease and health firmly in a functional analysis based upon the recognition of the importance of evolution has the best chance of succeeding.

The Proponents of Normativism

The critics of the view that health and disease are concepts that can be defined without reference to values of any sort are sometimes referred to as normativists.

Normativists believe that health and disease are concepts that are inherently value-laden. They believe that to understand exactly what it is that these concepts mean or refer to, it is necessary to realize that decisions have to be made about states of the body or mind that must involve considerations of what is desirable or undesirable, useful or useless, good or bad. Normativists argue that no matter how many descriptive facts are known about the body or about the functions of a particular cell or organ system, it is impossible to decide whether or not a particular state of affairs represents health or disease without some reference to a standard or criterion that contains explicit or implicit reference to values (Engelhardt 1986; Fabrega 1972; Margolis 1976; Sedgwick 1973).

Historically, the primary focus of philosophical attention on the part of physicians and others interested in health care has been the concept of disease. If disease could be adequately defined and interpreted then it was believed that all other questions about the aims, goals, and purposes of health care would be resolved.

Much of the historical debate within Western society about disease centered not on the question of whether values play any role in the definition of disease but, rather, on the seemingly unrelated question of the metaphysical causes of disease. While the Greeks and Romans developed an extensive literature on the subject of the definition of disease and the ontological status of disease, for hundreds of years diseases were seen as the products of supernatural forces, either divine or magical. It was only with the rise of the mechanical philosophy of Descartes, Boyle, Galileo, and Newton in the sixteenth and seventeenth centuries that attempts were made to recast disease in light of natural rather than supernatural causes.

To some extent the concern with establishing a value-free conception of disease derives from the attempt to locate a conception of health and disease consistent with a materialistic or scientific outlook within the practice of medicine. However, contemporary normativists usually have no interest in returning to the pre-scientific outlooks of the Middle Ages. While there are some exponents of normativism in the ranks of those who espouse holistic health or alternative forms of medical intervention such as spiritual or psychic healing, most normativists merely point out that values form an irreducible element in the definition of disease despite modern medicine's commitment to materialism.

Perhaps the clearest illustrations of the ways in which values influence the definition of health and disease emerge from the realm of mental health and mental illness. A cursory glance at nineteenth century American medical texts reveals that physicians asserted with all of the authority at their disposal that women who enjoyed sexual intercourse or engaged in masturbation were certainly afflicted with various forms of mental illness and, in all likelihood, a variety of corresponding physical ailments as well (Smith-Rosenberg and Rosenberg, 1973). Textbooks of the era were replete with diseases of the mind that seemed to afflict black men and women in astounding numbers. One of the most omnipresent disorders of the day was a condition labelled drapetomania, a horrible plague which, upon infecting some benighted black slave, put into his mind an obsessive desire to run away from his or her owner (Caplan, Engelhardt, and McCartney 1981).

Normativists are much impressed with illustrations of the ways in which values and cultural prejudices tacitly or even overtly influence medical determinations of health and disease (Sedgwick 1973). They point to contemporary disputes about the disease status of such conditions as homosexuality, premenstrual syndrome, and infertility and ask how anyone could possibly conclude that some particular state of physical or mental affairs as a diseased or healthy state involves nothing more than an empirical assessment of biological functioning (Bayer 1981).

Both historical and contemporary cases of shifts in beliefs or uncertainties as to the proper classification of various conditions make it clear that values play an inextricable but entirely appropriate role in defining health and disease. Moreover, as normativists point out, a key element of the definition of disease is that the states of the body and mind which are viewed as diseases in various cultures are so viewed only as a result of the fact that people disvalue them.

In a society burdened with overpopulation, infertility might be viewed as a healthy state. In a society wealthy enough to provide financial support for all newborns, infertility might be seen as a disease state meriting serious attempts at amelioration through surgical or pharmocological intervention.

One of the boldest attempts to formulate a normative definition of disease, which highlights the valuational dimension of this concept, is that of Charles Culver and Bernard Gert (1982). Culver and Gert argue that the core meaning of disease involves the recognition that something is wrong with a person. They argue that diseases are actually a subcategory of a more general category which they label "maladies." The members of this class include not only diseases but also injuries, disabilities, and death itself. They argue that what is common to all these conditions is that human beings universally view them as evils. Other things being equal, people disvalue these states and try to avoid them if they can do so unless they have some overriding reason for ignoring their adversions to these evils.

Unlike most non-normative analyses of health and disease which view disease and health in terms of deviations or nondeviations from various norms of species-typical functioning, Culver and Gert argue that it is not dysfunction but the perceived evil associated with the dysfunction that is at the heart of understanding health and disease. In the case of a myocardial infarct, it is not the deviation from normal functioning which makes us classify this event as a disease. Rather it is the loss of capacities, the onset of pain, and the risk to life itself which make us disvalue this particular deviation from functional normality.

While the members of different cultural groups or societies may not always agree on what constitutes an evil, every society, according to Culver and Gert (1982), recognizes certain states of the mind or body as evils to be avoided. While people may not always agree as to the identity of those mental or physical states that represent evils, they all recognize that a loss of abilities, a loss of freedom, pain, the loss of pleasure, or death are evils. Malady thus has the apparent advantage of unifying what may initially appear to be disparate states such as pain, injury, and death by allowing them to be grouped under the common criterion of states of the body or mind that people disvalue as evils.

A weakness in this approach to defining disease is that it makes the status of disease dependent upon the willingness of the members of society to recognize a particular state of affairs as evil. Those with hypertension may not feel any loss of capacity but the physician operating with a nonnormative sense of proper physiological functioning can say that disease is present even if the patient would not. Similarly a culture that has no written traditions may be unaware and unconcerned about the presence of dyslexia in some of its members. But a psychologist studying the group may be aware that a nondisvalued abnormal condition is present and may wish to try and intervene to modify the problem in order to allow such a person to learn to read should they move into another society.

Nevertheless, despite these problems, Culver and Gert's analysis provides a useful point of comparison to those of Boorse and other nonnormativists. Should those providing health care or seeking it be concerned as to which side of the argument is correct?

Normativism Versus Nonnormativism—What Is Really at Issue?

The debate about the role played by values in the definition of health and disease may appear to be nothing more than an abstract philosophical controversy having few if any consequences for either the clinical practice of health care or the formulation of health policy. However, once the underlying concerns motivating the debate are made clear it can readily be seen that what is at issue are understandings about the aims of medicine and the scientific status of its practices.

Normativists and nonnormativists are equally concerned with supplying a definition of health and disease that is capable of roughly capturing our intuitions about what ought be classified as a disease and who ought to be viewed as healthy. But those offering definitions are also concerned with providing a definition that can help classify ambiguous states of the body or mind or resolve uncertainty where disagreements exist as to the proper classification of a condition as a matter of health or disease.

Aside from the aesthetic appeal of living in a world where conceptual matters admit of neat and tidy resolutions, there are important reasons for undertaking these definitional efforts. Unless medicine and the other health-care professions use definitions of disease and health that are clear and univocal, there is a grave danger that uncertainties will exist on the part of both health-care providers and patients as to the aims, goals, expectations, and hopes they bring to medical encounters. If health and disease are nothing more than socially determined, culturally mediated and individually subjective concepts, then there will be little if any possibility of either placing medicine on a firm scientific footing or of finding consensus among experts and patients as to the proper limits of medical concern.

Objectivity, univocity of meaning, clarity, precision, and universality are at the heart of efforts to define health and disease. Since so much money is spent in our own country as well as other nations, on health care, and since there is so much controversy about the proper scope and responsibility of medicine in managing a host of human ailments that range from smoking, drinking, and obesity to infertility, appearance, and eligibility for a broad spectrum of social benefits, the determination that health and disease are nothing more than subjective concepts whose meanings change depending upon political, economic, and cultural exigencies would have reverberations far beyond the realms of the philosophy of medicine.

If the controversy over the role of values in defining health and disease can be seen as determining some rather high stakes in terms of the money spent on and power accorded to health-care professionals, then it should be obvious why so much hinges on the answer that is given to the normativist/nonnormativist debate. Putting the debate in this context makes it clear that more is at issue than whether values do or do not play a role in defining disease and health. It is the objectivity of values rather than the objectivity of health and disease as concepts that is at the heart of the debate.

If one doubts that judgments of value are in anyway objective, then the presence of values in the definition of health and disease will make it impossible for health care and medical science to rest upon an objective and universal foundation. If, on the other hand, value judgments are seen as amenable to objective reasoned argument, as Culver and Gert believe, then their presence in the definitions of health and disease will do nothing to undermine the objectivity or universality of medicine and health care.

My own sympathies lie with those who espouse normativism but at the same time I believe that dispute about values do admit of rational resolution. If it is possible to obtain agreement among rational human beings that some states of the body or mind are valuable and desirable while others are not, then it ought to be possible to accord an explicit role to values in the definition of disease and health without sacrificing objectivity, precision or universality. Since there would seem to be no lack of agreement among both patients and health-care providers that under ordinary circumstances life is preferable to death, ability is preferable to disability, and pleasure is more desirable than pain, then those committed to normativism would appear to have at least some grounds for optimism that an objective foundation can be found upon which to rest value-laden definitions of both health and disease. While this may be harder to do in other areas of life, it seems that the goods and evils that bring people into the health-care system and motivate others to want to practice the art and science of health care, form at least a rough area within which consensus can be reached about what is good and what is bad and therefore what is health and what is disease.

REFERENCES

Bayer, R. *Homosexuality and American Psychology: The Politics of Diagnosis.* New York: Basic Books, 1981.

Boorse, C. "On the Distinction Between Disease and Illness." *Philos and Public Affairs* 5 (1975):49–68.

Boorse, C. "What a Theory of Mental Health Should Be." *Philos of Science* 44 (1976):542–573.

Caplan, A. L., H. T. Engelhardt, Jr., and J. J. McCartney, eds. *Concepts of Health and Disease*. Reading, Mass.: Addison-Wesley, 1981.

Culver, C. M., and B. Gert. *Philosophy in Medicine*. New York: Oxford University Press, 1982.

Daniels, N. *Just Health Care*. Cambridge, England: Cambridge University Press, 1985.

Engelhardt, H. T. *The Foundations of Bioethics*. New York: Oxford University Press, 1986.

Engelhardt, H. T., and A. Caplan, eds. *Scientific Controversies*. New York: Cambridge University Press, 1987.

Fabrega, H. "Concepts of Disease: Logical Features and Social Implications." *Perspect Biol Med* 5 (1972):538–617.

Flew, A. "Disease and Mental Illness." In *Crime or Disease?* London: MacMillan, 1973, 38–48.

Fort, J. B. "Should the Morphine Habit Be Classed as a Disease?" *The Texas Courier Record of Medicine* 12 (1895):293–297.

Kass, L. R. "Regarding the End of Medicine and the Pursuit of Health." *The Public Interest* 40 (1975):11–42.

King, L. S. "What Is Disease?" *Philos of Science* 21 (1980):193–203.

Margolis, J "The Concept of Disease." *J Med Philos* 1 (1976):238–255.

Murphy, E. *The Logic of Medicine*. Baltimore: Johns Hopkins University Press, 1976.

Murray, T. "The Social Context of Workplace Screenings." *Hastings Center Report* 14 (1984):21–23.

Murray, T. H., W. Gaylin, and R. Macklin. *Feeling Good and Doing Better*. New York: Humana, 1984.

Parsons, T. "The Definitions of Health and Illness in the Light of American Values and Social Structures." In *Patients, Physicians and Illness*, edited by E. Jaco, 165–187. New York: Free Press, 1958.

President's Commission for the Study of Ethical Problems in Medicine and Biomedical and Behavioral Research. *Securing Access to Health Care*, Vol. 1. Washington, D.C.: Government Printing Office, 1983.

Rosner, D. *A Once Charitable Enterprise*. New York: Oxford University Press, 1981.

Scadding, J. G. "Diagnosis, the Clinician and the Computer." *Lancet* 2 (1967):877–882.

Sedgwick, P. "Illness—Mental and Otherwise." *Hastings Cent Rep* 1 (1973):19–40.

Smith-Rosenberg, C., and C. Rosenberg. "The Female Animal: Medical and Biological Views of Woman and Her Role in Nineteenth Century America." *J Amer Hist* 60 (1973):332–356.

Starr, P. *The Social Transformation of American Medicine*. New York: Basic Books, 1983.

Stone, D. *Disability and Illness*. Philadelphia: Temple University Press, 1980.

Susser, M. "Ethical Components of the Definition of Health." *Int J Health Serv* 4 (1974):1539–1548.

Weinstein, M. C., and W. B. Stason. "Allocating Resources: The Case of Hypertension." *Hastings Cent Rep* 7 (1977):24–29.

Whitbeck, C. "A Theory of Health." In *Concepts of Health and Disease*, edited by A. L. Caplan, H. T. Engelhardt, Jr., and J. J. McCartney, 611–626. Reading, Mass.: Addison-Wesley, 1981.

Whitbeck, C. "On the Aims of Medicine: Comments on Philosophy of Medicine as the Source of Medical Ethics." *Metamedicine* 2 (1981):35–41.

Whorton, J. *Crusaders for Fitness*. Princeton, N.J.: Princeton University Press, 1982.

DISCUSSION QUESTIONS

1. The World Health Organization defines health as total physical, mental, and social well-being. Does that make health the absence of disease? If so, what are the implications for deciding who has authority to make decisions affecting people's health?

2. Is health appropriately limited to physical well-being or does it include other dimensions as well? Are economic, educational, social, and spiritual well-being part of what is meant by health? If so, are professional counselors in these areas health professionals? Do physicians have responsibility for these dimensions of well-being or only organic well-being? Is mental well-being part of the health professional's responsibility or is it the task of a separate caring profession?

3. Is it more important for medicine to focus on curing disease or is it equally important to promote and preserve health? If a drug were available that would improve intelligence, would it be more ethical to use that drug to improve the intelligence of a severely retarded person rather than someone who was already mentally normal? If so, why?

4. To what extent is one making an ethical or other evaluative choice when one calls a condition a disease? Are there some conditions that are diseases simply because they are statistically unusual?

5. Is it possible to determine what constitutes health by analyzing what constitutes the normal functioning of members of the species? If so, would different assessments have to be made for persons of different ages? Of different genders? If not, is there any scientific way of determining that a person is sick or well?

4

The Physician/Patient Relationship

Howard Brody

SUMMARY

The physician-patient relationship prompts many basic questions in medical ethics. This chapter provides an overview of the roles of physicians and patients according to an "old" and "new" medical ethics. Under the old ethic, physicians often placed the moral principle of benefitting the patient (according to their own view of benefit) on a higher plane than the moral principle of autonomy. By doing this, physicians refused to acquiesce in the wishes or desires of their patients, often for the patient's own benefit. This is the ethic of paternalism.

The contractual method has often been proposed as an alternative to the physician paternalism that was increasingly being viewed as unacceptable. The specific requirements and features of the contractual model are outlined in this chapter, and problems which critics have noted to be associated with contractualism are delineated. A contractarian model of the physician-patient relationship is presented as a further refinement of the contractual concept. It is then compared to a virtue-based approach to ethics. Many supporters of virtue-based ethics find important elements to be lacking in a contractarian model. The characteristics of a virtue-based ethic are then discussed. Two basic expectations within the physician-patient relationship are truthful disclosure and confidentiality. The implications of these principles are also explored.

INTRODUCTION

What is a chapter about the physician-patient relationship supposed to accomplish? To answer this question, we need to understand a change that took place in the subject of medical ethics roughly between 1965 and 1970. At the risk of greatly oversimplifying a complex history, I will characterize an "old" medical ethics and a "new" medical ethics. The "old" medical ethics had the following features:

1. Ethics was generally thought of as a list of do's and don'ts for the physician.
2. Ethics was based on professional authority. Physicians would determine their own ethics. Nonphysicians did not know medicine and therefore could have nothing useful to say about medical ethics (Veatch 1979).
3. The primary ethical principle was benefit to the patient. So long as he was serving the patient's welfare, the physician could be justified in deceiving, coercing, and doing other things to the patient which would be impermissible in other human relationships.

This account is, again, historically oversimplified; but it will serve to highlight the features of the "new" medical ethics we will be examining below:

1. Ethics is thought of not merely as a list of rights and duties, but also as the study of the underlying reasons for those rights and duties.
2. People trained in moral reasoning, such as philosophers and theologians, can contribute to the subject. Physicians must be ready to give reasons for their ethical views that nonphysicians would find rational and reasonable. Medical ethics is no longer a privileged, in-house medical matter.
3. Patient benefit is only one moral principle among many. Of special importance is the principle of autonomy, often thought of as the right of self-determination.

The "old" ethics would have addressed the physician-patient relationship by compiling a list of how doctors should treat patients and vice versa (Benjamin

67

ct, the form of the first code of ethics adopted by the American n 1848. The "new" medical ethics approaches the physician-ith a more ambitious aim. We want, for practical guidance, to s of rights and duties. But we do not want to accept these habit or custom. We want an underlying theory of the ethical nship, so that the specific rights and duties can be seen as flowing logically from the more basic theory (Veatch 1981). And, in addition, we want that theory to fit well with two different considerations. One is general ethical theory that is pertinent to other human relationships; the other is the factual reality of medical practice. We want our underlying view of the physician-patient relationship to be both ethically valid and realistic.

One of the appeals of using the physician-patient relationship as a way to start looking at medical ethics is that a cluster of important ethical issues is linked closely to our understanding of that relationship. Two such issues will be taken up later in this chapter—truthful disclosure and confidentiality. A third, informed consent, is the subject of another chapter.

A few brief comments will further clarify the content we will be discussing. First, a focus on the physician-patient relationship suggests that our ethical inquiry is directed at the therapeutic practice of medicine. Physicians do many other things that are very important, but which frequently do not involve relationships with patients—public health and medical research are two examples. We will assume that these other activities raise different sorts of ethical issues. Second, we will ignore ethical issues arising in a health-team setting, where many professionals work together. While it would be an oversimplification to suggest that health-care-team issues may for practical purposes be reduced to the same issues encountered between a single physician and a single patient, we will not have the space here to deal with this complicating feature of health practice. Third, we note that the physician-patient relationship is also the subject of study of medical psychologists and medical sociologists (Bloom 1963; Parsons 1978); but both their purposes and their methods of study are somewhat different than ours in this chapter. Last, we should note that using the term *physician-patient relationship* is merely a matter of convenience and need not be taken to suggest that nurses and other health professionals will not reflect on precisely the same moral principles when determining how they ought to relate to their patients or clients, even though different role responsibilities may alter the precise nature of their relationships.

PATERNALISM AND CONTRACTUAL MODELS

The "old" medical ethics gives rise to a view of the physician-patient relationship which is *paternalistic*. The nature of paternalism has been discussed in great detail (Buchanan 1978; Gert and Culver 1976, 1979). For our purposes, we can use a definition by James Childress (1982): paternalism is refusing to acquiesce in the wishes or desires of another person for that person's own benefit. When we acquiesce in somebody else's wishes or desires, we recognize the moral principle of autonomy—seeing that person as entitled to make his own free choices. When we act paternalistically, we place the moral principle of benefitting that person (according to our view of benefit) on a higher plane than the moral principle of autonomy (Beauchamp and McCullough 1984).

Even before the era of the "new" medical ethics, paternalism in medicine was sometimes viewed with skepticism. Szasz and Hollender were two physicians who proposed early models for physician-patient relationships (1956). They suggested a range of possible relationships, from an extreme of total paternalism on one end to equal and mutual participation on the other, and argued that each of these models had utility for specific medical circumstances. (Obviously a mutual-participation model will not work for a patient in a coma, for instance.) But, to the critics who launched the "new" medical ethics, the "old" physician-patient relationship was too dependent upon a paternalistic stance and offered too few opportunities for alternatives. These critics sought to base an alternative to paternalism on a sound underlying theory, and not just in an unreflective distaste for paternalistic behavior. A possible way of establishing an underlying theory led to a label for this approach to the physician-patient relationship—the *contractual model.*

This label was fruitful and suggestive for philosophers because of an analogy with a similar concept in the history of Western political philosophy, social contract theory (Masters 1975). The "old" political theory stressed the divine right of kings; subjects were supposed to accept the established order and not object to the authority of their "betters;" the free consent or participation of citizens in political affairs played no part in establishing the legitimacy of the ruling system. By the time of the Enlightenment, such a theory seemed intolerably demeaning to the emerging idea of the dignity of the individual. Thus, philosophers began to explore an alternative theory of government, which relied explicitly on the idea of the free consent of the governed. Hypothetical people were viewed as having a choice to either remain outside of government altogether or else agree freely among themselves on ground rules for a just and decent state. By the social contract approach, to argue that a particular form of government is just is to argue that these hypothetical people would have been willing to choose freely that form of government rather than remain without any form of government at all. And presumably they would choose to do so only if that government respected their most basic and important human rights.

Similarly, the "old" medical ethics might be seen as one in which the patient's free consent counted for nothing. By the "old" theory, doctors could appropriately dictate to patients for a variety of reasons—the traditions of the medical profession; the individual physician's commitment to protect the well-being of his patients; and the helplessness and dependency that sickness can produce in the sick individual. If this theory and its paternalistic implications are insufficiently respectful to the patient's rights and dignity, then an obvious alternative is to ask what sort of relationship parties might freely and rationally consent to, assuming that they were placed in a position of equal power at the beginning. We can first look at the outlines of a contractual model of the physician-patient relationship, and then flesh out the model with a list of rights and duties implied by it.

An influential early description of a contractual model was provided by Veatch (1972). Veatch reviewed four possible models to govern the physician-patient relationship in evolving contemporary society. He rejected three of them. The "Priestly Model" was basically the "old" model of physician paternalism. The "Engineering Model" gave full decisionmaking power to the patient and reduced the physician to the role of technician. And the "Collegial Model" assumed shared decisionmaking in which the physician and patient would be regarded as equals on all counts.

The remaining model, the "Contractual Model," admitted differential decisionmaking capacity but respected both parties, physician and patient, as free moral agents with their own goals and interests. By this model, the physician would take responsibility for all purely technical decisions, of the sort for which one is specifically prepared for by medical training. The patient would retain control over decisions that involved personal moral values or life-style preferences, which she could be expected to know more about than the physician could. For example, in deciding the treatment of a newly discovered breast cancer which has not yet spread, the physician would decide the relative risks and benefits of a modified radical mastectomy as opposed to mere removal of the lump followed by radiation therapy. But the patient would ultimately decide which surgery to have, based on the impact of those risks and benefits on her own life preferences and goals. The physician might be competent to say, for instance, that the five-year survival rate for mastectomy would be 15 percent better than for lumpectomy in this particular sort of tumor; but only the patient could decide whether it is *worth it to her* to give up a breast in order to gain that extra 15 percent chance.

The Contractual Model envisions a process of information exchange and negotiation between the two parties as various decisions are encountered. It also includes the possibility that the patient may freely delegate some of her decisionmaking power back to the physician ("I'm confused by all these facts, Doctor. What do *you* think I ought to do?").

The Contractual Model can be fleshed out by listing some of the patient rights (and corresponding physician duties) that somebody negotiating this sort of "contract" would be likely to include. Fried (1974), in trying to explain what might be meant by "personal care," stated that a patient in this sort of ethical relationship should be regarded as having four "rights in personal care." Fried listed them as: *lucidity* (the right to a full disclosure of pertinent information); *autonomy* (the right to be regarded as a self-determining agent, to be consulted in one's own care); *fidelity* (the right to continuing service aimed toward one's own interests, and the rejection of possible conflicting interests); and *humanity* (the right to be treated with compassion, and to have one's own individual uniqueness taken into account). We could view this list as combining key elements of the "new" medical ethics (lucidity and autonomy) with preservation of the most desirable, nonpaternalistic strengths of the "old" professional ethics (fidelity and humanity). It is therefore reasonable to argue that a doctor and a patient, viewed as equally powerful contractors, could freely and mutually agree to this list of four rights as defining an ethically acceptable relationship.

In this way, contractual models can provide a nonpaternalistic alternative to the "old" ethics and, in the process, appeal to acceptable moral theory, including respect for the patient as being of equal moral worth despite the physician's superior technical knowledge. But contractual models have also been criticized for faults of their own. We can list the most important criticisms, and then see whether contractual models can be modified to meet them.

CRITICISMS OF CONTRACTUAL MODELS

While few critics of contractual models have attempted to resuscitate the "old" paternalist ethic, many have claimed nevertheless that contractual models have serious deficiencies as a positive account of what the physician-patient relationship should be. Compared to these flaws, the purely negative accomplishment of contractual models—undermining physician paternalism—may be insufficient justification for adopting such models.

One line of criticism is to reconsider the factual and moral assumptions which were thought to support the "old" ethic, to see if they can yield useful ethical guidance without necessarily forcing one into a paternalistic stance. Perhaps Pellegrino has been most articulate in defending these assumptions, by arguing that an ethic of medicine must be based on two features—the act of profession and the fact of illness. The former refers to the historical tradition of the physician's commitment to the welfare of the patient; and the latter refers to the patient's dependency and vulnerability in the face of serious illness. From this basis in the historical tradition of medicine (as opposed to a more superficial grounding in present-day "consumerism" or rights-talk), a more satisfactory and yet still nonpaternalistic medical ethic might emerge (Pellegrino 1979; Pellegrino and Thomasma 1981).

Contractual models have also been faulted for mistaking certain important but limited features of an ideal physician-patient relationship for the core or essence of the relationship (Siegler 1981). For example, Twiss (1977) has argued that a satisfactory ethical account of the physician-patient relationship ought to explain two special features. First, the fact that the needs of the patient constitute the major criteria for correct decisions and actions. Second, the importance of the ongoing integrity of the relationship, and the fact that a good physician-patient relationship evolves and grows over time in such a way that both physician and patient have an even greater stake in it and a deeper commitment to it. Contractual models, it could be charged, fail to explain either of these two aspects satisfactorily.

To go into more detail on this point, contractual models have been charged with these specific shortcomings:

1. Contractual models are based on a factually incorrect assumption, as it is generally not the case that a physician and a patient begin their relationship by explicitly negotiating a contract of any sort.
2. Contractual models focus attention on explicitly stated and shared expectations of the patient and the physician and ignore the fact that much of the relationship is based on implicit expectations.
3. Contractual models focus attention on financial aspects of the physician-patient encounter rather than on its deeper ethical content (Masters 1975).
4. Contractual models focus narrowly on rights, and neglect equally important moral concepts such as duties and goals (Masters 1975; Siegler 1980).
5. Contractual models envision the physician-patient relationship as a socially isolated dyad, when in fact both physicians and patients are embedded in social systems and reflect this in their behavior (Masters 1975).
6. Contractual models are legalistic. Since contract is more of a legal than an ethical notion, such models would have us replace medical ethics with medical law (Ladd 1979; May 1975).
7. Contractual models focus narrowly on one moral principle, that of respect for patient autonomy, and ignore other important moral principles such as patient benefit and avoidance of harm (Beauchamp and McCullough 1984).
8. Contractual models encourage "minimalist" thinking. Instead of asking, "How may I cultivate and nourish this relationship over the longterm for better service to the patient's welfare?," the models encourage the physician to ask, "What's the least I can get away with in the short run without violating any explicit rights of the patient?" (Callahan 1981; May 1975; Siegler 1980).

Some of these criticisms can be quickly brushed aside by referring back to models such as Veatch's and Fried's. It is, for example, readily apparent on sympathetic reading that these models do not assume explicit "contracting" as the primary mode of interaction, that they allow for implicit as well as explicit expectations, and that they are in no way limited to the fiscal aspects of the relationship. Further, Fried's four rights in personal care make clear that autonomy is only one important principle and that beneficence is specifically encouraged rather than excluded. The "minimalist" criticisms, however, seem to strike closer to the mark. So long as one's view of oneself as a free, self-interested negotiator is the *primary* moral conception that one brings into a relationship, one is unlikely to "go the extra mile" for the other party in ways likely to make the relationship grow and flourish over time. Thus May (1975, 1983) was led to suggest that the religious ideal of "covenant" captured the core notion of the physician-patient relationship better than "contract."

One way to respond to these criticisms is simply to abandon the contractual model and look for some other way to describe the ethical features of the physician-patient relationship. (One possible candidate, a virtue-based model, will be discussed below.) But first we might ask whether the contractual model can be rescued by refining it to meet these objections.

A CONTRACTARIAN REPLY TO CRITICISMS

One way to defend patient autonomy and participation in decisionmaking, while avoiding a narrow model that seems to ignore beneficence and compassion, is to turn to a *contractarian* approach. To understand what this means, we have to go back to the origins of the contractual model in social-contract theory to see that the role that "contracting" plays in our account may be ambiguous. We could confuse two very different theories. One theory is that the contracting is done by real people in a particular social setting. These real people are seen as having the attributes of contractors—they are rational in choosing their options; they are free to make the best choice; they want to promote their own ends and not necessarily anyone else's, and so on. But another possibility—which is closer to the way that one political philosopher (Rawls 1971) has refined social-contract theory—is that we view some imaginary or hypothetical people as doing the actual contracting and having the idealized attributes of free and rational contractors. These hypothetical people would contract for the basic ground rules that would govern the social relationship. But they would do so bearing in mind the fact that this would be a real world relationship, and that the real world people that would have to follow those ground rules would have all the usual and normal human limitations and failings.

Rawls added one other feature to this second theory of contracting. He noted that one thing that causes real-world people to ignore rules agreed upon by previous negotiation is the idea that those rules are *unfair*. We suspect that some people may have agreed to those rules because the rules gave special advantages to those persons or their friends and associates. Now, to agree on unfair rules, it seems necessary that we know just how we are placed with respect to our fellow humans. If, for instance, we wanted to have an unfair society in which one race of people would be enslaved by another race, we would clearly have to know which race we and our friends belonged to before we would be willing to set the rules. But suppose that that information could somehow be hidden. Since we would (Rawls assumes) never take a chance that our own race would be the victims of slavery, we could have no choice but to contract for a social scheme in which slavery was prohibited. We could repeat this exercise for every bit of information that could lead to unfair contracting—sex, religion, social class, and so on. If we hid all the information that could lead to unfair advantages, and if the hypothetical people are ideally free and rational, then we would have grounds for thinking that any rules agreed to in this hypothetical contracting exercise must be fair. And so, if real world people want to follow fair rules and avoid unfair rules, our ability to argue that some set of rules would have been agreed to by people in this hypothetical contracting exercise would be a powerful argument to get people to abide by those rules.

To review these two contract theories, we can see that the first is open to all the criticism lodged against the contractual model of the physician-patient relationship. It sees doctors and patients as having unrealistic qualities, and focuses on contracting sorts of behaviors to the exclusion of other important human functions. But the second theory does not commit any such error. The unrealistic features are explicitly labeled as a hypothetical exercise, not as a real-life description of how physicians and patients act. Yet, if it yields any rules for the doctor-patient relationship, we have good reason to think that those rules would be *fair* rules. To contrast the second theory with the first, let us call it a *contractarian* model.

Now, a quick summary of Rawls' idea for how the hypothetical contracting exercise would proceed shows that we need to be very clear on three things. First, we have to describe the hypothetical contractors and how they behave. Second, we need a lot of facts about the real world; otherwise the rules those contractors agree to will have no relation to reality and would be useless for us. But third, we need to hide those real-world facts that would give any contractor an unfair advantage in picking rules that favor one group over another. That is, the information provided in this hypothetical exercise needs to be general information, and specific information about individuals needs to be hidden.

Table 4–1 lists the details we might provide, under these three headings, to modify Rawls' idea to make it applicable to the physician-patient relationship.

One idea in Table 4–1 may need some explaining—that of "life plans" and "conceptions of the good." The contractarian model assumes that each person values certain things and tries, as much as possible, to plan for a life that would maximize the chances that one will actually get those things. However, what those things are will vary quite a bit among people. Some may value physical fitness; some material wealth; others artistic creativity or intellectual contemplation; most of us will want some mix of many of these. To a large extent we choose our schools, or jobs, our spouses, and other things we have control over with an eye toward having a better chance to carry out the life plan that best includes our preferred values. Knowing our own life plan, in the contracting exercise, could produce unfairness. If we knew that we would choose to be fitness nuts, we might, for instance, vote for a rule that states that if health care is scarce or expensive, those who exercise regularly will get first dibs. If we knew that we would rather be sedentary university professors, we might vote for a very different rule. So specific information about each person's life plan is kept hidden for the exercise, while general information about the sorts of life plans people normally have, and how illness and medical care might affect them, is included.

A full explication of the contractarian model would require a detailed discussion of how contractors in this hypothetical exercise would go about selecting a group of ground rules to govern the physician-patient relationship. This would take a long time and cannot be described in detail here. But I would suggest that if Fried's four rights in personal care were presented to this hypothetical contracting convention as a proposal, the people would, after careful reflection, approve of the four rights, at least as a starting point.

Table 4–1. A Modified Hypothetical Contracting Exercise to Choose Guidelines for the Physician-Patient Relationship

I. Description of the "Contractors"
A. Specifically motivated to choose basic moral principles to govern the physician-patient relationship
B. Motivated to choose rules that will be binding in the "real world"
C. Rational (in the sense of choosing most efficient means to one's ends)
D. Mutually disinterested; dedicated to furthering own interest only
E. Possessed of a variety of different life plans and conceptions of the good (value pluralism)

II. Knowledge Available to the "Contractors"
F. The general nature of medicine and health care
G. The state of medical science and technology in the real-world society, including relevants costs and resource availability
H. The nature of illness and its impact on individual life plans
I. The psychology of illness, including effect on rational choice
J. Other key social institutions and arrangements that impinge on health care

III. Knowledge Hidden from the "Contractors" to Assure Fairness
K. Each one's own specific life plan and conception of the good
L. Each one's relative status in society (position and wealth)
M. Each one's specific real-world role (physician, patient, etc.)
N. Each one's state of health (generally healthy, occasionally acutely ill, seriously or chronically ill, etc.)

What makes us think that the people would contract this way? First, if they could know they were going to be doctors and not patients, they might vote for physician paternalism as a rule; but not knowing for sure which role they might occupy, they would have to protect their own rights and interests by favoring a rule of autonomy. Second, the knowledge they have about the psychology of illness, and how it makes people behave, would guarantee that they would never approve autonomy as the only rule. Knowing that severe illness could interfere with their acting in a fully autonomous way, they would want to include the rules of fidelity and humanity to make sure that the physician provided humane and compassionate care in any case (Brody 1985). Finally, since autonomy is not much use to somebody who is unaware of his options, they would see the right of lucidity as necessary also.

Obviously this is just a sketch of how the discussion would go; but it indicates in general outline form the way the contractarian model could be used to start with a hypothetical description, as in Table 4–1, and end up with a set of practical guidelines which are rational, realistic, and fair. If we proceed like this, we can give strong reasons to avoid physician paternalism, describe a set of alternative rules to

ian-patient relationship, and still avoid most of the criticisms that
_ model provoked (Brody 1981, 38–41; Miller and Brody 1983).

CONTRACT VERSUS VIRTUE

While many criticisms might be turned aside by going from a contractual to a contractarian model, the latter still arises from a particular philosophical tradition in ethics (the social contract approach). If one rejects that entire tradition as being a good way to do ethics, then one must reject the contractarian model also. Lately, among those interested in ethical theory, this is exactly what some authors have proposed. MacIntyre (1981) has been especially interested in replacing that philosophical tradition with one more like Aristotle's system of ethics, which stressed the idea of virtue.

MacIntyre's arguments are very complex and we can present here only a crude sketch of them. We can view MacIntyre as contrasting a "bottom line" method of applying ethics with an ethics of virtue, which is based much more on ongoing human activity. In "bottom line" ethics, all that matters is what comes out at the end—how you behave or what you do or what the consequences are. In virtue ethics, the way you do things along the way matters as well. To be quite simplistic about it, "bottom line" ethics is only concerned with whether you win or lose, while virtue ethics is also concerned about how you play the game.

Virtues, as Aristotle saw them, are sorts of excellences in human activity. If we use playing a game as a metaphor, virtue requires learning the rules of the game carefully, developing one's skills and talents over time by careful practice, and using whatever creativity one has eventually to put the stamp of one's own individuality on the way the game is played. To really understand what virtues are all about, our observation point has to be the way one's life unfolds over an extended period, not how one carries out one specific action.

Smith and Newton (1984) endorse a virtue ethic when they point out that our philosophical tradition has encouraged us to think about the physician-patient relationship only in terms of rules and rights—purely "bottom line" thinking. By reducing everything to rules, it is almost as if we thought we could make the relationship "doctor-proof." It is as if we thought you could ignore whether the doctor is a saint, a sinner, a sophisticate, a nerd, a humanitarian, a technician—just get him to follow the rules, and you will have a good doctor-patient relationship. But Smith and Newton feel this is unrealistic; any really deep description of the relationship must include some picture of what sort of person the doctor ought to be. And this picture will reveal certain excellences, or virtues, that we ought to expect and promote among physicians. For example, in an ethics of virtue, the quality of sympathy would probably be singled out as a central excellence of the physician's role. But in "bottom line" ethics we do not know what to do with sympathy, as it is hard to reduce it to a right or a rule. "Bottom line" thinking reduces qualities like sympathy to frosting on the cake instead of seeing them as central excellences.

A virtue-based ethics contributes to our understanding of the physician-patient relationship by focusing attention on integrity and character, which tend to get left out of "bottom line" or contractual discussions. In "bottom line" ethics, what I do this week is assessed as right or wrong by whether it fits with the rules, rights, duties, or whatever method my ethical theory stipulates to determine the rightness or wrongness of individual actions. What I do next week is assessed the same way; but there is no necessary connection between the two actions. However, with the virtue theory, this is a peculiar and perverted way of looking at human existence and human morality. It is not enough to say that we desire, as a moral person, to follow the rules. This may be fully sufficient if somebody is going to have very limited contact with us and simply expects predictable and appropriate behavior in that one instance. But it is insufficient if we are going to look at our lives as a whole. "He followed the rules" is not what most of us would want our friends to say about us after we die. Instead, we would like our friends to see a life that was connected, that made sense, as a whole. We would like to think that the ideals and values we felt most strongly about would be revealed to anyone who took the time to look at how we lived our lives over time. We feel most proud of ourselves when our actions, over time, steadfastly adhere to those values; and we feel least proud when we deviate from those values simply because some individual act is the easy thing to do at the time. Looked at this way, "living a life" can be seen as something quite different, and more basic to our human identity, than "following the rules" or "exercising our rights."

A virtue model of the physician-patient relationship would ask what sort of character an ideal physician ought to have, and what virtues or excellences go to make up that character (Shelp 1985). It would also view the relationship as growing and evolving, in such a way that no set of rules set out at the beginning could fully determine its future (an idea similar to "covenant," as argued in May 1975; Twiss 1977). If it is to grow, both physician and patient must find rewards in seeking a common goal, which must be centered on the patient's welfare. And, as the patient grows older and perhaps moves into different social settings, what that welfare consists of may change and the relationship will have to be altered to take this into account. For this relationship to grow and be nurtured in this way, Smith and Newton (1984) suggest that "dialogue" is one critical feature it must include. To keep the relationship going and to keep it focused on the common goal, the physician and patient will have to exchange information in a regular and explicit way. It will not do for each person to assume that she can read the other's mind and know what she is thinking. And it will not do to reduce communication to a cold and legalistic catalogue of medical facts, options, risks, and benefits. Real dialogue lies between these two extremes, but exactly where, for each relationship, is a tricky question. There are no rules of dialogue that guarantee the physician and patient will always get it right. In a somewhat similar vein, Katz (1984) has discussed the problem of informed consent under the rubric of "conversation," where he means a conversation that includes at least the possibility that the patient will become involved in making decisions.

We are left with many unanswered questions about the physician-patient relationship, and medical ethics will proceed in the future to try to answer many of them. To those who favor a contractarian approach, answers may come from refining and using Table 4–1 and seeing which ground rules emerge from the exercise. To those favoring a virtue approach, answers may come from more in-depth studies of the sorts of "dialogue" or "conversation" that best suit various relationships in various circumstances, and an elaboration of the virtues that mark the ideal physician or the ideal patient. Hopefully, each approach will supplement the other. In the remainder of this chapter, we need to look at two more specific features of the physician-patient relationship, truthful disclosure and confidentiality. As more basic theoretical issues remain unresolved, it will help to use Fried's four rights of personal care.

TRUTHFUL DISCLOSURE

The models of the physician-patient relationship discussed above have important implications for what physicians are obligated to tell patients about their illnesses and treatment. According to the contractarian model, the hypothetical choosers would pick as a right of the patient what Fried called "lucidity," which involves the right to know the truth about one's medical condition. The issue of truth-telling in medicine is both closely linked to, but is also distinguishable from, the issue of informed consent. Informed consent involves two of Fried's rights, lucidity and autonomy—the patient has the opportunity both to know the truth and to use that information in deciding upon her own strategy of care. We will see below that the concept of autonomy is important in understanding both why truthful disclosure is important for patients, and also what legitimate exceptions may exist to the physician's duty to disclose (Sheldon 1982). But patients themselves readily distinguish between receiving truthful information and involving themselves in their own medical decisions. An intensive study of hospitalized patients revealed that nearly all of them wanted information, for a variety of reasons ranging from simple courtesy to a desire to better follow the doctor's advice. But only about 10 percent of these patients wanted to participate in the choosing of medical treatment along with the physicians (Lidz et al. 1983).

The right of lucidity runs into some of the same problems that contractual models encounter when contrasted with the long, historical tradition of medical practice. It is very hard to find anyone, in the last decade or so, arguing seriously in the American medical literature for routine deception of patients or arguing against the right of lucidity. (Lucidity is not, however, accepted in other countries to the same extent, as some British literature suggests; and in the Soviet Union it is generally rejected; Veatch 1981.) However, the entire history of medicine before about

1960 is the history of routine deception and withholding of information, for fear that frank truth would frighten or harm the patient; voices calling for more disclosure were distinctly in the minority (Reiser 1980). There were some good reasons for the shift, such as new research suggesting that the truth is nowhere near as harmful to patients as physicians had previously feared (Kubler-Ross 1969). But the very radical nature of the shift is at least puzzling; when about 90 percent of cancer physicians favor nondisclosure of the diagnosis in 1960 (Oken 1961) and yet, in a similar survey 20 years later, 90 percent favor full disclosure (Novack et al. 1979), we might naturally wonder whether this represents new ethical insight or a temporary fad.

One of the deepest analyses of information disclosure by physicians appears in a recent book by Jay Katz, a psychiatrist interested in medical law (1984). Katz is interested primarily in informed consent, but his observations apply equally to the disclosure issue. He suggests that the long history of nondisclosure can be explained by powerful psychological forces in the physician-patient relationship. These forces feed into each other so that blame cannot be assigned to either doctor or patient alone. A great deal of the problem is the natural human fear of uncertainty, especially when one is facing serious illness and really wants a magical cure rather than a scientific analysis of probabilities and statistics. In most cases of serious illness, a frank conversation would quickly reveal that important facts are unknown or are understood only as statistical probabilities. A cancer patient may naturally wonder, "How long have I got, Doc?" But the physician knows that any information beyond something like, "There is a 34 percent chance that you will survive for five years," would require a crystal ball which no physician possesses. Medical science cannot tell this patient whether he is in the 34 percent group or the 66 percent group.

Thus, both physician and patient have a psychological interest in maintaining a mutual charade that medicine is much more certain and powerful than we know it to be—the patient so that he can retain hope in miracles, and the physician so that she can think of herself as meriting the great faith and trust that the patient places in her. Further, the more severely ill patient may regress psychologically, so that the relationship is more like a child-parent than an adult-adult relationship; and the parent usually does not feel that full disclosure of information to the child is needed or helpful. As a result of these and similar forces, both physician and patient may find strategies to dodge real lucidity, and these strategies, over time, will become embedded in customary medical practice and the usual expectations that patients have of physicians.

Now Katz personally favors recognizing the right of lucidity and promoting increased patient autonomy. He argues, however, that this can be achieved in medicine only if we study and take very seriously the strong psychological forces that drive us in the other direction. He also argues that medicine scientifically is in a much better position to do this now than at any previous time in its history. To Katz, medicine always was and still is characterized by a great deal of uncertainty and ignorance; but what is different today is our ability to describe and demarcate our uncertainty in scientific terms (such as probability, statistics, and quantitative decision analysis; Weinstein et al. 1980). Since we can talk more accurately and more meaningfully with our patients about medical uncertainty, we have much less reason to waver on the right of lucidity.

Even if we can accept truthful disclosure as a historically neglected right of patients whose time has finally arrived, we need an analysis of why it should be important in the physician-patient relationship. Gadow (1981) provides such an analysis, which has the additional virtue of indicating the reasons why physicians may, on occasions, legitimately limit disclosures to patients. Gadow notes two competing principles, which we have discussed above in defining the issue of paternalism—benefit and autonomy. The benefit principle justifies truth-telling on the grounds that disclosure is generally better for patients than nondisclosure or deception. However, the way that the benefit principle is generally viewed in medicine, what counts as "better" is usually seen as a matter for the physician's judgment, not the patient's. This principle can be quite powerful with reference to some of the research cited above that shows that patients who are told the truth often seem to be helped and not harmed by the disclosure. But, at the same time, it suggests a series of exceptions to the general rule of lucidity—namely, those situations in which the physician thinks the patient will be harmed by the disclosure. In the law of informed consent this is generally referred to as "therapeutic privilege," and is recognized by some courts (with a variety of stringent safeguards) as a legitimate reason for the physician to withhold the truth. Katz (1984), however, argues that such court rulings really undermine the right of lucidity, and err in giving too much weight to the benefit principle and not enough to the autonomy principle.

The other principle that might justify a policy of lucidity is what Gadow calls the autonomy principle. The focus is not on benefit or harm, but on respectfully treating another individual as a person, in the same way we would want to be treated by others. The autonomous person has at least the opportunity to make free choices about his fate. Such choices, to be meaningful, must be based on a true picture of the world and of the real options open to that person. Withholding that information, because it shortcircuits any possibility of meaningful free choice, is a very special and strong way of displaying a basic disrespect for the moral dignity and personhood of someone else. In the language of the philosopher Immanuel Kant, it is an especially egregious example of treating someone as a means only rather than an end-in-himself. This is not to say that the principle of autonomy is unconcerned with benefits and harms. But it does differ from the benefit principle as Gadow characterizes it in insisting that the patient himself should be the first to decide what counts as benefit and harm from his own point of view.

Therefore, the autonomy principle suggests a very different set of exceptions to the duty of lucidity. Legitimate nondisclosure or deception can occur only when an autonomous patient requests this of the physician. The patient himself may, for example, feel that in the past he has been terribly upset and anxious whenever he received medical "bad news," and that his suffering on that count outweighs any corresponding increase in his ability to make free choices. Assuming that this is his true wish, and not just a way of accommodating what he thinks the physician expects of him, he might autonomously request his personal physician not to disclose such information in the future. Such restrictions might be more limited—for example, the patient might say, "Don't tell me any bad news if my family isn't around; make sure you wait until they arrive before you tell me."

A further extension of this is possible, but dangerous. Suppose the physician observes for herself that a particular patient, when certain sorts of medical information is disclosed, becomes anxious, confused, or otherwise less able to make autonomous choices. The physician might decide on her own to withhold such information, and instead to release other sorts of information which make the patient better able to make free choices. In this way, the physician acts in a way normally classed as paternalistic, but cites the goal of patient autonomy rather than patient benefit as the underlying justification (Komrad 1983). Now, if this sort of thinking is used simply to change the wording or the precise timing of disclosure, so long as the same basic facts are transmitted in the end, it is fully consistent with the "rights in personal care" described above. Nothing in the right of lucidity suggests that the way the truth is told ought to be insensitive or brutal; such behavior would obviously violate the patient's right of humanity (Cousins 1980). However, if significant truths are withheld or if the patient is substantially deceived, the fact that this is being done in the name of patient autonomy cannot reassure us that the behavior is not really a simple return to the "old" and unacceptable paternalism.

If the two principles, benefit and autonomy, give us different reasons why lucidity is important and if they point to different practical policies (since they point to different exceptions to the rule), which should we choose, if the two come into conflict? Gadow (1981) argues that the autonomy principle is more basic and more inclusive. She points out that some patients may be harmed by the truth while most will benefit from it, most of the time. If we adopt the autonomy principle, we tell the truth to those who will benefit, while those most likely to be harmed can autonomously choose nondisclosure. Thus, benefit is really maximized under the principle of autonomy.

Another reason can be given for avoiding use of the benefit principle when it comes to possible justifications of deception and nondisclosure. The benefit principle works fairly well when we imagine one person possessing some goods that a second person wants, and making decisions about whether to hand over those goods or not. (Imagine a parent, an adolescent, and the keys to the family car.) Suppose that person #1 refuses to hand over the goods on the grounds that harm would come to #2 if the goods were obtained. Person #2 knows exactly what was withheld and why. If #2 thinks that #1 was mistaken in guessing as to the harmful outcome, she can try to argue with or reason with #1 to get her to see her mistake. Assuming that both parties are rational and are open to new information and evidence, the system is self-correcting over time; mistakenly paternalistic behavior will be identified and criticized so that it will not be repeated.

But this model falls down when applied to truth as a "good" to be either handed over or held back. It is part of the very idea of nondisclosure or deception that #2 never finds out that any good was withheld at all, let alone what it was or why it was withheld. Thus, there is no opportunity for longterm self-correction; if mistaken judgments are made about harms and benefits, they are likely to be perpetuated. Indeed, one may argue that this is what happened in the history of medicine. Physicians decided that patients were happier not knowing the truth, and patients, who never had the opportunity to experience full disclosure, could never lodge a disagreement. But the autonomy principle does a better job of dealing with truth-telling, because it makes it clear that there is a close link between truthful disclosure and one's basic dignity as a person. The benefit principle, by treating truth merely as a "good" to be handed back and forth, misses this point entirely.

Before leaving the issue of lucidity, we might note one interesting way that a physician may deceive a patient or practice incomplete disclosure. The physician may administer a placebo pill or treatment that is intended for symbolic purposes only, while the patient is allowed to think that the treatment has a pharmacologic or physiologic potency. While experiments and experience have shown that occasionally placebos can be powerful healing tools, the right of lucidity and respect for the principle of autonomy suggests that their use in medicine should be strictly limited (Brody 1982). Indeed, a proper analysis of lucidity and its implications shows that the physician who is tempted to use a placebo in order to help the patient is almost always guilty of a limited imagination. For one thing, there are a great many ways in which the powerful symbolism of the physician-patient relationship can be used to promote healing, without using a sugar pill or a similar deceptive device (Benson and Epstein 1975). For another, in some situations where a placebo may actually be beneficial, the patient may be able to give explicit permission for its use. Suppose, for example, that a patient is sure that a pill with possible serious side effects is necessary to relieve his symptoms; the physician thinks the pill works by suggestion only. They may jointly agree on a trial in which the patient will take unmarked pills, some active drug and some placebo, and keep a diary of his symptoms over time to see if the active drug has any advantage. In this example, a placebo has been used but the patient was not deceived and gave free consent (Vogel et al. 1980).

To conclude, while the history of medicine reveals a record of deception and nondisclosure, there are sound reasons, referring back to the features of the physician-patient relationship discussed above, to favor a policy of truthful disclosure unless the autonomous patient requests a different approach. The rare exceptional case, when telling the truth may produce great harm, must be dealt with under the question of when paternalism may be justified (Childress 1982), a question we cannot analyze here.

CONFIDENTIALITY

Traditionally, the patient's right to fidelity (as Fried uses the term) has included a right to have her privacy respected and not to have any information about herself disclosed to other parties without her permission. One version of the Hippocratic oath states, "What I see or hear in the course of the treatment . . . , which on no account one must spread abroad, I will keep to myself . . ." (Beauchamp and Childress 1983, 330). This sentence suggests two things. One is that, historically, physicians have been expected to maintain confidentiality and patients have been encouraged to take this for granted. The other is that, on occasion, the physician must use individual judgment to decide "what ought to be spoken of abroad" and what should not. That is, occasionally other important moral considerations may override a duty to confidentiality.

The historical basis of confidentiality can, however, be misleading. The old model for confidentiality, which is the picture that many patients still carry in their minds (Weiss 1982), assumes one physician, one patient, and information which is largely kept in the physician's memory and which is solely his to disclose or not. The current health-care situation is radically different, with dozens of physicians and health-care professionals commonly involved in care, the unquestioned need for written records to which many people must have access, the need to transmit information to insurance companies and others with a financial interest to assure payment for services, and the increasing computerization of all this information. If, under these pressures, confidentiality is not to become a "decrepit concept" (Siegler 1982), we need a careful analysis of what it is and why it is basic to the physician-patient relationship, as well as a sense of its limits.

Privacy and confidentiality should be seen as closely linked with basic human dignity and respect for persons, just as with lucidity. It will clearly not do, for example, to tie confidentiality with solely material harms that could befall the patient. Suppose that I find out a patient is a homosexual, I tell his employer, and he is fired. Being fired is a material harm, and I could be blamed for having caused it. But suppose, in another case, I know that the employer is a very liberal and tolerant sort of person, and so it is certain that the patient will not be fired or harmed in any material way. Yet the moral duty to keep my mouth shut is not altered by this change in the circumstances of the case.

A more subtle and satisfactory reason is that patients are routinely called upon to disclose private and embarrassing information to physicians, and yet patients are also routinely helped by their physicians' care. If they could not trust physicians to keep the embarrassing information private, many patients might be discouraged from seeking medical help, and this could, over time, lead to both individual and social harm.

This second reason gives a better account of why confidentiality is basic to the physician-patient relationship. Yet it is also unsatisfactory, in ways analogous to our discussion above of why the benefit principle ultimately fails to do justice to truth-telling. By appealing to patient benefit, this argument undermines itself. In those cases where physicians think that violating confidentiality would benefit the patient in some way, they would be encouraged to seek that benefit at the expense of patient privacy. But that would encourage precisely the state of affairs—patient mistrust in physicians—that the argument seeks to avoid. Thus, even though patients benefit in a variety of ways from having their privacy honored, we may conclude that benefit is not the most basic moral value that explains the importance of confidentiality.

A deeper explanation of why confidentiality is central to respecting the patient's human dignity can be sketched only briefly. We assume that who we are, as individual persons, is centrally bound up with a series of human relationships, roughly depicted by a set of concentric circles with the individual in the middle. The smallest circles represent the few, most intimate relationships while the largest circles depict chance acquaintances and those with whom we have no personal stake or commitment. To a large degree, we define and control this system of relationships by choosing what information about ourselves to reveal to various people. We reveal very minimal information to those on the outermost circles, usually just enough to get some specific task done, like using a credit card to purchase clothing. We reveal a great deal more (though still not everything) to those on the smallest inner circles. Controlling these relationships constitutes a large part of what it means for us to have control over our lives and our identities (Beauchamp and Childress 1983, 228–237).

If someone now proceeds to violate our confidentiality by revealing private information about us without our consent, that person has effectively taken control of our lives and our identities away from us in one important sense. If that person chooses to reveal that information to others, that person, not us, is determining who shall be (to some extent) in a relationship of intimacy with us. If that person uses that information toward some goal that is his, not ours, we and our very identities are being made use of in an undignified and disrespectful way. This account, better than any benefit analysis, shows why fundamental human dignity hinges upon confidentiality. As the term "fidelity" implies, violating confidentiality is a particularly gross example of breaking faith with someone who has trusted you.

Thus, confidentiality is central to preserving the human dignity of patients. Occasionally, however, some other important moral considerations can cause us to disclose information without the patient's consent. We may next ask which sorts of moral considerations, and under what circumstances, might be sufficiently strong to override this aspect of the duty of fidelity. But before we take up this question, it will be useful to dispense with some cases that appear at first glance to be potential violations of confidentiality, but which do not, on analysis, call for this careful weighing of competing moral claims. Health professionals are required by law to report certain information to appropriate authorities; this includes communicable diseases (including sexually transmitted diseases), gunshot wounds, and suspicions of child abuse or neglect. These are all examples of information that a patient may have strong reasons for keeping private, and where harm can come to the patient if the information is revealed. But it is possible to see these cases as instances where the physician can report the information, even without the patient's consent, without major moral qualms. The reason is that the laws requiring this are (theoretically) in the public domain, passed by the representatives of the people, and thus fully in the public knowledge. Patients (theoretically) have already consented to disclosure of this sort of information, if they choose to go to a physician, because of their presumed awareness of the law (Marsh 1979). Obviously the patient may not see it this way. And the physician may certainly desire, as a matter of courtesy, not to reveal the information without warning the patient that the disclosure is about to occur. But this argument suggests that the disclosure of this sort of information, covered by law, need not engender a major moral controversy.

With the "easier" cases set aside, we can look at the tough decisions that balance confidentiality against other major moral principles. These might be of two general types. First, we could envision the other moral principle being the well-being of the same patient who demands privacy. Imagine a patient who suffers from an alcohol or other drug dependence problem, which so far he has succeeded in hiding from his family and work associates. You know that if you reveal the seriousness of his problem to his friends or family, they might put effective pressure on him to seek definitive treatment; but he refuses to consent to this disclosure. Your desire to respect confidentiality (the right of fidelity) is in conflict with your desire to save him from harm (the right of humanity). As we discussed above, this would be a good example of a paternalistic interference with his liberty. Thus, the basic arguments about when, if ever, paternalism is justified apply to this case (Beauchamp and McCullough 1984; Childress 1982).

Another general type of dilemma around confidentiality involves conflicting fidelities. The harm threatened by not disclosing some information will strike not the patient, but someone else. If the someone else is someone to whom the physician feels a justified duty of fidelity, aside from and in addition to the fidelity owed the patient within the physician-patient relationship, then a moral dilemma will arise.

The easiest competing duty of fidelity to imagine is one's faithfulness as a member of society, which engenders a duty to save the public, or specific individuals, from grave and immediate harm. This duty arose in one of the most widely discussed recent court cases on confidentiality, the Tarasoff case (Beauchamp and Childress 1983, 281–284). A psychologist learned from a patient of the latter's intent to murder a former girlfriend who had jilted him. The legal dispute, which obscured the ethical issue, was whether it was enough to tell the police (which the psychologist did) or whether there was also an obligation to tell the girl or her family (which was not done). But the central moral conclusion, which was not really in dispute, was that the grave harm threatened to a specific individual was sufficient to override the moral duty to protect confidences.

Deciding when confidentiality may be overridden is one of the most difficult problems in medical ethics (Jonsen et al. 1982, 153–154). To summarize very quickly, and without supporting reasons, what many authors have said on the subject, we can distinguish three sorts of situations:

1. Revealing the information would produce some considerable public good.
2. Revealing the information would prevent some possible risk of harm to someone, but we cannot identify with certainty who that would be.
3. Revealing the information would prevent some very likely harm to specific and identifiable individuals.

As we go from #1 to #3, the justification for overriding confidentiality becomes progressively stronger.

A duty to the public at large is not, however, the only duty of fidelity that a physician may feel. As medical practice becomes more complex, and as health care institutions become more multifaceted and pervasive, several competing loyalties may be encountered. The family physician, for example, may owe a duty to respect privacy to a patient, but also feel a duty to other family members of that patient, who are also members of that physician's practice, and who may have a strong interest in knowing that information. An adolescent who does not want her parents to know she is asking for birth control pills is a common example (Eaddy and Graber 1982). The physician employed by an industrial firm may feel loyalty both to the employee who seeks help, and also the firm that pays her. She may wish to reveal to the employer any patient information that would prevent financial losses to the company—like the patient's alcohol problem, or the fact that the patient's disability may be due not to a work-related injury but to some previously existing medical problem. Other situations that may create similarly divided loyalties are physicians employed by the military, by prisons (Thorburn 1981), or by athletic teams (McKeag et al. 1984).

These divided-loyalty settings may cause a physician to become too attentive to who signs the paycheck and too unconcerned about the rights of patients. On the other hand, some of the moral problems may be sidestepped by a frank disclosure of possible competing loyalties. If the company physician is forthright with the employee about the circumstances in which he will feel obligated to report information to the firm, the employee can freely choose what to reveal and what to keep secret. But the "patient's free choice" argument also has its limits. Take the increasingly common practice of requiring employees to undergo blood tests, such as screens for drug use, which threaten to reveal private information. The company may claim that anyone working for them has given their free consent; after all, if they do not want to participate, they can always find another job. But most of us would find threatened loss of employment so serious a risk that our consent could not be said to be truly voluntary under these circumstances (Graebner 1984).

A glance at the newspapers will show that medicine is not the only domain of modern life where confidentiality and privacy are at issue. A public debate is currently taking place over a proposal to link together various governmental and nongovernmental computer systems for a nationwide data linkup. The goals of this effort, such as preventing welfare fraud or defaulting on government loans, are laudable. But the inevitable consequence would be a loss of control over who has access to which private information about each citizen. Increasingly, health providers will become involved in such issues, at the public policy level as well as on the individual level, and will have to take an ethical stance on them.

CONCLUSION

Our understanding of the physician-patient relationship has been aided by a constructive give-and-take among physicians and philosophers interested in developing sound theoretical models that can guide clinical practice. Contractual models were proposed as an alternative to the physician paternalism that was increasingly being viewed as unacceptable. Critics then listed a number of problems that seemed to arise from contractual models. In reply to those critics, one might suggest a contractarian model as a further refinement of the contractual concept. In turn, those advocating a virtue-based alternative approach to ethics generally might find important elements lacking in a contractarian model. However, for our present purposes, we can note that a contractarian model can be used to answer two questions about two basic expectations within the physician-patient relationship, truthful disclosure and confidentiality: first, why these expectations are important to the basic human dignity of the patient, and second, what legitimate exceptions exist to the more general duties to tell the truth and to respect confidences.

Case 1. A 38-year-old paraplegic white male is admitted to the community hospital for treatment of a urinary tract infection, causing high fevers and prostration. The presumed source of infection is an indwelling suprapubic catheter. The patient suffered a spinal cord injury in an accident approximately four years previously. Since his rehabilitation he has worked as a public relations manager for a radio station. The week prior to hospitalization, he was informed abruptly that he would be laid off in just a few weeks. He has been extremely upset about how he will support his family, which consists of his wife and two young adopted children, and what he will do when his medical benefits lapse when he loses his job.

In the hospital, the patient appears as an extremely anxious man who appears insecure and fearful. Additional history reveals that he is being bothered by flashbacks to his previous hospitalization for the spinal cord injury, and that many unresolved emotional problems relating to that injury and the resulting life crises are coming back to haunt him at this time. As part of his anxiety, he indicates an insistence that he be kept fully informed of all developments and that no significant information about his illness be withheld from him. The family physician gives him this assurance, since this is in fact routine procedure for this physician regarding all patients. However, the physician is worried about the patient's emotional response to illness and the multitude of emotional risk factors that may complicate the patient's response to treatment.

A rare gram-negative organism is identified as the source of the urinary tract infection and an intravenous antibiotic, amikacin (brand name: Amikin) is ordered. The next morning on rounds, the family physician notes that the patient has begun to respond to antibiotic and feels a little better and has a lower temperature. However, there is also an incident report in the chart. Because of a pharmacy error which was not discovered in time by the nurses in the unit, the patient initially received 500 mg of aminocaproic acid (brand name: Amicar), a drug which is used to treat a disorder of blood coagulation. As the appropriate dose of Amicar is in the range of 4 to 5 grams, the 500 mg dose represents an almost insignificant amount. No side effects were noted from the medication, and in fact nothing of consequence occurred to the patient other than a brief delay in receiving the amikacin. However, the amikacin appears to be working and the delay does not seem to have hindered the patient's response.

The family physician wonders whether he should inform the patient, who is feeling a little bit better but still acts very anxious and ill at ease, about the medication error. He reasons that the information is totally unrelated to the course of management of the patient's illness, since the patient does not appear to have been jeopardized and nothing about the patient's treatment need be changed in order to respond to the error. Furthermore, the likely result of imparting this knowledge will be to increase the suspicion and vigilance with which the patient watches nursing staff in administration of all his medication; this is unlikely to provide the kind of relationship with staff that is needed for the patient's care, and is also very likely to worsen all of the patient's emotional risk factors which may hinder a good response to treatment. On the other hand, the physician feels that he has made a promise which he would be breaking if he withheld this information.

DISCUSSION QUESTIONS

1. Should the family physician tell the patient about the medication error?

2. If the family physician is entitled to withhold this information, would it have made a difference if the patient had actually suffered harm from the medication error, or if the patient's treatment was significantly changed as a result of the error?

3. If the family physician decides that it is justifiable to withhold this information now, is the physician nevertheless required to inform the patient of what he has done at a future time when the patient might be in a better emotional state?

4. Does the fact that the error was made by other health team members require that the physician get their consent before disclosing it?

Case 2. When the hospital nurse reports for duty at 7:00 AM, she discovers that one of the new patients admitted last evening is Mr. Turner, a 46-year-old male. As she is uncertain of the details and will be responsible for Mr. Turner's care during this shift, she takes out his chart and begins to review it. She notices that Mr. Turner is currently under the care of Dr. Brown, who came into the emergency room to see him and then admitted him and wrote the orders.

As she is reading the chart, Dr. Green walks up. "I see Bill Turner's name is on the board under Dr. Brown's case list. I've been Turner's family doctor for ten years now. I wonder why he didn't call me for this illness, and how he came in under Dr. Brown's care. Just let me see his chart, will you?"

The nurse knows that the hospital has recently had a staff conference on confidentiality. One point emphasized was that access to charts should be restricted to staff members who have a "need to know" because they are actually involved in caring for the patient during that hospital stay. Curiosity or personal acquaintance with the patient were cited as common but indefensible reasons for looking at the chart. By this stated policy, Dr. Green has no right to see Mr. Turner's chart. But it would be highly unusual for a nurse to refuse to give a doctor a chart, especially when the doctor has provided care for the patient in the past. Dr. Green could easily complain to her supervisor and get her into trouble.

DISCUSSION QUESTIONS

1. Assess the "need to know" policy. Does Dr. Green's long-established relationship with the patient provide such a "need to know?" Do you agree with the nurse's assessment that the chart should be withheld?

2. The case description gives us no clue *why* Mr. Turner might not want Dr. Green to see his chart. Can you imagine some circumstances in which Mr. Turner *would* want Dr. Green to see his chart? Can you imagine circumstances in which Mr. Turner would not want Dr. Green to see his chart? How could you determine which set of circumstances actually existed?

3. What should the nurse in this case say to Dr. Green?

REFERENCES

Beauchamp, T. L., and J. F. Childress. *Principles of Biomedical Ethics*, 2d ed. New York: Oxford University Press, 1983.
Beauchamp, T. L., and L. B. McCullough. *Medical Ethics: The Moral Responsibilities of Physicians.* Englewood Cliffs, N.J.: Prentice-Hall, 1984.
Benjamin, M. "Lay Obligations in Professional Relations." *J Med Philos* 10 (1985): 85–103.
Benson, H., and M. D. Epstein. "The Placebo Effect: A Neglected Asset in the Care of Patients." *JAMA* 232 (1975): 1225–1227.

Bloom, S. W. *The Doctor and His Patient.* New York: Russell Sage Foundation, 1963.

Brody, H. *Ethical Decisions in Medicine,* 2d ed. Boston: Little, Brown, 1981.

———. "The Lie That Heals: The Ethics of Giving Placebos." *Ann Intern Med* 97 (1982): 112–118.

———. "Autonomy Revisited: Progress in Medical Ethics." *J Roy Soc Med* 78 (1985): 380–387.

Buchanan, A. "Medical Paternalism." *Philos and Public Affairs* 7 (1978): 370–390.

Callahan, D. "Minimalist Ethics." *Hastings Cent Rep* 11, no. 5 (1981): 19–25.

Childress, J. F. *Who Shall Decide? Paternalism in Health Care.* New York: Oxford University Press, 1982.

Cousins, N. "A Layman Looks at Truth-Telling in Medicine." *JAMA* 244 (1980): 1929–1930.

Eaddy, J. A., and G. C. Graber. "Confidentiality and the Family Physician." *Am Fam Physician* 25, no. 1 (1982): 141–145.

Fried, C. *Medical Experimentation: Personal Integrity and Social Policy.* New York: American Elsevier, 1974.

Gadow, S. "Truth: Treatment of Choice, Scarce Resource, or Patient's Right?" *J Fam Pract* 13 (1981): 857–860.

Gert, B., and C. M. Culver. "Paternalistic Behavior." *Philos and Public Affairs* 6 (1976): 45–57.

———. "The Justification of Paternalism." In *Medical Responsibility,* edited by W. L. Robison and M. S. Pritchard. Clifton, N.J.: Humana Press, 1979.

Graebner, W. "Doing the World's Unhealthy Work: The Fiction of Free Choice." *Hastings Cent Rep* 14, no. 1 (1984): 28–37.

Jonsen, A. R., M. Siegler, and W. J. Winslade. *Clinical Ethics.* New York: Macmillan, 1982.

Katz, J. *The Silent World of Doctor and Patient.* New York: Free Press, 1984.

Komrad, M. S. "A Defence of Medical Paternalism: Maximising Patients' Autonomy." *J Med Ethics* 9 (1983): 38–44.

Kubler-Ross, E. *On Death and Dying.* New York: Macmillan, 1969.

Ladd, J. "Legalism and Medical Ethics." *J Med Philos* 4 (1979): 70–80.

Lidz, C. W., A. Meisel, M. Osterweis, et al. "Barriers to Informed Consent." *Ann Intern Med* 99 (1983): 534–543.

MacIntyre, A. *After Virtue.* Notre Dame, Ind.: University of Notre Dame Press, 1981.

Marsh, F. H. "The 'Deeper Meaning' of Confidentiality Within the Physician-Patient Relationship." *Ethics in Science and Med* 6 (1979): 131–136.

Masters, R. D. "Is Contract an Adequate Basis for Medical Ethics?" *Hastings Cent Rep* 5, no. 6 (1975): 24–28.

May, W. F. "Code, Covenant, Contract, or Philanthropy?" *Hastings Cent Rep* 5, no. 6 (1975): 29–38.

———. *The Physician's Covenant: Images of the Healer in Medical Ethics.* Philadelphia: Westminster Press, 1983.

McKeag, D., D. Hough, and H. Brody. "Medical Ethics in Sport." *The Physician and Sportsmedicine* 12, no. 8 (1984): 145–150.

Miller, B. L., and H. Brody. "Contracting the Principles of Medical Ethics: A Critique of Veatch's 'A Theory of Medical Ethics.'" *Westminster Institute Review* 2, no. 3 (1983): 11–13.

Novack, D. H., et al. "Changes in Physicians' Attitudes Toward Telling the Cancer Patient." *JAMA* 241 (1979): 897–900.

Oken, D. "What to Tell Cancer Patients." *JAMA* 175 (1961): 1120–1128.

Parsons, T. "Health and Disease: A Sociological and Action Perspective." In *Encyclopedia of Bioethics,* edited by W. T. Reich. New York: The Free Press, 1978.

Pellegrino, E. D. "Toward a Reconstruction of Medical Morality: The Primacy of the Act of Profession and the Fact of Illness." *J Med Philos* 4 (1979): 32–56.

Pellegrino, E. D., and D. C. Thomasma. *A Philosophical Basis of Medical Practice.* New York: Oxford University Press, 1981.

Rawls, J. *A Theory of Justice.* Cambridge, Mass.: Harvard University Press, 1971.

Reiser, S. J. "Words as Scalpels: Transmitting Evidence in the Clinical Dialogue." *Ann Intern Med* 92 (1980): 837–842.

Sheldon, M. "Truth Telling in Medicine." *JAMA* 247 (1982): 651–654.

Shelp, E. E., ed. *Virtue and Medicine.* Boston: D. Reidel, 1985.

Siegler, M. "A Physician's Perspective on the Right to Health Care." *JAMA* 244 (1980): 1591–1596.

———. "Searching for Moral Certainty in Medicine: A Proposal for a New Model of the Doctor-Patient Encounter." *Bull NY Acad Med* 57 (1981): 56–69.

———. "Confidentiality in Medicine—A Decrepit Concept." *N Engl J Med* 307 (1982): 1518–1521.

Smith, D. G., and L. Newton. "Physician and Patient: Respect for Mutuality." *Theor Med* 5 (1984): 43–60.

Szasz, T. S., and M. H. Hollender. "The Basic Models of the Doctor-Patient Relationship." *Arch Intern Med* 97 (1956): 585–592.

Thorburn, K. M. "Croaker's Dilemma: Should Prison Physicians Serve Prisons or Prisoners?" *West J Med* 134 (1981): 457–461.

Twiss, S. B. "The Problem of Moral Responsibility in Medicine." *J Med Philos* 2 (1977): 330–375.

Veatch, R. M. "Models for Ethical Medicine in a Revolutionary Age." *Hastings Cent Rep* 2, no. 3 (1972): 5–7.

———. "Professional Medical Ethics: The Grounding of Its Principles." *J Med Philos* 4 (1979): 1–19.

———. *A Theory of Medical Ethics.* New York: Basic Books, 1981.

Vogel, A. V., J. S. Goodwin, and J. M. Goodwin. "The Therapeutics of Placebo." *Am Fam Physician* 22, no. 1 (1980): 105–109.

Weinstein, M. C., H. V. Fineberg, A. S. Elstein, et al. *Clinical Decision Analysis.* Philadelphia: Saunders, 1980.

Weiss, B. D. "Confidentiality Expectations of Patients, Physicians and Medical Students." *JAMA* 247 (1982): 2695–2697.

ACKNOWLEDGEMENTS

Tom Tomlinson, Kenneth Howe, Leonard Fleck, and Robert Veatch made helpful suggestions for revising an earlier draft of this chapter. Tom Tomlinson provided Case 2.

5

Limiting Procreation

Judith Areen

SUMMARY

This chapter examines the development of controls on contraception, sterilization, and abortion. In the first stage, limitations on procreation in marriage were prohibited by religious authorities. Sexuality was also discouraged, not only outside of marriage but also to a great extent within marriage. With the rise of the modern secular state, civil law was increasingly employed to regulate marriage and procreation. In the United States, the first national law restricting access to contraception, the Comstock Act, was passed in 1873. Increasingly, however, the right of secular authorities to regulate private behavior came under attack. Debate increased about whether the law should regulate the use of contraception, sterilization, or abortion.

In the second stage, the use of sterilization to limit procreation was not only permitted but also was mandated at least for certain mental patients and criminals. Mandatory sterilization laws were passed in a number of states by the early twentieth century, only a few decades after medical science first developed safe procedures for sterilizing men and women. The United States Supreme Court upheld the constitutionality of such statutes in 1927 in Buck v. Bell. *That decision has never been overruled.*

In the third stage, some governmental restrictions on limiting procreation have been struck down as unconstitutional. The modern era began in 1965 when the United States Supreme Court announced in Griswold v. Connecticut *that there is a right of privacy protected by the Constitution of the United States and that the right empowers a married couple to decide whether to use contraception. A later decision of the Court extended the right to use contraceptives to single individuals. In 1973 in* Roe v. Wade, *the Court held that the right of privacy includes the right of a pregnant woman to seek an abortion at least during some stages of pregnancy. The Court has extended the right to seek an abortion to some pregnant minors but has not yet addressed the issue of whether a state may intervene in a pregnancy for the benefit of the fetus over the objection of the pregnant woman.*

Abortion remains the most controversial method of limiting procreation because the interests of another living being—the fetus—are at stake. The intensity of disagreement about the morality of abortion as well as the complex interrelationship in this country between morality and constitutional rights are underscored by the fact that the Supreme Court is more closely divided than in 1973 as to whether Roe v. Wade *was correctly decided.*

Knowledge of ways to limit procreation has existed for millennia. Egyptian papyri from between 1900 and 1100 BC contain recipes for contraceptive preparations (Noonan 1966, 9). Religious prohibitions on the use of contraception, sterilization, or abortion to limit procreation are also very old. Consider the biblical account of Onan. Er, Onan's older brother, had been killed:

> Then Juda [Onan's father] said to Onan, "Go to your brother's wife, perform your duty as brother-in-law, and raise up seed for your brother." Onan knew that the descendants would not be his own, so whenever he had relations with his brother's wife, he let the seed be lost on the ground, in order not to raise up seed for his brother. What he did displeased Yahweh, who killed him also (Genesis 38:8–10).[1]

With the rise of the modern secular state, restrictions on marriage and procreation were incorporated into the civil and criminal law. But the right of secular authorities to regulate the private behavior of individuals later came under challenge. John Stuart Mill, for example, argued that "[t]he only purpose for which power can rightfully be exercised over any member of a civilized community, against his will, is to prevent harm to others. His own good, either physical or moral, is not a sufficient warrant" (1859, 9). In turn, the argument has gained force that contraception, abortion, and sterilization are a form of private conduct that should not be regulated by the law.

Mill might well have objected to this extension of his position. He made clear that his conception of liberty did not extend to giving parents unlimited power over children. He criticized the fact that parents were not required to sacrifice or to secure an education for their children. He also supported population control mea-

---

[1] The passage has sometimes been interpreted to condemn masturbation. The text provides no support for this position. Indeed, the text arguably does not support the widespread interpretation that the passage condemns contraception as opposed to Onan's failure to carry out a levirate marriage, that is, marriage with the wife of a deceased brother. The objective was to maintain the family line in a society that set great store by blood ties and, consequently, had little use for adoption. [The Anchor Bible: Genesis 300 (E. A. Speiser intro., trans. and notes 1964).]

sures such as laws forbidding marriage unless the parties can show that they have the means of supporting a family. Thus, if the birth rate had fallen low enough to threaten the economic viability of a society, Mill himself might have supported restrictions on contraception, sterilization, or abortion.

The extent to which contraception, sterilization, and abortion should be regulated by public authorities continues to be the subject of much debate. Of the three, abortion is the most controversial method of limiting procreation because the interests of another living being—the fetus—are at stake. The debate about whether abortion is morally wrong is thus complicated by a more basic debate over whether a fetus is entitled to the same moral or legal protection as any citizen.

This chapter is organized into three sections. Each is devoted primarily to a historical stage in the development of controls on contraception, abortion, and sterilization. In the first stage, any limitation of procreation by married couples was prohibited, first by religious and later, by secular authorities. Sexuality was also discouraged, not only outside of marriage, but to a great extent within marriage as well. The second stage, mandatory sterilization of individuals for eugenic purposes, began in the late nineteenth century when medical science first developed procedures for safely sterilizing men and women. The third stage, constitutional protection of the right of individuals to decide whether or not to limit procreation, began in 1965 with the decision of the Supreme Court in *Griswold v. Connecticut*[2] to protect the use of contraceptives by married couples. In 1973, this right of privacy, as it was denominated, was extended to the decision to seek an abortion, at least during some stages of fetal development.

CONTRACEPTION, VOLUNTARY STERILIZATION, AND THE DUTY TO PROCREATE

The Legacy of the Past

There was little discussion of procreation by secular philosophers before this century. Aristotle approved of abortion early in pregnancy when a couple had too many children, but otherwise devoted little attention to the subject (Politics 7.16). By contrast, procreation has always been a central concern of the major Western religious traditions.

The early Christian church opposed any limits on procreation. This position was derived in part from the belief that marriage is a state inferior to celibacy. In St. Paul's language, marriage is for those who "cannot exercise self-control;" therefore, "it is better to marry than to burn" (7 Cor. 9–10). Even within marriage, sexual liberty was discouraged by holding that the only acceptable purpose for sexual relations is procreation. St. Paul accordingly denounced abortifacient and contraceptive drugs (5 Gal. 20) (Noonan 1978, 206–207).

---

[2]381 U.S. 479 (1965).

The early Christian moralists appear to have been strongly influenced in their views on sexuality by the Stoics, who sought to control bodily desires by reason. Epictetus, for example, considered immoderation in bodily activities irrational, for it made a man dependent on his own body (Manual 41). Seneca, the first-century Stoic and statesman, proclaimed:

> All love of another's wife is shameful; so too, too much love of your own. A wise man ought to love his wife with judgment, not affection. Let him control his impulses and not be borne headlong into copulation. Nothing is fouler than to love a wife like an adulteress (Seneca, Fragments no. 84).

In the fourth century, St. Augustine distinguished between lust and sexual relations for the purpose of procreation. He took the position that in marriage only the former is sinful. He therefore explicitly condemned the use of contraception by married couples (401) (Wilcox 1955).

The Protestant reformation brought no change in position on contraception. Because he relied heavily on Augustine for his theology, Martin Luther followed him on marriage. Luther taught that God created man and woman differently "not for lewdness but to be true to each other, be fruitful, beget children, and support and bring them up to the glory of God" (Fischer 1959, 37).

In the Jewish tradition, the duty of procreation is considered the first "mitzvah" or obligation. Most commentators derive the duty not solely from the admonition to "increase and multiply" (Genesis 1 : 22), but also from the charge to the sons of Noah (Genesis 9 : 1 and 7) or to Jacob (Genesis 35 : 11) (Feldman 1968, 46). The duty, however, has been interpreted to apply only to men. Thus although the story of Onan was interpreted to prohibit coitus interruptus, the Talmud prescribed two contraceptive methods—a potion called the Cup of Roots and a vaginal sponge— that women could employ, although only in limited circumstances (Feldman 1968; Gordon 1976, 5).

Secular legal restrictions on interference with procreation date back at least to the first century BC. Contraception appears to have been lawful in the early Roman Empire, but concern about the falling birth rate of the upper classes led to the passage of legislation in 18 BC and AD 9 prohibiting the childless from holding certain high offices and restricting their rights of inheritance (Noonan 1966, 21).

Secular regulation of marriage in England was not established until well into the middle ages (Helmholz 1974). In Roman law, marriage had been a relatively private matter. No special formula or ceremony was required to contract a valid marriage. There was no requirement of intervention by any sort of public official, and there was no registration of marriages. Divorce was allowed without a decree by any court. It was against this background of freedom in marriage practice that the Christian view of marriage developed. Not surprisingly, the establishment of control over marriage by the Church was a "long and disputed process," which was not accomplished even as late as the thirteenth century (Helmholz 1974, 5). Ultimately, the civil law came to reflect the positions of the Church:

"As the first cause and reason of matrimony," says Ayliffe, "ought to be the design of having an offspring;" so the second ought to be the avoiding of fornication. And the law recognizes these two as the "principal ends of matrimony," namely, "a lawful indulgence of the passions to prevent licentiousness, and the procreation of children according to the evident design of Divine Providence" (Bishop 1852, 175).

In addition to legal restrictions on childlessness and marriage, procreation was controlled indirectly by sanctions imposed on having children outside of mar-riage—both the kind of community sanctions for adultery immortalized in *The Scarlet Letter* and legal disabilities placed on children conceived out of wedlock.

In the nineteenth century, the law began to regulate access to contraceptives directly. In the United States, the first national law restricting access to contracep-tion, the Comstock Act, was passed in 1873. Its passage may have been in part a reaction to an increasing use of contraceptives that was reflected in the sharp decline in the national birth rate. It is estimated, for example, that in the year 1800, white women in the United States had an average of 7.04 children. By 1870, the number was down to 4.55 (by 1940 it had dropped to 2.10) (Gordon 1976, 48).

The Comstock Act bears the name of the young man most responsible for securing its passage, Anthony Comstock, who was secretary of the New York Society for the Suppression of Vice. He has been described as a "deeply religious man with a strong sense of personal sin" (Haney 1960, 19). Born in 1844, he believed that his mission was to improve the morals of other people by ridding the country of obscene literature and photographs (Smith 1964, 275).

The Comstock Act prohibited the use of the mails for the sending of any "obscene . . . book or other publication of an indecent character, or any article or thing designed or intended for the prevention of conception." Importation of these items was also forbidden by the Act (Smith 1964, 276). The reasons identified by historian Carl Degler for passage of the law are remarkably similar to those ad-vanced by early Christian moralists:

> . . . The reasons . . . fell into two categories. One was a fear that if people
> practiced contraception they might overindulge in sex, a practice that
> seemed fraught with unknown consequences. The sexual urge might get
> out of control. Even an advanced feminist like Charlotte Perkins Gilman
> had doubts about contraception in the 20th century because she thought it
> would lead to overindulgence. The second category of argument against
> contraception was that it represented an interference with nature's as well
> as God's intentions. According to this line of thought, sexuality presum-
> ably had been tied to reproduction for a purpose; to sever that connection
> was to oppose the natural and religious order as people of the 19th century
> perceived it (Degler 1980, 191).

The Beginning of the Modern Era

The seeds of change were sown in the nineteenth century when use of contracep-tives spread. By midcentury, the women's rights movement in the United States was pressing for "voluntary motherhood." They did not support contraception, however, but favored abstinence as the preferred method for limiting the number of children:

> The Voluntary Motherhood advocates' . . . concern for all the needs of women . . . led them to recognize a number of contradictions. First, they realized that while women needed freedom from excessive childbearing, they also needed the respect and self-respect motherhood brought. . . . Second, they understood that while women needed freedom from pregnancy, they also needed freedom from male sexual tyranny, especially in a society that had almost completely suppressed accurate information about female sexuality and replaced it with information and attitudes so false as to virtually guarantee that women would not enjoy sex. Abstinence as a form of birth control may well have been the solution that made most sense in the particular historical circumstance. Abstinence helped women strengthen their ability to say no to their husbands' sexual demands, for example, while contraception and abortion would have weakened it (Gordon 1982, 45).

Most feminists did not change their minds about contraception until the early twentieth century when Margaret Sanger organized and led the modern movement for birth control. Influenced initially by Emma Goldman, a leading radical, and later by Havelock Ellis and other sexual-liberation theorists, Sanger ultimately drew most of her political support by turning from working class issues to eugenics (Gordon 1976). In 1919, for example, she announced: "Birth control is nothing more or less than the facilitation of the process of weeding out the unfit, or preventing the birth of defectives or of those who will become defectives" (Kennedy 1970, 115).

During the twentieth century, a number of religious groups altered their position on the subject of contraception. In 1930, the bishops of the Anglican church voted to accept methods other than sexual abstinence to avoid parenthood. By 1959, when the World Council of Churches endorsed contraception, the Protestant consensus in its favor was considered overwhelming (Fagley 1960).

The Catholic Church, by contrast, did not change its position at least with respect to "artificial" contraception, although by the end of the eighteenth century the Catholic theological consensus no longer insisted on procreative purpose in marital intercourse. In the nineteenth century, Jean Gury, a French jesuit, taught that intercourse might "manifest or promote conjugal affection." His view was very influential (Noonan 1978, 213). In Casti Connubi, an encyclical letter issued in 1930, Pope Pius XI approved marital intercourse at times when the wife would be unlikely to conceive because "there are . . . secondary ends, such as mutual aid, the cultivating of mutual love, and the quieting of concupiscence which husband and wife are not forbidden to consider so long as these are subordinated to the primary aim [of begetting children]." A papal commission appointed just after the Second Vatican Council (1963–1965) recommended the approval of contraceptives in marriage (Noonan 1978, 213). Pope Paul VI nonetheless reaffirmed the traditional condemnation of artificial birth control in 1968:

[Consider] how wide and easy a road would thus be opened up towards conjugal infidelity and the general lowering of morality. Not much experience is needed in order to know human weakness, and to understand that men—especially the young, who are so vulnerable on this point—have need of encouragement to be faithful to the moral law, so that they must not be offered some easy means of eluding its observance. It is also to be feared that the man, growing used to the employment of anti-conceptive practices, may finally lose respect for the woman, and, no longer caring for her physical and psychological equilibrium, may come to the point of considering her as a mere instrument of selfish enjoyment, and no longer as his respected and beloved companion (Paul VI 1968, 11).

He also reaffirmed approval of recourse to infecund periods:

If [there] are serious motives to space out births, which derive from the physical or psychological conditions of husband and wife, or from external conditions, the Church teaches that it is then licit to take into account the natural rhythms immanent in the generative functions, for the use of marriage in the infecund periods only, and in this way to regulate birth without offending . . . moral principles (Paul VI 1968, 10).

Significant legal change first occurred in the United States in 1936 when a federal court held that the Comstock Act did not prohibit the distribution of contraceptives prescribed by doctors.[3] By this time, however, a number of states had passed "little Comstock laws" that in some instances were even more restrictive than the original act. These were not successfully challenged until 1965, when the Supreme Court, in *Griswold v. Connecticut*,[4] held unconstitutional as applied to a married couple a Connecticut statute that prohibited the use of contraceptives. The basis for the decision was not that the Constitution provides a right of access to contraceptives, but that it provides married couples with a right of privacy. This privacy right was found to be impermissibly infringed by the Connecticut statute.

It is worth spending some time on *Griswold* and the way it linked procreation and privacy because the opinion laid the foundation for far more controversial Court decisions in the 1970s and 1980s involving abortion and the rights of pregnant minors.

The word privacy does not appear anywhere in the U.S. Constitution. How then did the Court find a right of privacy? Justice Douglas, writing for the Court, explained:

The association of people is not mentioned in the Constitution nor in the Bill of Rights. The right to educate a child in a school of the parent's choice—whether public or private or parochial—is also not mentioned. Nor is the right to study any particular subject or any foreign language. Yet the First Amendment has been construed to include certain of those rights.

•   •   •

---

[3]United States v. One Package, 86 F.2d 737 (2nd Cir. 1936).
[4]381 U.S. 479 (1965).

The foregoing cases suggest that specific guarantees in the Bill of Rights have penumbras, formed by emanations from those guarantees that help give them life and substance. Various guarantees create zones of privacy. The right of association contained in the penumbra of the First Amendment is one, as we have seen. The third amendment in its prohibition against the quartering of soldiers "in any house" in time of peace without the consent of the owner is another facet of that privacy. The Fourth Amendment explicitly affirms the "right of the people to be secure in their persons, houses, papers, and effects, against unreasonable searches and seizures." The Fifth Amendment in its Self-Incrimination Clause enables the citizen to create a zone of privacy which government may not force him to surrender to his detriment. The Ninth Amendment provides: "The enumeration in the Constitution, of certain rights, shall not be construed to deny or disparage others retained by the people."

Emphasizing that the Connecticut statute before the Court prohibited the *use* of contraceptives, including use by married couples, Justice Douglas linked procreation and privacy by adding, "Would we allow the police to search the sacred precincts of marital bedrooms for telltale signs of the use of contraceptives? The very idea is repulsive to the notions of privacy surrounding the marriage relationship."

Recognition by the Supreme Court of rights not explicitly protected by the Constitution (such as the right of privacy announced in *Griswold*) has been criticized by many legal scholars as placing too much power in the hands of unelected judges. Professor John Ely, for example, notes that "appeal to some notion to be found neither in the Constitution nor . . . in the judgment of the political branches, seems especially vulnerable to a charge of inconsistency with democratic theory" (Ely 1980, 5). By contrast, Professors Heymann and Barzelay contend:

> [The] family unit [is] an integral part of [our constitutional system.] . . . [The] immensely important power of deciding about matters of early socialization has been allocated to the family, not to the government. . . . For the Court to have declined strict review of state legislation that limits the private right to choose whom to marry and whether to raise a family, or to decide within wide bounds how to rear one's children, would have been to leave the most basic substructure of our society and government [to] political whim (Heymann and Barzelay 1973, 772–773).

Professor Charles Black has said that *Griswold* is not so much a case that the law tests as a case that tests the law:

> If our constitutional law could permit such a thing to happen then we might almost as well not have any law of constitutional limitations, partly because the thing is so outrageous in itself, and partly because a constitutional law inadequate to deal with such an outrage would be too feeble, in method and doctrine, to deal with a very great amount of equally outrageous material. Virtually all the intimacies, privacies and autonomies of life would be regulable by the legislature . . . (Black 1970, 32).

Whether or not the Court was justified in finding a right of privacy in the Constitution, it is important for our purposes to notice the way *Griswold* became a stepping stone to the establishment of a right of *access* to contraceptives. In 1977, in *Carey v. Population Services International*,[5] the Supreme Court decided a case involving a New York statute that regulated access to contraceptives. The statute prohibited anyone other than a licensed pharmacist from distributing contraceptives to persons over 16 years of age, and prohibited anyone from selling or distributing contraceptives to anyone under the age of 16. A restriction on sale, of course, would not have to be enforced by the kind of offensive methods that led the Court in *Griswold* to overturn a prohibition of use. The Court nevertheless struck down the first restriction:

> . . . *Griswold* may no longer be read as holding only that a State may not prohibit a married couple's use of contraceptives. Read in light of its progeny,[6] the teaching of *Griswold* is that the Constitution protects individual decision in matters of childbearing from unjustified intrusion by the State.

By the 1980s, the legal right to limit procreation through the use of contraceptive measures was so firmly established that private suits began to reach the courts in which women sued sexual partners for deceiving them about their infertility.

Consider the facts in one recent California case.[7] Barbara A. hired John G., a lawyer, to represent her in a family law matter. On two occasions they had sexual intercourse with each other. Before they engaged in sexual intercourse the first time, Barbara demanded that John use a condom because she did not want to become pregnant. He assured her, "I can't possibly get anyone pregnant." Relying on this representation, Barbara A. proceeded. She did become pregnant. It was a tubal pregnancy; and, as a consequence, Barbara was forced to undergo surgery to save her life. Her Fallopian tube was removed and she was rendered sterile by the surgery. She sued John G. for physical, emotional, and financial injuries resulting from the pregnancy, and won.

The Supreme Court had more difficulty in *Carey v. Population Services* with the issue of whether to uphold the restriction on distribution of contraceptives to minors. A majority of the justices could not agree on a single opinion. A plurality of four[8] argued that because the Court in an earlier case had struck down a blanket requirement of parental consent on the choice of a minor to terminate her pregnancy, a blanket prohibition on the distribution of contraceptives had to be unconstitutional as well. They reasoned: "The State's interests in protection of the mental and physical health of the pregnant minor, and in protection of potential life are clearly more implicated by the abortion decision than by the decision to use a nonhazardous contraceptive." As to the claim that access to contraceptives would lead to increased sexual activity among the young, the four justices replied, "The same

---

[5]431U.S. 678 (1977).
[6]The primary case the Court cited was *Roe v. Wade*, discussed in the text at note 17, infra.
[7]Barbara A. v. John G., 145 Cal. App. 3d 369 (Cal. Ct. App. 1983).
[8]Justices Brennan, Stewart, Marshall and Blackmun.

argument . . . would support a ban on abortions for minors, or indeed support a prohibition on abortion, or access to contraceptives, for the unmarried. . . . Yet, in each of these areas, the Court has rejected the argument, noting in *Roe v. Wade,* that 'no court or commentator has taken the argument seriously.'"

Justice White agreed that the statute at issue in the case was unconstitutional, but only because the State had failed to prove that the prohibition "measurably contributes" to the deterrent purposes the State advanced as justification for the restriction. He agreed with Justice Stevens who said "I would describe as 'frivolous' the argument that a minor has the constitutional right to put contraceptives to their intended use, notwithstanding the combined objection of both parents and the State." Justice Powell also concurred to make clear that he too would uphold a requirement of prior parental consultation. Chief Justice Burger and Justice Rehnquist dissented. According to Justice Rehnquist:

> Those who valiantly but vainly defended the heights of Bunker Hill in 1775 made it possible that men such as James Madison might later sit in the first Congress and draft the Bill of Rights to the Constitution. The post-Civil War Congresses which drafted the Civil War Amendments to the Constitution could not have accomplished their task without the blood of brave men on both sides which was shed at Shiloh, Gettysburg, and Cold Harbor. If those responsible for these Amendments, by feats of valor or efforts of draftsmanship, could have lived to know that their efforts had enshrined in the Constitution the right of commercial vendors of contraceptives to peddle them to unmarried minors through such means as window displays and vending machines located in the men's room of truck stops, notwithstanding the considered judgment of the New York Legislature to the contrary, it is not difficult to imagine their reaction.

The division on the Court continues a longstanding debate over how much minors' rights are limited and how to implement the limits. Even John Stuart Mill, perhaps the leading proponent of the principle of autonomy, qualified his position with respect to minors:

> It is, perhaps, hardly necessary to say that this doctrine is meant to apply only to human beings in the maturity of their faculties. We are not speaking of children or of young persons below the age which the law may fix as that of manhood or womanhood. Those who are still in a state to require being taken care of by others must be protected against their own actions as well as against external injury (Mill 1859, Chapter 1).

Although there seems to be widespread agreement that minors must be protected from their own imprudence, there is less agreement on when protection is needed and on whether the ultimate power to protect minors should be vested in their parents or in the state.

Consider the challenge brought in 1981 in federal court in New York[9] to state restrictions on marriage and illegitimacy. At bottom, the case was about whether

---

[9]Moe v. Dinkins, 533 F. Supp. 623 (S.D.N.Y. 1981), affirmed 669 F.2d 67 (2d Cir. 1982).

the state should permit minors to marry in order to legitimize the birth of their child despite the opposition of their parents. The plaintiffs, Maria Moe, age 15, and Raoul Roe, age 18 (the names are fictitious, reflecting the willingness of the judicial system to protect the privacy of minors who litigate on personal matters) wanted to marry. The law in New York provided at that time that all male applicants for a marriage license between ages 16 and 18 and all female applicants between ages 14 and 18 had to obtain "written consent to the marriage from both parents of the minor or minors." Maria, who was pregnant, requested consent from her mother, a widow, to marry Raoul, but her mother refused, apparently because she wanted to continue receiving welfare benefits for Maria. Maria then challenged the New York law as a violation of the constitutional right to marry. The court denied her request and upheld the statute on the basis that the right to marry does not protect the rights of minors to the same extent it protects the rights of adults.

Case 1. In 1981, the right of parents to oversee the reproductive activities of their adolescent children was also at issue in the decision of the United States Department of Health and Human Services to issue regulations requiring any family planning program that received federal funds to notify within ten working days the parents or guardians of any minor who was given contraceptives. The regulations were later invalidated by a federal judge, who found that they were not consistent with the expressed intent of Congress in authorizing funding for family planning programs.[10] Can the result in this case be squared with the holding in the case of Maria Moe and Raoul Roe? Assume you have been asked to advise your Congressman on whether to vote for proposed new legislation that would legalize the notification requirement. What are the strongest arguments for and against such legislation? What would you advise, and why?

There has been almost no litigation over the use of (voluntary) sterilization to limit procreation despite the fact that by 1977, sterilization had become the contraceptive measure used most by married couples in the United States. One partner in each of some six million couples, constituting one-third of all couples practicing birth control, has undergone sterilization (Areen 1985, 820).

This relative absence of public controversy does not reflect greater consensus on the ethics of sterilization as religious objections to contraception generally also apply to sterilization. There are additional religious objections, moreover, that apply only to sterilization. Pope Pius XI's 1930 encyclical on marriage, for example, holds: "[p]rivate individuals have no other power over the members of their bodies than that which pertains to their natural ends; and they are not free to destroy or to

---

[10]Planned Parenthood Federation of America v. Heckler, 712 F.2d 650 (1983).

multilate their members, or in any other way render themselves unfit for their natural functions, except where no other provision can be made for the good of the whole body" (Pius XI 1930).

The fact that sterilization is generally irreversible distinguishes it from other contraceptive measures. Its irreversible character also makes it particularly important to ensure that any consent to sterilization is both informed and voluntary. To prevent abuse in the wake of publicized reports of young black girls being sterilized in circumstances that suggested deceit or coercion, the federal government has taken the position that federal funding may not be used to pay for the sterilization of minors of mentally incompetent adults.[11] Federal money can be used to fund voluntary sterilization for competent adults, but only after they have given informed consent in writing. They must also be informed that their right to future care or treatment or to other federally funded benefits will not be affected if they reject sterilization.

MANDATORY STERILIZATION FOR EUGENIC PURPOSES

No medically safe method of sterilizing men or women was developed until almost the end of the nineteenth century (O'Hara and Sanks 1956, 20). Once the new technology was available, a period of widespread governmental intrusion on reproductive choice began with the passage of eugenic legislation that authorized mandatory sterilization designed to "save" society from the offspring of "defective" citizens. The first such state sterilization law was passed in 1907, in Indiana, where Dr. Sharp of the State Reformatory mounted a campaign for the measure. His purpose was not only eugenic, but "to reduce sexual overexcitation in delinquent boys" (Kevles 1985, 108). Between 1907–1917, fifteen more states enacted eugenic sterilization laws. Most of these laws gave the state the power to compel the sterilization of habitual or confirmed criminals, epileptics, and the "insane" (Kevles 1985, 100).

In 1927, the Supreme Court considered the constitutionality of one of these statutes in *Buck v. Bell.*[12] In an opinion by Justice Oliver Wendell Holmes, Jr., the Court upheld a Virginia law that authorized the forcible sterilization of 18-year-old Carrie Buck, who was alleged to be "feeble minded," and who had already given birth to one daughter. Holmes' opinion reflects the social Darwinism that was popular at the time:

> . . . We have seen more than once that the public welfare may call upon the best citizens for their lives. It would be strange if it could not call upon those who already sap the strength of the State for these lesser sacrifices, often not felt to be such by those concerned, in order to prevent our being swamped with incompetence. It is better for all the world, if instead of waiting to execute degenerate offspring for crime, or to let them starve for their imbecility, society can prevent those who are manifestly unfit from

---

[11]42C.F.R. sections 50.201 to 50.210.
[12]274 U.S. 200 (1927).

continuing their kind. The principle that sustains compulsory vaccination is broad enough to cover cutting the Fallopian tubes. Three generations of imbeciles are enough.

The Supreme Court has never overruled *Buck*.[13] Seventeen states, moreover, currently authorize the involuntary sterilization of some persons (Areen 1985, 833). It is estimated that some 70,000 people have been subjected to compulsory sterilization in this country since the beginning of the century (Id.).

The rationale provided by the Supreme Court in *Buck* for mandatory sterilization does not stand up well in the light of modern scientific knowledge. First, no hereditary basis has been established for criminal behavior. Science has found no genetic basis for murder or stealing, for example. Second, although there is evidence of a genetic component to intelligence, great debate exists over the relative influence of heredity and environment (Jensen 1972; Layzer 1974). Finally, errors can be made in attempting to measure a person's intelligence. It is striking that mistakes appear to have been made in the very case that went to the Supreme Court. Carrie Buck's daughter Vivian, who died at the age of seven, was considered a "bright child" by her second grade teachers. A physician who examined Carrie Buck in the 1970s reported that she also was not mentally retarded. He judged that she had been sterilized because her infant daughter was considered "slow" and because she was the unwed daughter of an "antisocial" woman some thought was a prostitute (Areen 1985, 835). Thus, there were not "three generations of imbeciles."

In recent years, a growing number of state courts have established standards that must be met before a retarded person may be sterilized:

1. Those advocating sterilization bear the heavy burden of proving by clear and convincing evidence that sterilization is in the best interests of the incompetent.
2. The incompetent must be afforded a full judicial hearing at which medical testimony is presented and the incompetent, through a guardian appointed for the litigation, is allowed to present proof and cross-examine witnesses.
3. The judge must be assured that a comprehensive medical, psychological, and social evaluation is made of the incompetent.
4. The judge must determine that the individual is legally incompetent to make the decision whether to be sterilized, and that this incapacity is in all likelihood permanent.
5. The incompetent must be capable of reproduction and unable to care for offspring.
6. Sterilization must be the only practicable means of contraception.

---

[13]It was arguably narrowed by *Skinner v. Oklahoma*, 316 U.S. 535 (1942), where the Court held unconstitutional a statute that authorized the involuntary sterilization of certain, rather arbitrary, categories of criminals. The Court explained: "We are dealing here with legislation which involves one of the basic civil rights of man. Marriage and procreation are fundamental to the very existence and survival of the race. The power to sterilize, if exercised, may have subtle, farreaching and devastating effects. In evil or reckless hands it can cause races or types which are inimical to the dominant group to wither and disappear. There is no redemption for the individual whom the law touches. Any experiment which the State conducts is to his irreparable injury. He is forever deprived of a basic liberty."

7. The proposed operation must be the least restrictive alternative available.

8. To the extent possible, the judge must hear testimony from the incompetent concerning his or her understanding and desire, if any, for the proposed operation and its consequences.

9. The judge must examine the motivation for the request for sterilization (Areen et al. 1984, 1283).

Do you think these safeguards are sufficient to protect against possible abuse of the power to sterilize? What justifications, if any, might there be for sterilizing a mentally impaired person? Consider the case of Sonya F.[14]

Case 2. Sonya is a severely retarded 13-year-old with an IQ of about 25 to 30 (the equivalent of a mental age of 1 to 2 years), blind, and with pronounced neurological problems. She was born a normal child. At the age of five months, she was severely injured in an automobile accident, which caused brain damage and temporary paralysis. Unable to cope with the event, Sonya's mother took her to live with her grandmother, who is 61-years-old. Sonya, her two sisters, and her aunt have been living with her grandmother ever since. Sonya regularly attends a special school but has missed many sessions lately because of her physical problems. Sonya has reached puberty and is experiencing pain connected with menstruation. She is unable to care for her most basic hygienic needs and is irritable and disoriented during the menstruation process. Her grandmother, wanting to free Sonya from her pain and disorientation during her periods, as well as to protect her from the consequences of rape, seeks to have a hysterectomy performed, which would both terminate Sonya's menstrual cycle and sterilize her. If you were the judge, would you authorize sterilization? Why or why not? Do you find the reasoning in *Buck v. Bell* helpful? Why or why not?

ABORTION, FETAL RIGHTS, AND THE RIGHT OF PRIVACY

Once constitutional protection was granted for the use of contraceptives, it was inevitable that the question of the constitutional status of abortion would arise. Abortion and infanticide have often been used to limit procreation when contraceptive measures fail. Abortion, from this perspective, is simply another form of birth control, and one that should be entitled to the same constitutional protection.

On the other hand, infanticide is condemned both legally and morally as murder. If a fetus is entitled to the same protection as an infant, then abortion

---

[14]Wentzel v. Montgomery General Hospital, 293 Md. 685, 447 A.2d 1244, certiorari denied, 103 S. Ct. 790 (1983).

should also be considered murder. The resolution of the moral and legal status of abortion, in short, appears to be closely tied to the moral status of the fetus.

The Status of the Fetus

Unfortunately, there is no agreement in our society on the moral status of a fetus. Many hold that from the moment of conception, a fetus should have the same moral status as a (born) human being. Philip Devine, for example, begins with the rule against infanticide. He argues there are two possible justifications for the rule: (1) the infant is a member of the human species (species principle); and (2) the infant will, in due course, think, talk, love and have a sense of justice (potentiality principle). Because principles (1) and (2) are also true of fetuses, it follows that, from conception on, fetuses should also be protected and abortion considered murder (Devine 1978).

What if the life of the pregnant woman is at stake? Baruch Brody argues that the principle of self-defense does not permit abortion even in this instance because the fetus is not attempting to take the woman's life. He suggests considering the situation in which A needs a medicine to stay alive. C owns some but will give it to A only if A kills B. He concludes that just as it is not permissible for A to kill B in this instance, it is not right for a woman to abort a fetus even when her own life is at stake (Brody 1975, 6–8).

Nancy Davis has challenged the position taken by Brody and others that a pregnant woman has no right to abort even when her life is at stake. Davis argues that the pregnant woman has a stronger claim to life than the fetus when the two are in conflict because there is "a morally relevant asymmetry between the woman and the fetus" (Davis 1984):

> [I]f we ask ourselves what is plausible in the view that [the fetus] does owe a debt to the woman who carries it, [we would note that a] pregnant woman provides life-support to the developing fetus through her body, and the fetus is, in turn, parasitic upon her: a fetus thus survives off a woman (that is, at her expense), not in partnership with her. Since the life and well-being of the fetus are sustained through its physical dependence on the woman's body, the very fact of being pregnant undermines a woman's autonomy. She cannot choose what she shall do without thereby choosing for someone else, and she must therefore take into account the possible risks of even the most mundane sorts of activities: driving a car, lifting a bucket, taking an aspirin. While providing assistance to a post-fetal person may involve a significant reduction of a benefactor's freedom of choice and action, pregnancy involves a physical invasion of the body. . . . The relationship between the pregnant woman and the dependent fetus can thus be seen to be inherently asymmetrical. . . . The supposition that the asymmetry is of moral significance may well underlie the widespread conviction that abortion is defensible whenever the pregnancy poses a threat to the woman's life. . . . It may [also] have considerably more permissive implications. . . . If the woman's claims are strong enough to justify abortion—with the assistance of a third party—when it is undertaken to preserve her life, then they *may* be strong enough to justify it in other cases as well.

Others take the position that fetuses should not have the same moral status as persons, including pregnant women. H. Tristam Engelhardt, for example, argues:

> Even if the fetus is a human organism that will probably be genetically and organically continuous with a human person, it is not yet such a person. Simply put, fetuses are not rational, self-conscious beings—that is, given a strict definition of persons, fetuses do not qualify as persons. One sees this when comparing talk about dead men with talk about fetuses. When speaking of a dead man, one knows of whom one speaks, the one who dies, the person whom one knew before his death. But in speaking of the fetus, one has no such person to whom one can refer. There is not yet a person, a "who" to whom one can refer in the case of the fetus (compare: one can keep promises to dead men but not to men yet unborn). In short, the fetus in no way singles itself out as, or shows itself to be, a person. . . . (Engelhardt 1982, 96)

Suppose we had a social practice of naming fetuses once a woman knew she was pregnant. Would that affect your view as to how the fetus should be regarded? What significance, if any, should we attach to the fact that no such practice exists? Even if one concludes that fetuses are not entitled to the same respect as (born) persons, however, it does not follow that we can be indifferent to their well-being. Engelhardt cautions, "It is one thing to say that an entity lacks the dignity of being a person strictly, and another thing to say that it does not have great value" (Engelhardt 1982, 100). A person who believes that abortion is always morally permissible, for example, might nonetheless think punishment appropriate for a person who wantonly kicked a pregnant woman in an effort to injure the fetus.

A third group takes an intermediate position on the moral status of the fetus. Judith Jarvis Thomson states, "we shall probably have to agree that the fetus has already become a human person well before birth. By the tenth week, for example, it already has a face, arms and legs, fingers and toes; it has internal organs, and brain activity is detectable" (Thomson 1971, 3–4). Warren Quinn favors what he terms a "process theory" of the fetus:

> [T]he fetus is a being to some extent capable of losing a fully human future life, the very kind of life we now enjoy. [I]t is hard for me to see how the loss of an object of this significance, the loss of the very thing that for ourselves we hold most important in the world, could have no moral weight. In any case, there is surely no precedent for thinking that it could be ignored, for there are simply no other situations in which such losses are at issue where a morally sensitive agent ignores them. The fetus, I feel, must have a right that its future welfare counts for something and thus that there be a sufficiently strong moral case for sacrificing its good. And to the extent that the ties of biological kinship themselves add special weight, it will have an especially strong version of this right against its parents. [A]s the fetus becomes more fully human the seriousness of aborting it will approach that of infanticide. In this way the process theory . . . validates the . . . moral intuition that later abortions are more objectionable than earlier ones (Quinn 1984, 53–54).

Can the Morality of Abortion Be Separated from the Status of the Fetus?

Judith Jarvis Thomson has argued that abortion may be morally acceptable even if a fetus is granted the same moral status as an adult. Imagine that you wake up one morning to find yourself in a hospital bed next to a famous, unconscious violinist. He was found to have a fatal kidney ailment. The Society of Music Lovers canvassed all the available medical records and found that you alone had the right blood type to help. They therefore kidnapped you and plugged the violinist's circulatory system into yours, so that your kidneys can be used to extract poisons from his blood as well as your own. The director of the hospital says "We're sorry the Society did this to you—we would never have permitted it if we had known. But still, they did it, and the violinist is now plugged into you. To unplug you would be to kill him. But never mind. It's only for nine months. By then he will have recovered from his ailment and can be safely unplugged from you."

Thomson concludes that to allow the violinist to use your kidneys is a "kindness on your part" but not "something you owe him." She explains, "the right to life consists not in the right not to be killed, but rather in the right not to be killed unjustly. [This is how] to square the fact that the violinist has a right to life with the fact that you do not act unjustly toward him in unplugging yourself, thereby killing him. For if you do not kill him unjustly, you do not violate his right to life. . . . [Now] the gap in the argument against abortion stares us plainly in the face: it is by no means enough to show that the fetus is a person, and to remind us that all persons have a right to life—we need to be shown also that killing the fetus violates its right to life, i.e., that abortion is unjust killing." She adds that this is not an argument that abortion is always moral. On the contrary, if it would take only one hour to save the life of the violinist, for example, then it would be "indecent" to refuse (Thomson 1971). The point is that a person should not be required to be more of a Good Samaritan when pregnant than at other times.

The analogy used by Thomson has been criticized for overlooking the responsibility that the pregnant woman has for placing the fetus in a vulnerable position. Except in the case of pregnancy due to rape, the woman did indulge in intercourse and thus is "among those who are at least partially responsible [for] the fetus being in need of a life-support system" (Tooley 1983, 45). Thomson replies:

> [Suppose] people-seeds drift about in the air like pollen, and if you open your windows, one may drift in and take root in your carpets or upholstery. You don't want children, so you fix up your windows with fine mesh screens, the very best you can buy. As can happen, however, [one] of the screens is defective, and a seed drifts in and takes root. Does the person-plant who now develops have a right to the use of your house: Surely [not] (Thomson 1971).

Donald Regan has also attempted to expand the good samaritan analogy to pregnancies that do not result from rape (Regan 1979). He concedes that except in cases of rape the pregnant woman has done something that provides some reason to compel her to aid the fetus. But she has not done as much as has a parent to establish a relationship with a child, nor a voluntary rescuer to establish a relationship with the object of the rescue. In addition, no other potential samaritan is required to bear burdens as physically invasive as the burdens of pregnancy and childbirth. He concludes that laws forbidding abortion are at odds with the general principles of good samaritan law.

To what extent can moral disagreement about abortion be resolved by appeals to analogies, by appeals to our moral instincts or judgment about other situations and circumstances, or by refining our concept of a "person" or a "human being?" Is our collective concept of a "person" or "human being" a determining influence on our moral view of abortion, or is our moral view of abortion, supported on other grounds, the determining factor, to which our concept of a "person" or "human being" is adapted?

The Constitutional Status of Abortion

In 1973, in *Roe v. Wade*,[15] the Supreme Court invalidated a Texas statute that made it a criminal act to perform most abortions. Justice Blackmun's opinion for the Court contains a long historic section devoted to proving that most restrictions on abortion are not ancient, but originated in the latter half of the 19th century. A major obstacle to his thesis was the Hippocratic Oath which prohibits giving an "abortive remedy" to any woman (Edelstein 1943, 3). Justice Blackmun turned to scholarly sources to demonstrate both that the Oath was the code of a minority medical group and that most Greek thinkers approved of abortion, at least early in the pregnancy. Aristotle, for example, thought that the fetus did not become animate until about the fortieth day after conception if male, and about the ninetieth day after conception if female (Hist. Anim. 7.3.583b). His views were later adopted by early Christian writers including St. Augustine.

The Romans shared many of the Greeks' attitudes. The Stoic philosopher Seneca wrote without apology, "We destroy monstrous births, and drown our children if they are born weakly and unnaturally formed." There was, in the code of Justinian, an attempt to limit abortion, but the reason was to protect the right of the father to his children—the child's interests do not seem do have mattered (Rachels 1986, 8).

At common law, abortion was not a crime prior to "quickening," i.e. the point when the pregnant woman first feels fetal movement. Even after quickening, abortion was punished less harshly than the murder of a (born) person.

As late as 1800, there was no legislation in the United States on abortion, yet by 1900 virtually every state made most abortion a crime due in large part to an aggressive campaign against abortion launched by physicians affiliated with the American Medical Association begun at the end of the civil war (Mohr 1978).

The basis for the decision of the Supreme Court in *Roe* was the right of privacy first announced in *Griswold*. Although the Court in *Roe* held that a right of privacy belongs to the pregnant woman, it also stated that the right does not include an unlimited right to "do with one's body as one pleases." In summarizing its holding, the Court added that during the first trimester of pregnancy the abortion decision "must be left to the *medical judgment of the pregnant woman's attending physi-*

---

[15]410 U.S. 113 (1973).

cian" (emphasis added). The *Roe* decision thus grants women only a conditional power to decide whether to have an abortion, a power that may be vetoed by the medical profession. The Court never explained what it meant when it invoked a medical judgment standard, moreover. In practice, a physician is likely to decide on the basis of his or her own moral judgment. Is this an appropriate basis on which to make an abortion decision? Will it encourage women to shop for a physician whose moral judgment is compatible with their own? Is that bad?

The Court in *Roe* also made clear that the right of privacy is to be balanced against other rights. Thus the Court held that after the end of the first trimester of pregnancy, states are free to regulate the abortion procedure in ways that are "reasonably related to maternal health." The Court stated that states might, for example, require that late-term abortions be performed in hospitals rather than in out-patient settings.[16]

The Court also held that a fetus is not a "person" as that term is used in the Fourteenth Amendment of the Constitution. States nonetheless are free to legislate to protect the life and health of fetuses, just as they can (and do) legislate to protect other nonpersons, such as animals or personal property. States may not regulate or proscribe abortion, however, in pursuing their interest in "the potentiality of human life" until after the fetus is "viable."

The Court defined a viable fetus as one "potentially able to live outside the mother's womb, albeit with artificial aid." Thus the Court did not set viability at the end of the second trimester as sometimes reported. Rather, it explicitly drew a technology-dependent line; one that will advance closer to conception as medical science increases its ability to save ever younger fetuses. Is this an appropriate line for protecting fetuses? It could be argued that viability is the modern equivalent of birth in the sense that it is the time when, at least in theory, the fetus could survive being separated from the mother and thus is the point when the fetus should be given the same moral deference as an infant. Would it be preferable to have a line that is linked to brain capacities or other characteristics of the fetus?

The holding in *Roe* permits states to proscribe the abortion of viable fetuses; it does not mandate that result. The Court added that the abortion of even viable fetuses may not be proscribed by state law "where it is necessary, in appropriate medical judgment, for the preservation of the life or health of the mother." Only about half the states have acted to limit late abortions (Areen 1985, 181).

In 1983, in *Akron v. Akron Center for Reproductive Health,*[17] the Court reaffirmed the *Roe* decision. The Court noted that new medical knowledge made some second trimester abortions as safe as earlier ones had been in 1973. Thus, what has been referred to as the trimester framework of *Roe* has already changed; both the time when states can regulate to protect maternal health and the time when they can regulate to protect potential life are in flux.

---

[16]In Akron v. Akron Center for Reproductive Health, 462 U.S. 416 (1983), the Court held that such a requirement was not constitutional before well into the second trimester of pregnancy because early abortions have become so safe.
[17]462 U.S. 416 (1983).

In 1986, *Roe* was again reaffirmed but by a more closely divided Court (5 to 4), in *Thornburgh v. American College of Obstetricians and Gynecologists*.[18] The opinion held unconstitutional a Pennsylvania statute that, among other things, provided that before an abortion could be performed, a pregnant woman had to be told of the availability of materials that describe the fetus and list agencies offering alternatives to abortion. The materials had to describe fetal characteristics at two week intervals. The majority of the Court held that this information was not always relevant to the woman's decision and might serve only "to confuse and punish her and to heighten her anxiety, contrary to accepted medical practice." The opinion also revealed a split on the Court on the status of the fetus. Justice White focused on unique genetic information present from conception on:

> . . . However one answers the metaphysical or theological question whether the fetus is a "human being" or the legal question whether it is a "person" as that term is used in the Constitution, one must at least recognize, first, that the fetus is an entity that bears in its cells all the genetic information that characterizes a member of the species *homo sapiens* and distinguishes an individual member of that species from all others, and second, that there is no nonarbitrary line separating a fetus from a child, or indeed, an adult human being. Given that the continued existence and development—that is to say, the *life*—of such an entity are so directly at stake in the woman's decision whether or not to terminate her pregnancy, that decision must be recognized as *sui generis*. . . . Accordingly, the decisions cited by the Court both in *Roe* and in its opinion today as precedent for the fundamental nature of the liberty to choose abortion do not, even if all are accepted as valid, dictate the Court's classification.

Justice Stevens, by contrast, adopted a process view:

> Justice White is . . . surely wrong in suggesting that the governmental interest in protecting fetal life is equally compelling during the entire period from the moment of conception until the moment of birth. Again, I recognize that a powerful theological argument can be made for that position, but I believe our jurisdiction is limited to the evaluation of secular state interests. I should think it obvious that the state's interest in the protection of an embryo—even if that interest is defined as "protecting those who will be citizens", increases progressively and dramatically as the organism's capacity to feel pain, to experience pleasure, to survive, and to react to its surroundings increases day by day. The development of a fetus—and pregnancy itself—are not static conditions, and the assertion that the government's interest is static simply ignores this reality.

Is Justice White persuasive when he argues that because the life of an entity is at stake, the decision is *sui generis?* On the other hand, can Justice Steven's position be squared with the significance the Court has attached to viability. Notice that the constitutional status of abortion may change now that Justice Powell, who was one

---

[18]476 U.S. 747 (1986).

of the five justices who voted with the majority in *Thornburgh*, has retired from the Court. What does this reveal about the relationship between morality and constitutional rights in our system of government?

Examining the Relationship Between Law and Morality

The existence in our society of profound disagreement on the moral status of the fetus as well as the moral status of abortion makes it extremely difficult to decide how the law should treat abortion. Any law will be in conflict with the strongly held moral position of parts of the society. Such a law is likely, therefore, to be strongly resisted. Some contend that in such a situation, the law should tolerate different views by leaving the decision to individuals. Mario Cuomo, the Governor of New York, believes abortion to be morally wrong, for example, yet argues the law should not forbid abortion:

> I believe that legal interdicting of abortion by either the federal government or the individual states is not a plausible possibility and even if it could be obtained, it wouldn't work. Given present attitudes, it would be "Prohibition" revisited, legislating what couldn't be enforced and in the process creating a disrespect for law in general (Cuomo 1984).

Is the danger of disrespect sufficient reason to eschew prohibiting abortion? Are you more persuaded by the arguments of Thompson and Regan that legal prohibitions on abortion impose a disproportionate burden on pregnant women to be good samaritans?

A third argument against a legal prohibition of abortion rests on the claim that an accurate understanding of our constitutional heritage dictates that abortion as well as other limits on procreation should be left to private rather than public control:

> The Constitution was consecrated to the blessings of liberty for ourselves and our posterity—yet it contains no discussion of the right to be a *human* being; no definition of a person; and, indeed, no express provisions guaranteeing to persons that right to carry on their lives protected from the "vicissitudes of the political process" by a zone of privacy or a right of personhood. . . . But the Constitution is not a totalitarian design, dependent for its success upon the homogenization or depersonalization of humanity. The judiciary has thus reached into the Constitution's spirit and structure, and has elaborated from the spare text an idea of "human" and a conception of "being" not merely contemplated but required. [This conception recognizes] the fundamental personal character of a right to reproductive autonomy (Tribe 1978, 893, 923).

The argument for leaving abortion to private choice is buttressed for some by recognition that pregnancy is a burden imposed only on women. Because women's interests have not often been protected in the political system, according to this view, it was appropriate for the Court to protect their interests by removing the debate from the political arena.

On the other hand, to those who think abortion immoral, the argument that the abortion decision should be a matter of individual choice is equivalent to saying that murder should not be a crime simply because some people think it proper.

Additional Legal Issues Concerning Abortion

Three important legal issues were explicitly not decided in *Roe,* but have been addressed in subsequent Supreme Court cases: the rights, if any, of fathers; the rights of pregnant minors; and public funding of abortion. A fourth issue, the right to intervene for the benefit of a fetus over the objection of the pregnant woman, has not been addressed by any federal court although there are several state court decisions on the point.

THE RIGHTS OF FATHERS

In *Planned Parenthood of Central Missouri v. Danforth,*[19] in 1976, the Supreme Court considered a Missouri statute that required a pregnant woman to have the consent of her spouse before an abortion could be performed. Faced with having to empower one spouse or the other to make the decision in the event of conflict, the Court reasoned, "Since it is the woman who physically bears the child and who is the more directly and immediately affected by the pregnancy, as between the two, the balance weighs in her favor." The right of privacy first announced in *Griswold* as grounded in the marital relationship thus has evolved into an individual right that permits a wife to limit procreation by aborting a fetus even in the face of an objection from the man who is her husband and the father of the fetus.

Although the logic of the Court's decision is clear, its broader implications are more fully illustrated by an example posed by George Harris. Imagine a wife, Michelle, who discovers she is pregnant and who decides to have an.abortion because a child would interfere with her career. She has never told her husband Steve of her feelings because she knows that he wants a family, but believes she will eventually talk him out of it. That very day Steve is in an automobile accident that leaves him sterile. He tells Michelle that if she will not have the abortion, he will assume full economic and parental responsibility for the child, who is the only biologically-related child he will ever be able to father. *Danforth* means Michelle is legally free to refuse. Is her refusal moral? Harris contends that it is not:

> Due to the fact that both men and women have a morally legitimate interest in procreation, couples have an obligation to be forthright and informative about their desires and reservations about family planning. . . . [It] is understandable, though neither mature nor laudable, for a person who is deeply in love with someone with significantly different life plans, perhaps as a result of self-deception, to think that the other person can be brought around to seeing things the other way. But it is not

---

[19]428 U.S. 52 (1976).

excusable. . . . [It] would be wrong to Steve for Michelle to have the abortion (Harris 1986).

Conversely, consider a woman who deliberately deceives a man with whom she has a sexual relationship by telling him that she is taking birth control pills. When she gets pregnant, he again makes clear that he does not want to be a father and offers to pay for an abortion. She refuses, and later sues him for child support. In the judgment of all courts that have ruled on this issue, he must pay.[20] The rationale generally given is that any other result would harm the child. One lower court suggested that a better resolution in the face of maternal deceit would be to require the mother to provide as much child support as she possibly can, and to hold the father liable only for the difference, if any, between what the mother can afford and the needs of the child. That court was overruled on appeal, however.[21]

RIGHTS OF MINORS

In 1979, the Supreme Court in *Bellotti v. Baird*,[22] considered the right of a pregnant minor to obtain an abortion. As a general rule, except in emergencies parents must consent before any medical procedure can be performed on their child. The issue in *Bellotti* was whether a state statute that embodied that traditional legal rule with respect to abortions was constitutional. A majority of the Court decided the statute was unconstitutional, but no rationale for the decision was supported by a majority of the Justices. A plurality of four Justices held that "mature minors" must be able to decide for themselves whether to have an abortion. Because the term is a new one in constitutional law, it is very unfortunate that the Justices provided only a sketchy definition. They explained that a "mature minor" is one who is "mature enough and well enough informed to make her abortion decision." The plurality also stated that the determination of who is a "mature minor" need not be made by a court, but can be made by an administrative agency or officer. Finally, they cautioned that it is a determination that must be made on a case-by-case basis; thus, a state cannot pass a law that declares all 17-year-olds to be "mature minors."

The Justices next held that even a minor who does not qualify as mature must be able to have a court order an abortion, even in the face of parental objections, if the court determines it would be in her best interests.

The principle of carving out an exception for mature minors to age-based legal standards is not only new, but potentially extremely far-reaching. Should Maria Moe, for example, have been able to attempt to convince the court that she was mature enough to decide to marry the father of their son?[23] Should a seventeen year

---

[20]See, e.g., People in Interest of S.P.B., 651 P.2d 1213 (1982).
[21]In re Pamela P. v. Frank S., 110 Misc.2d 978, 443 N.Y.S.2d 343 (1981), reversed 88 A.D.865, 451 N.Y.S.2d 766 (1982), affirmed 59 N.Y.2d 1, 462 N.Y.S.2d 819, 449 N.E.2d 713 (1983).
[22]443 U.S. 622 (1979).
[23]The problem is presented on page 104 of the text.

old be able to convince a court that he or she is mature enough to vote in a presidential election? Is abortion different? If so, why?

PUBLIC FUNDING

In a series of cases the Supreme Court has repeatedly held that public funding of abortions is not required by the Constitution. In *Harris v. McRae*,[24] for example, the Court upheld the Hyde Amendment, a law passed by Congress that prohibits federal funding of even medically necessary abortions:

> [R]egardless of whether the freedom of a woman to choose to terminate her pregnancy for health reasons lies at the core or the periphery of the due process liberty recognized in [*Roe v.*] *Wade,* it simply does not follow that a woman's freedom of choice carries with it a constitutional entitlement to the financial resources to avail herself of the full range of protected choices. [A]lthough government may not place obstacles in the path of a woman's exercise of her freedom of choice, it need not remove those not of its own creation. Indigency falls in the latter category. The financial constraints that restrict an indigent woman's ability to enjoy the full range of constitutionally protected freedom of choice are the product not of governmental restrictions on access to abortions, but rather of her indigency. Although Congress has opted to subsidize medically necessary services generally, but not certain medically necessary abortions, the fact remains that the Hyde Amendment leaves an indigent woman with at least the same range of choice in deciding whether to obtain a medically necessary abortion as she would have had if Congress had chosen to subsidize no health care costs at all.

Compare the rationale of the three dissenting Justices, Brennan, Marshall, and Blackmun:

> *Roe* and its progeny established that the pregnant woman has a right to be free from state interference with her choice to have an abortion—a right which, at least prior to the end of the first trimester, absolutely prohibits any governmental regulation of that highly personal decision. The proposition for which these cases stand thus is not that the State is under an affirmative obligation to ensure access to abortions for all who may desire them; it is that the State must refrain from wielding its enormous power and influence in a manner that might burden the pregnant woman's freedom to choose whether to have an abortion. The Hyde Amendment's denial of public funds for medically necessary abortions plainly intrudes upon this constitutionally protected decision, for both by design and effect it serves to coerce indigent pregnant women to bear children that they would otherwise elect not to have.

---

[24]448 U.S. 297 (1980).

Feminist Catherine MacKinnon has criticized the rationale of *Roe v. Wade* for ignoring the needs of women. In her view, *Harris v. McRae* follows logically from *Roe,* but for reasons quite different from those articulated by the Court:

> Most [women who seek abortion] did not mean or wish to conceive. In contrast to this fact of women's experience, the abortion debate has centered on separating control over sexuality from control over reproduction. . . . Liberals have supported the availability of the abortion choice as if the woman just happened on the fetus. The political Right imagines that the intercourse which precedes conception is usually voluntary, only to urge abstinence, as if sex were up to women. . . . Continuing this logic, many opponents of state funding of abortions, such as supporters of the Hyde Amendment, would permit funding of abortions when pregnancy results from rape or incest. Thus they make exceptions for those special occasions during which they presume women did not control sex. From all this I deduce that abortion's proponents and opponents share a tacit assumption that women significantly do control sex.
>
> Feminist investigations suggest otherwise. . . . Under conditions in which women do not control access to our sexuality, [the decision in *Roe v. Wade*] facilitates women's heterosexual availability. The availability of abortion removes the one remaining legitimized reason that women have had for refusing sex besides the headache. . . . It is not inconsistent, then, that framed as a privacy right a woman's decision to abort would have no claim on public support and would genuinely not be seen as burdened by that deprivation. Privacy conceived as a right from public intervention and disclosure is the opposite of the relief that [*Harris* and other abortion funding cases] sought for welfare women. State intervention would have provided a choice women did *not* have in private. [Indigent] women, women whose sexual refusal has counted for particularly little, needed something to make their privacy effective. The logic of the court's response resembles the logic by which women are supposed to consent to sex. Preclude the alternatives, then call the sole remaining option "her choice." The point is that the alternatives are precluded *prior* to the reach of the chosen legal doctrine. They are precluded by conditions of sex, race, and class—the very conditions the privacy frame not only leaves tacit, but which it exists to *guarantee* (MacKinnon 1984).

If you were a member of Congress, would you support or oppose use of public funds for abortions for indigent women? How would—or should—the fact that many citizens think that abortion is a serious moral wrong affect your choice?

MEDICAL INTERVENTIONS FOR FETUSES

A final issue that *Roe v. Wade* did not resolve is whether the Constitution limits judicial or legislative action intended to protect fetuses when the action also poses risk to, or restrictions on the liberty of, the pregnant woman. Consider the facts of a recent Georgia case.[25]

---

[25]The facts are based on Jefferson v. Griffin Spalding County Hospital Authority, 247 Ga. 86, 274 S.E.2d 457 (1981).

Case 3. A woman came into the hospital in her thirty-ninth week of pregnancy. She was diagnosed as having a complete placenta previa, a condition in which the placenta blocks the opening of the womb. In the judgment of the examining physician, there was a 90 percent certainty that the child could not survive vaginal delivery and a 50 percent chance that the mother would also die if vaginal delivery were attempted. A caesarian section was recommended, as it normally is in such circumstances. The woman, for religious reasons, refused to consent to the recommended procedure. The hospital then sought a court order. The trial court granted temporary custody of the fetus to the state. It also ordered the mother to submit to a caesarian in the event that a sonogram confirmed that her condition made vaginal delivery too dangerous. If you were asked to review the decision of the trial court on appeal, how would you decide the matter?

In reaching your decision it is important to notice that the woman was not seeking an abortion. Thus *Roe v. Wade* arguably has no bearing on the matter. On the other hand, one could argue that because the woman has a constitutional right to have an abortion (because her life is at stake), surely she also has the right to subject the fetus to vaginal delivery, whatever the risks. This argument raises the question of what is an abortion. When the Court in *Roe* held that a woman has a right, at least early in the pregnancy, to have an abortion, did that mean a right to have the fetus killed, or only a right to terminate the pregnancy by having the fetus removed from her body, in which case the fetus might survive? If *Roe* is read narrowly as granting only a right to terminate the pregnancy, then it does not empower a woman to have the fetus killed except when fetal death is a necessary result of the removal procedure.

But to conclude that *Roe* does not empower the woman to refuse a caesarian does not mean that she does not have other principles to invoke to justify her refusal. She might, for example, invoke the principle of respect for autonomy. In addition to overriding her autonomous refusal, implementing the trial court's decision would involve a physical invasion of her body. Surely the right of privacy protects against coerced surgery—or does it? Recall that the Supreme Court has never overruled *Buck v. Bell*, which upheld forcible sterilization for eugenic purposes. Does it follow that a woman could be forced to undergo surgery for the benefit of her fetus (e.g., implantation of a shunt to offset a blocked ureter) although the surgery posed some risk and no benefit to the woman herself?

SUMMARY

The first restrictions on contraception, sterilization, and abortion were religious in origin. With the rise of the modern secular state, civil law was increasingly employed to regulate marriage and procreation. As the view gained strength that private behavior, including procreation, should not be subject to secular regulation, debate increased as to whether, and if so, to what extent, the law should govern contraception, sterilization, and abortion.

By the late nineteenth century, there were stringent legal restrictions on access to contraceptives or abortion in most states. By the early twentieth century, a number of states had passed statutes authorizing the involuntary sterilization of certain mental patients and prisoners. The legal pendulum then began to swing toward individual choice. In 1965, a decision of the Supreme Court of the United States established that the right of privacy embodied in the Constitution includes the right to decide whether or not to use contraception. In 1973, the Court held that the right of privacy also encompasses a woman's decision to seek an abortion, although later decisions made clear that poor women have no constitutional right to public funds to pay for an abortion. Although the *Roe* decision has been reaffirmed by the Court on several occasions, the Court is now more closely divided than ever on the issue. A number of difficult related questions remain unresolved, moreover, including the extent to which the law can coerce a pregnant woman to act, or not to act, in order to benefit the fetus.

REFERENCES

Areen, J. *Cases and Materials on Family Law*, 2d ed. New York: Foundation Press, 1985.
Areen, J., P. King, S. Goldberg, and A. Capron. *Law, Science and Medicine.* New York: Foundation Press, 1984.
Aristotle, The Complete Works of (Revised Oxford Translation). Edited by J. Barnes. Princeton, N.J.: Princeton University Press, 1984.
Augustine, St. 401. *The Good of Marriage* (De bono coniugali) (Wilcox trans.). New York: Fathers of the Church, 1955.
Bishop, J. P. *Commentaries on the Law of Marriage and Divorce and Evidence in Matrimonial Suits*, Vol. I. London, 1852.
Black, C. "The Unfinished Business of the Warren Court." *Wash. L. Rev.* 46 (1970): 3–45.
Brody, B. *Abortion and the Sanctity of Human Life: A Philosophical View.* Cambridge, Mass.: MIT Press, 1975.
Callahan, D. *Abortion: Law, Choice and Morality.* New York: MacMillan, 1970.
Cuomo, M. "Religious Belief and Public Morality: A Catholic Governor's Perspective." Paper Delivered at the University of Notre Dame, September 13, 1984.
Davis, N. "Abortion and Self-Defense." *Philos and Public Affairs* 13 (1984): 175–207.
Degler, C. *At Odds: Women and the Family in America from the Revolution to the Present.* Oxford, England: Oxford University Press, 1980.
Devine, P. *The Ethics of Homicide.* Ithaca, N.Y.: Cornell University Press, 1978.
Edelstein, L. *The Hippocratic Oath.* Baltimore: Johns Hopkins Press, 1943.
Ely, J. *Democracy and Distrust: A Theory of Judicial Review.* Cambridge, Mass.: Harvard University Press, 1980.
Engelhart, H. T. "Medicine and the Concept of Person." In *Contemporary Issues in Bioethics*, 2d ed., edited by T. Beauchamp and L. Walters, 94–101. Belmont, Calif.: Wadsworth, 1982.
Fagley, R. *The Population Explosion and Christian Responsibility.* New York: Oxford Press, 1980.

Feldman, D. M. *Marital Relations, Birth Control and Abortion in Jewish Law*. New York: Schocken, 1968.

Gordon, L. *Woman's Body, Woman's Right*. New York: Penguin, 1976.

———. "Why Nineteenth-Century Feminists Did Not Support 'Birth Control' and Twentieth-Century Feminists Do: Feminism, Reproduction, and the Family." In *Rethinking the Family: Some Feminist Questions*, edited by B. Thorne with M. Yalom. New York: Longman, 1982.

Haney, R. *Comstockery in America*. Boston: Beacon Press, 1960.

Harris, G. W. "Fathers and Fetuses." *Ethics* 96 (1986): 594.

Helmholz, R. *Marriage Litigation in Medieval England*. Cambridge, Mass.: Cambridge University Press, 1974.

Heymann, R., and D. Barzelay. "The Forest and the Trees: *Roe v. Wade* and Its Critics." *B.U.L. Rev.* 53 (1973): 675–784.

Jensen, A. *Educability and Group Differences*. London: Methuen, 1972.

Kennedy, D. *Birth Control in America: The Career of Margaret Sanger*. New Haven, Conn.: Yale University Press, 1970.

Kevles, D. J. *In the Name of Eugenics: Genetics and the Uses of Human Heredity*. New York: Knopf, 1985.

Layzer, D. "Heritability Analysis of IQ Scores: Science or Numerology?" *Science* 183 (1974): 1259–1266.

Luther, M. *The Large Catechism*. (R. E. Fischer, Trans.) Philadelphia: Fortress Press, 1959.

MacKinnon, C. "*Roe v. Wade*: A Study in Male Ideology." In *Abortion: Moral and Legal Perspectives*, edited by J. Garfield and P. Hennessey. Amherst, Mass.: University of Massachusetts Press, 1984.

Mill, J. S. *On Liberty* (Rapaport ed. 1978). Indianapolis: Hackett Publishing, 1859.

Mohr, J. C. *Abortion in America: The Origins and Evolution of National Policy, 1800–1900*. Oxford, England: Oxford University Press.

Noonan, J. *Contraception: A History of Its Treatment by Catholic Theologians and Canonists*. Cambridge, Mass.: Harvard University Press, 1966.

———. *The Morality of Abortion: Legal and Historical Perspectives*. Cambridge, Mass.: Harvard University Press, 1970.

———. "Contraception." In *I Encyclopedia of Bioethics*, edited by W. Reich, 204–216. New York: Free Press, 1978.

O'Hara, J., and T. Sanks. "Eugenic Sterilization." *Georgetown L J* 45 (1956): 20–24.

Paul VI. "Humanae Vitae." Trans. as "Humanae Vitae (Human Life)." *Catholic Mind* (Sept. 1968): 35–48.

Pius XI. "Casti Connubi." Trans. as "On Christian Marriage." *Catholic Mind* (1930): 21–64.

Quinn, W. "Abortion: Identity and Loss," *Philos and Public Affairs* 13 (1984): 24–54.

Rachels, J. *The End of Life*. Oxford, England: Oxford University Press, 1986.

Regan, D. "Rewriting *Roe v. Wade*." *Mich. L. Rev.* 77 (1979): 1569–1646.

Seneca. *Fragments*, edited by F. Haase No. 84, quoted in Noonan, 1966.

Smith, P. "Comment: The History and Future of the Legal Battle Over Birth Control." *Cornell L Rev* 49 (1964): 275–303.

Speiser, E. A. *The Anchor Bible: Genesis*. New York: Doubleday, 1964.

The Stoic and Epicurean Philosophers: The Complete Writings of Epicurus, Epictetus, Lucretius and Marcus Aurelius, edited by W. Oates. New York: Random House, 1940.

Thomson, J. "A Defense of Abortion." *Philos and Public Affairs* (1971): 47–66.

Tooley, M. *Abortion and Infanticide*. Oxford, England: Clarendon, 1983.

Tribe, L. *American Constitutional Law*. Mineola, N.Y.: Foundation Press, 1978.

Veatch, R. *Case Studies in Medical Ethics*. Cambridge, Mass.: Harvard University Press, 1977.

Warnock, M. *A Question of Life*. London: Blackwell, 1985.

CASE LIST

Akron v. Akron Center for Reproductive Health, 462 U.S. 416 (1983).
Barbara A. v. John G. 145 Cal. App. 3d 369 (Cal.Ct.App. 1983).
Bellotti v. Baird, 443 U.S. 622 (1979).
Buck v. Bell, 274 U.S. 200 (1927).
Carey v. Population Services International, 431 U.S. 678 (1977).
Griswold v. Connecticut, 381 U.S. 479 (1965).
Harris v. McRae, 448 U.S. 297 (1980).
Jefferson v. Griffin Spalding County Hospital Authority, 247 Ga. 86, 274 S.E.2d 457.
Moe v. Dinkins, 533 F. Supp. 623, affirmed, 669 F.2d 67 (2d Cir. 1982).
In re Pamela P. v. Frank S., 110 Misc.2d 978, 443 N.Y.S.2d 343 (1981), reversed 88 A.D. 865, 451 N.Y.S.2d 766 (1982).
People in Interest of S.P.B., 651 P.2d 1213 (1982).
Planned Parenthood Federation of America v. Heckler, 712 F.2d 650 (D.C.Cir. 1983).
Planned Parenthood of Central Missouri v. Danforth, 428 U.S. 52 (1976).
Roe v. Wade, 410 U.S. 113 (1973).
Skinner v. Oklahoma, 316 U.S. 535 (1942).
Thornburgh v. American College of Obstetricians and Gynecologists, 476 U.S. 747 (1986).
United States v. One Package, 86 F.2d 737 (2d Cir. 1936).
Wentzel v. Montgomery General Hospital, 293 Md. 685, 447 A.2d 1244. certiorari denied, 103 S.Ct. 790 (1983).

DISCUSSION QUESTIONS

1. Should minors have the same right of access to contraceptives as adults? Should parents be notified if contraceptives are provided to their minor children?

2. Should government-sponsored limitations on procreation for the purpose of limiting the size of the population ever be permitted? When? Is there a morally relevant difference between direct limitations (such as mandatory sterilization) and indirect limitations (such as limiting the amount of welfare available to poor families who have more than three children)?

3. At what point during fetal development does a fetus achieve the status of a full member of the moral community? What is the moral significance of each of the following: conception, implantation, the development of central nervous system tissue, measurable brain activity, the ability to survive outside the womb albeit with mechanical aid, quickening (perception of fetal movement by the mother), birth, ability to use language, ability to reason?

4. No court has ever ordered a parent to give a kidney to a child, yet more than twenty courts have ordered pregnant women to undergo surgical procedures that pose risks to the life of the woman for the sake of a

fetus. Is it appropriate to impose greater obligations on pregnant women than on parents? Should a court order a pregnant women to stop using heroin during the pregnancy for the sake of her fetus? Should a court order a pregnant woman not to drink? Should a court order a pregnant woman not to go skiing? Should physicians be required to report when pregnant women are engaged in activities that may harm the fetus they carry? Should such court orders be enforced by jailing pregnant women who refuse to comply? If the obligations of pregnancy become too onerous, will more women avoid seeking medical care or elect to have abortions?

Human Experimentation

A. M. Capron

SUMMARY

We often think of the German concentration camp experimentation as the epitome of unethical research, yet the regulations governing research in Germany at the time were as advanced as any in existence. The German experience is compared with the development of research ethics in the United States beginning with criticism of the ethically questionable American research in the 1960s.

Key terms such as "research" and "therapy;" "therapeutic" and "nontherapeutic;" and "benefit," though commonly employed, are characterized by a host of subtle nuances that make their meanings unclear. The very definitions of these terms carry ethical freight.

Research involving human subjects needs to be justified by appealing to ethical principles. Such principles include respect for persons (regardless of competence), beneficence, nonmaleficence, and justice. The emergence of ethical and legal guidelines for human experimentation and the participation of the government in the establishment of such standards mark important developments in bioethics. This chapter outlines the steps involved in the regulatory process, and explores such documents as the Nuremburg Code and the Declaration of Helsinki, as well as federal and state regulation of research with human subjects.

Next, the discussion turns to current ethical issues such as highly risky research, risky behavior and beneficence, randomization, disclosure of the null hypothesis, double-blind studies, placebos, waiver of consent, research design, and the use of fetuses and abortuses. Each are analyzed within a theoretical framework that emphasizes the interplay of two central factors—risk and consent.

Evaluating research involving human beings is a difficult and puzzling task. Such research is at once both necessary and problematic, both socially laudatory and ethically dangerous. On the good side, it has enabled physicians to exercise the highest form of beneficence by creating tools with which they can truly do good for their patients. On the bad side, some of the darkest moments in medical annals have involved abuses of human research subjects. Even ignoring such extreme instances of maleficence, the whole practice of exposing human beings to risk for the sake of knowledge collides with the traditional Hippocratic injunction, "First, do no harm."

Historically, scientific investigation has been central to advances in modern health care because it is only through such research that medicine—which for thousands of years relied upon magic, superstition, and unproven remedies—has been transformed into a powerful (albeit imperfect) force for human betterment. Well within the memory of physicians still practicing today, the stethoscope was the major piece of medical technology, and quinine, digitalis, and aspirin were the major drugs. Biomedical scientists have totally transformed that picture in the past forty-five years—and the transformation has been so rapid and so total that those who have grown up in this new world may well take it for granted. Nonetheless, risking the health or even the life of one person to gain knowledge is potentially very dangerous. It can destroy the moral position of physicians and, worse yet, the well-being of those who have entrusted them with their lives.

Despite such risks, American society continues to allow and indeed to encourage human experimentation, perhaps from the realization that as amazing as the changes that have occurred in the field of medicine may be, much remains to be learned. The need for knowledge extends beyond the discovery and perfection of new diagnostic and therapeutic methods—from human gene therapy to artificial organs to effective cancer cures—to encompass, perhaps even more importantly, the development of means to validate and calibrate existing therapies. There is a critical need for data that would establish the relative safety and effectiveness of perhaps most of what is now done in medicine, done without proof of efficacy, done out of tradition or habit, done often very differently from town to town or hospital to hospital, or even physician to physician, without proof of which approach, if any, is really the best.

Plainly, these moral tensions make the subject of human research pivotal in any study of bioethics. Yet today the subject is often naïvely viewed as one of settled ethical principles, detailed statutory and regulatory requirements, and multifaceted procedures. History suggests that such claims must be viewed skeptically: the principles may be less conclusive and the guidelines less protective than they appear.

AN HISTORICAL COMPARISON

Consider two historical examples. In each case, a government, abetted by a physician's revelations of shocking experiments, promulgated general guidelines, followed by detailed regulations. In the first case, the official rules did not prevent horrible abuses; the second case is still unfolding.

German Regulations, 1900–1945

The first story begins in 1900 when the Prussian government issued a directive to the heads of clinics and similar establishments "absolutely prohibiting" medical interventions "for purposes other than diagnosis, therapy, and immunization" when:

1. the person in question is a minor or is not fully competent on other grounds;
2. the person concerned has not declared unequivocally that he consents to the intervention;
3. the declaration has not been made on the basis of a proper explanation of the adverse consequences that may result from the intervention (Der Minister der geistlichen 1900).

The directive also specified that interventions required the explicit approval of the director of each medical institution and the keeping of records to show that the subject met the three qualifications.

This document is notable for many reasons. First, it did not speak directly of research; instead, it implied its coverage by what it excluded thereby blurring the boundary lines around practices that mix diagnosis, therapy, or immunization with investigation. Second, it gave special protection to vulnerable persons who are unable to consent on their own behalf. Third, it required not merely consent but disclosure. Fourth, it placed responsibility on the institution where the research was conducted, not merely on the individual investigator.

Why did the Prussian government attend to this issue at this time? Professor Erwin Deutsch (1979, 23) suggests that "unethical, rough and even criminal experiments were taking place and being reported in [biomedical] journals." This gave rise to "a countercurrent" in journals and books, of which the best known is the turn-of-the-century pseudonymous memoir of Vikenty Veressayev (1901, 365), a

Russian physician who provided a "martyrology of the unhappy patients offered up [by his fellow physicians] as victims to science." Many of the studies he described involved venereal diseases because these conditions had to be studied in humans in the absence of an appropriate animal model. For example, one physician, in order to establish that a specific microorganism was the cause of gonorrhea, inoculated unwitting patients and repeatedly showed that infection (painful and not always curable) occurred. The memoirist also described experiments involving transplanting cancers, exposing people to typhoid and scarlet fever (sometimes through injections), and manipulation of the brain of a woman who then had seizures, lapsed into a coma, and died shortly thereafter. With the exception of this last case, Veressayev wrote, "these bizarre disciples of science proceeded upon their way without encountering any effective opposition, either from their colleagues or the medical press."

The 1900 directive was followed up by even more detailed German regulations in 1931; these distinguished between "new therapy" which is "therapeutic experimentation and modes of treatment which serve the process of healing . . . even though the effects and consequences . . . cannot yet be adequately determined," and "human experimentation" which consists of "operations and modes of treatment . . . carried out for research purposes which are nontherapeutic" (Sass 1983).[1] The horrible events of the following fourteen years in the Nazi prison camps demonstrate, however, that neither official endorsement nor high aspirations—embodied here by requirements for consent and risk-limitation—are necessarily enough to guarantee that an ethical code will protect subjects from abuse or worse.

American Regulations, 1966–

The second story follows a remarkably similar sequence. In September 1965, James A. Shannon, the Director of the U.S. National Institutes of Health, sought the advice of the National Advisory Health Council (NAHC) concerning the ethical implications of the changes that were occurring in biomedical research which had moved from mere observation of patients to "manipulation [of] not only the diseased

---

[1]The guidelines for new therapy required: (a) cost/benefit balancing, (b) prior animal testing, where possible, (c) consent or proxy consent after appropriate information has been provided, (d) use without consent only to save lives or prevent severe harm or because of special circumstances, (e) special consideration in cases involving minors, (f) rejection of the exploitation of the needy, (g) special care in use of live microorganisms, (h) acceptance of full responsibility by the facility's chief physician, (i) written documentation, and (j) publication which respects the patient's dignity.

In addition to these requirements, the guidelines for human experimentation also specified: (a) no human experimentation without consent, (b) no human experimentation until laboratory and animal research has been completed, and therefore no unfounded or random use of humans, (c) no use of minors if they are endangered, and (d) no use of dying persons.

Physicians were charged with the duties of introducing new therapy in suitable cases and conducting human experimentation in order to promote the progress of medicine. They were also charged with the "grave responsibility . . . for the life and health of each individual undergoing New Therapy or Human Experimentation." The importance of these factors was reiterated in the mandate given to teachers in medical schools to stress these special duties (Sass 1983).

individual but also [of] normal individuals" (Frankel 1972, 30). Dr. Shannon stressed that

> since such investigation departs from the conventional patient-physician relationship, where the patient's good has been substituted for by the need to develop new knowledge, . . . the physician is no longer in the same relationship . . . and indeed may not be in a position to develop a purely or wholly objective assessment of the moral nature or the ethical nature of the act which he proposes to perform (National Advisory Health Council 1965).

At its next meeting, in December 1965, the NAHC resolved that the Public Health Service should support clinical research involving human beings "only if the judgment of the investigator is subject to prior review by his institutional associates to assure an independent determination of the protection of the rights and welfare of the individual or individuals involved, of the appropriateness of the methods used to secure informed consent, and of the risk and potential medical benefits of the investigation." This recommendation became the basis for an order by the Surgeon General on February 8, 1966, mandating prior peer review of federally supported research (U.S. Public Health Service 1966a).[2] In December 1966, the order was further modified, in light of comments from the American Psychological Association and the American Sociological Association; certain behavioral science experiments were to be exempted from the requirement of informed consent or even awareness of the people being studied (U.S. Public Health Service 1966b).

As in Germany, the governmental directive coincided with criticism of existing research practices by a physician who had compiled a list of unethical experiments which likewise included operations performed without consent, exposure of patients to infections, and the transplantations of cancers from one patient to another (Beecher 1966). The twenty-some examples published by the physician were drawn from a larger group in excess of one hundred, all appearing during a single year in a single, prestigious medical journal. Despite the horrifying nature of the revelations, he concluded that the best protection for patients lay in the conscience of the investigator. This article—which the author followed with a book on the same subject (Beecher 1970)—caused quite a stir and probably contributed to Dr. Shannon's goal of creating a more profound sense of research institutions' ethical responsibilities (Frankel 1972, 36).[3] (Only later—with the discovery of other, even larger

---

[2]A revision was issued on July 1, 1966, to make clear that the "assurance" of review by a peer panel could be submitted for an entire research institution rather than for each individual project. An assurance had to include (1) agreement with the principles of the policy; (2) a description of the method of review; (3) the competencies represented in the review committee; (4) the administrative mechanism for surveillance and advice; and (5) the manner in which the institution would assure itself that the advice of the committee would be followed. John F. Sherman, NIH Deputy Director, recalls that NIH officials also "hoped that the use of a single but institutionally oriented assurance would, in most, if not in all situations, stimulate consideration also of reviews by a similar process of projects not supported by PHS grants" (Frankel 1972, 35).

[3]This was only reinforced by the publication shortly thereafter of another detailed examination of human

experiments that had been conducted by American physicians, both before and after World War 2, involving lack of knowledge or actual deception of subjects—would the degree of need for attention to such responsibilities become fully apparent.)

Over the years, the initial PHS policy statement has evolved into detailed regulations based upon a statutory requirement (National Research Act 1974) for prior review of research protocols at each institution, no longer just by an investigator's scientific peers but by a multidisciplinary group at least one of whom must not be affiliated with the institution. The regulations of the Department of Health and Human Services (HHS 1983), the government department with the greatest involvement in research with human subjects, form the basis for oversight by most of the other two dozen departments and agencies that conduct or support such research (President's Commission 1981).

It is the existence of these federal rules, as well as the extensive scrutiny the issues have received (Levine 1986, 365–391), that gives rise to the sense that the problems in human experimentation have all been neatly cabined if not totally resolved. Ought the horrible abuses perpetrated by distinguished physicians during the Nazi era in Germany, despite that nation's similar (indeed, in some ways even stronger) official rules, disturb this complacent view of the present American situation? Deutsch (1979, 25) suggests that the German guidelines did not arouse public interest and had "ein obskurses Dasein" (an obscure existence), whereas in the United States, the guidelines interact closely with public opinion. There is no question that the requirements for ethically and legally acceptable human studies are widely accepted among researchers and that the rules and procedures are applied even in cases where they are not mandatory (for example, in studies not supported by federal funds). Are such differences between the present situation and that which prevailed when subjects were misused—in the United States as well as abroad—sufficient to conclude that that research with human subjects is now no longer ethically problematic? Or, even when professional codes and governmental rules are perfectly applied, do certain difficult issues remain, as inherent features of this enterprise?

DEFINITIONS

Taxonomy seems important to students of many fields, and writers on human experimentation have devoted a great deal of attention to drawing categories. In the end, of course, an ethicist will want to know: what is the moral significance of such differences? Is the matter simply a procedural one? For example, formal review by a committee (such as an Institutional Review Board, or IRB) may be required for

---

experimentation by M. H. Pappworth (1968, 200) who also drew on reputable journals (emphasizing British over American) but who reached a less tolerant conclusion: "the voluntary system of safeguarding patients' rights has failed and new legislative procedures are absolutely necessary."

"research" but not for "therapy." Or are substantive differences also implied? By labeling something "therapy," does a physician claim to have wider leeway to proceed without as much disclosure of risks or even without consent, on the ground that the intervention is "routine?" Are physicians less obligated to provide, and patients to accept, "experimental" interventions? Such questions are raised rather than resolved by the framing of definitions.

Two, Three, or Many Categories?

In medicine, every intervention by a physician could be regarded as an experiment, because each person is different and the exact outcome of medical interventions must therefore remain somewhat uncertain (Blumgart 1969, 253; Ivy 1948, 2). Further compounding the confusion, the practice of medicine does involve a mixture of techniques (the well-proven, the merely historically accepted, and the truly novel) and a mixture of motives (to help the individual, but also to teach the practitioner things of value for future cases). The same is also true in research outside the biomedical arena; for instance, policy analysts and behavioral scientists are interested both in present practices and in developing and testing new ones.

Nonetheless, some rough lines can be drawn. As concluded by a governmental commission that for several years in the mid-1970s examined research with human subjects, "the term 'practice' refers to interventions that are designed solely to enhance the well-being of an individual patient or client and that have a reasonable expectation of success" (National Commission 1978a, 2). In the medical sphere, practices usually involve diagnosis, preventive treatment, or therapy; in the social sphere, practices include governmental programs such as transfer payments, education, and the like.

"By contrast, the term 'research' designates an activity designed to test a hypothesis, permit conclusions to be drawn, and thereby to develop or contribute to generalizable knowledge (expressed, for example, in theories, principles, and statement of relationships)" (National Commission 1978a, 3). In the polar cases, then, practice uses a proven technique in an attempt to benefit one or more individuals, while research studies a (usually novel) technique in an attempt to increase knowledge.

These definitions have several implications. First, use of an unproven technique is not necessarily research unless the way in which it is used is designed to permit generalizable knowledge to be gained—not just to see what results from using the technique in a particular instance. Conversely, not each intervention carried out with the intent of benefitting the patient (or other subject) automatically qualifies as "practice;" adequate information must exist to provide a reasonable basis for believing it will achieve the intended result.

Of course, distinctions between research and therapy are not solely matters of intellectual curiosity; the label "research" carries with it requirements for protocol review. Consequently, a tension arises between an investigator's desire to design a formal research program that will yield scientifically valid results and the desire simply to do some experimentation or innovation that, not being cast in the form of "research," seems more like "treatment." Jay Katz tells of listening at a national meeting

> to an interesting paper on the treatment of leukemia in young children. The investigator reported that he had performed more than half a dozen bone marrow biopsies during a two-week interval in order to monitor the efficacy of the anti-leukemic drugs employed. During the discussion period I expressed surprise that he had been able to receive IRB committee approval for a project that exposed infants to considerable discomfort. He responded that committee review had been unnecessary because his was not a research project, but a therapeutic intervention (Katz 1987, 5).

Cases of this sort suggest a need to recognize a region—between pure instances of research and of practice—of "innovative therapy" (National Commission 1978a, 4) or "nonvalidated practices:"

> A practice might be nonvalidated because it is new; i.e., it has not been tested sufficiently often or sufficiently well to permit a satisfactory prediction of its safety or efficacy in a patient population. It is equally common for a practice to merit the designation "nonvalidated" because in the course of its use in the practice of medicine there arises some legitimate cause to question previously held assumptions about its safety or efficacy. . . . At the time of the first substantial challenge to the validity of an accepted practice, . . . subsequent use of that modality should be considered nonvalidated. . . . (Levine 1986, 4).

Since nonvalidated practices are not carried out according to a research plan (or "protocol"), they cannot be justified by their benefit to science; since they lack a valid basis in science, they cannot be defended for the benefit they will provide to those with whom they are used. The more unproven the procedure and the more risk its use creates, the more troublesome is this state of affairs. The solution, of course, is to employ a nonvalidated practice in the context of an appropriate research plan or to substitute a proven treatment.

This will not always be possible, especially when attempting to cure problems (such as life-threatening conditions) for which no satisfactory therapy exists and when the need to intervene is too urgent to allow a formal research plan to be adopted. But the failure to convert situations of nonvalidated practice into either real research or pure practice occurs much more frequently than is justified by the number that are truly on the frontiers of biomedical and behavioral science. Rather, there are other impediments—practical and psychologcal—that stand in the way.

Testing a new practice requires much more effort than simply trying it out on an individual. The average practitioner's outlook differs from a researcher's; physicians feel justified in using a nonvalidated treatment because the general uncertainty of much of medical practice makes it acceptable to proceed with good intentions rather than face the lack of proof. Moreover, "human experimentation" has strongly negative connotations. The suggestion that physicians enroll their patients in a research project rather than use a nonvalidated practice is resisted because physicians see this as a request to sacrifice patients' well-being for the good of science or they fear that their patients would, at least, perceive the request that way.

Nonetheless, the resistance to experimenting should not be lightly dismissed. Danger can arise when professionals have conflicting loyalties—both to the goals of science and their obligations as care-givers to protect and enhance their clients' well-being. Because of this tension, society has adopted (as will be explored later) means of overseeing the relationship of practitioner-qua-researcher and patient-(or citizen)-qua-research subject in order to minimize the harmful effects on the interests of the latter, as well as to augment the beneficial effects both to subject and to society. The existence of such safeguards has probably done much to legitimate the place of human research in society; by reassuring the public, these safeguards make it more acceptable for practitioners to ask for participation in an "experiment." Yet procedures and delays entailed in these safeguards tar "experimentation" anew with unfavorable connotations for practitioners, who argue that what they are doing is "just practice" (even if unvalidated), and hence they ought not to be subjected to the rigors of formal research review.

"Therapeutic" Versus "Nontherapeutic" Research

A further example of the ways in which mere definitions can carry ethical freight is found in the terms "therapeutic" and "nontherapeutic" research. These terms are commonly employed to distinguish research that is carried out as a part of patient-care from that which involves subjects for whom the procedure being examined is not expected to have any value. In revising its 1964 code for biomedical investigators, *The Declaration of Helsinki*, in 1975 the World Medical Association proposed the phrase "clinical research" for medical research combined with professional care, and "non-clinical biomedical research" for nontherapeutic research.

Whatever terminology is used, the distinction is certainly clear, though not without danger. Modifying "research" with "therapeutic" may well lull an investigator and any persons called upon to review the research into treating the project as inherently more justified than "nontherapeutic" research because of the assumed intention to provide a benefit to the patient-subject. Yet, in order to be justified as research, the project must aim to answer questions about the intervention being tested (such as whether it is safe and provides a net benefit). Thus, there can be no assumption that patient-subjects will derive any benefit (i.e., "therapeutic" results).

The risk of being led to misevaluate the research because of the benign label "therapeutic" is at least as great for patients as for practitioners. Although many codes suggest that greater protection is needed for participants in nonclinical research than in research combined with professional care, the reverse may be the case, especially regarding the standards for informed consent because patients are less likely than "normal volunteers" to be in a good position to consider the physical, psychological and monetary risks and benefits in consenting to participate. A patient's emotional ties to the physician, his or her need for treatment (especially when conventional methods have proved ineffective), and the human tendency to overrate the benefits and underestimate the risks of a research technique, justify setting higher requirements for consent and imposing additional safeguards when therapy is combined with experimentation, lest investigators even unwittingly expose "consenting" patient-subjects to unreasonable risks (Capron 1972, 151–52).

Benefits to Others

Part of the definition of "practice" as opposed to "research" is that it involves interventions "designed solely to enhance the well-being of an individual. . . ." (National Commission 1978a, 2). Yet there are some activities (such as vaccination) that, while accepted practices because of their expectation of success, are not intended "solely" to benefit the individual, and there are others (quarantine, organ and tissue donation) that are intended solely to benefit others and not the individual. While appearing to fall outside the definition of "practice," such activities clearly are not "research" either.

Faced with this definitional problem, the National Commission insisted that this apparent inconsistency not be allowed "to confuse the general distinction between research and practice" (National Commission 1978a, 3). The reason given, however, seems disingenuous:

> Even when a procedure applied in practice may benefit some other person, it remains an intervention designed to enhance the well-being of a particular individual or group of individuals; thus, it is practice and need not be reviewed as research.

This rationale is either tautological (a "procedure applied in practice" is a "practice") or unpersuasive (if only a few people suffer from a disease, an intervention aimed at discovering a cure for that disease would be "designed to enhance the well-being of a particular . . . group of individuals," but it would still be "research," not "practice"). It would be better simply to recognize that sometimes practices of proven value are carried out for the purpose of benefitting someone other than the persons immediately subjected to the intervention.

This recognition yields an important ethical conclusion: "practice" sometimes shares an important feature with "research," namely benefitting others. In research, the benefit to others is a benefit to "science" from an increase in generalizable knowledge, while in the case of certain practices, the benefit flows to other individuals (the recipient of donated blood) or to society at large (protected by a quarantine from an infectious person). The willingness of society to accept the gift of such benefits—and sometimes even to extract them from an unwilling person—in the context of biomedical, as well as behavioral or social, practices and programs is a point worth remembering when evaluating the legal and ethical issues posed by research (Fox 1974, 5–39).

JUSTIFICATIONS AND PRINCIPLES

In an era as dependent upon science and technology as ours, it may seem unnecessary to examine the justifications for research with human subjects, since such research is an indispensable link between theory or initial observations and the application of scientific findings and technology developments to benefit people and society at large. But in ethical terms, such scrutiny is needed because the question is not whether to have all possible research or none at all but rather how much research to have at what cost, when "cost" includes possible harm to values other than the advancement of knowledge.

Research: Necessary or Optional?

As philosopher Hans Jonas eloquently argued nearly two decades ago, these value conflicts do not occur when science employs inanimate objects, but once feeling beings "become the subjects of experiment, as they do in the life sciences and especially in medical research, this innocence of the search for knowledge is lost and questions of conscience arise" (Jonas 1969, 219). The promotion of progress is a valid social goal but not, in his view, one to which individuals must be committed simply as members of society and beneficiaries of the current state of scientific knowledge.

Those who take the contrary view, that there is a "social imperative" in medical research, do not actually disagree with the view that other values must enter into the evaluation of research projects and the enterprise as a whole. Instead, they point to the enormous harm that is caused by well-meaning but misinformed biomedical (and social) interventionists using methods that have never been adequately tested, and they stress "the necessity for controlled trials to determine whether what is traditional does harm rather than good" (Eisenberg 1977).

Since the risks of medical research are small—comparable to the rates for accidental injury in the general population (Cardon, Dommel, and Trumble 1976)—there is a strong argument that patients should participate in evaluation studies on the risks and benefits of the practices to which they are routinely subjected, at least as to those practices whose morbidity and mortality exceed those encountered in research. However, this justification is insufficient for treatments on the frontiers of knowledge, especially those that contribute to some far-off goal of eventual understanding (or even cure) and those that involve more than minimal risks. For the latter, support of, and involvement in, research is a noble choice rather than a moral obligation. Progress is, after all, an optional not a mandatory goal, and its pursuit must take place within limits established by other values, including the value of individual autonomy.

Basic Ethical Principles in the History of Human Research

The bioethical principles that get the most attention in the context of human subjects research are respect for persons, beneficence, and justice (National Commission 1978).

RESPECT FOR (COMPETENT) PERSONS

Respect for persons has two rather different implications for research; the first emphasizes respect for the personhood or personal rights of research subjects, the second their personal well-being. To respect personal rights in either Kantian or utilitarian terms implies that those in charge of a project must provide prospective subjects with information that will enable them to decide whether it is acceptable according to their own values and goals and must then permit the subjects to choose whether or not to participate, rather than manipulating the information or coercing the choice.

This requirement may seem so basic as to require no comment, but it has presented problems both in historical experience and in theory. Deviations from the requirement of consent have sometimes been so shocking that it is well to remember that there have also been fine examples of physicians throughout history who respected the freedom and dignity of the subjects with whom they conducted research, such as the nineteenth century American pioneer physician William Beaumont, who made a true collaborator of the patient whose internal workings he observed for many years through the opening left from an injury, and Walter Reed, who sought the consent of subjects for his yellow fever study not merely in English but also in Spanish for the Spanish-speaking.

Such respect was, of course, horribly absent in the work of the Nazi physicians in the concentration camps. The terrors inflicted upon unconsenting subjects in experiments in which numerous inmates died in low-pressure environments (designed to simulate the effects on pilots of flying at, or falling from, high altitudes), from exposure to freezing air or water, from being used as human incubators and vaccine subjects for typhus, and from being given poisons—to name just a few categories of "research"—so blinded the investigators that in many instances they missed important scientific findings. The horror of the civilized world at what was revealed during the trial of twenty-three Nazi physicians at Nuremberg is embodied not only in the conviction of sixteen of them of war crimes and crimes against humanity (with seven condemned to death) but also in the judges' statement of principles, commonly called the Nuremberg Code, which begins: "The voluntary consent of the human subject is absolutely essential."

A similar fate did not await Japanese researchers who had carried out similarly barbarous experiments in Manchuria during World War 2. Indeed, the existence of these abuses was not even generally known for more than thirty-five years because, in exchange for not being publicly tried and punished, the Japanese investigators agreed to cooperate with their American captors and share the information they had gathered about biological warfare through their experiments with Chinese captives (Gomer, Powell and Roling 1981).

Between 1930–1945 Japan conducted human experiments in biological warfare and physical response to infection both through controlled research on prisoners of war and through field trials on mainland China. The main research installation was Unit 731, located near Harkin, which was operated by Lieutenant-

General Ishii. At least 3000 people were reported killed; some died as a result of the experiments, others were killed to observe the progression of the experiment, and others were killed when they became too weak to continue. At least two other sites were in operation, one near Changchun and one near Nanjing. Complaints from the People's Republic of China have identified at least eleven cities believed to be the targets of "field tests." A reported seven hundred victims contracted the plague as a result of these attacks.

Unit 731 was "a large, self-contained installation with sophisticated germ—and insect—breeding facilities, a prison for the human experimentees, testing grounds, an arsenal for making germ bombs, an airfield, its own special planes and a crematorium for the human victims." It was capable of producing eight tons of bacteria per month. Experiments were conducted on the human response to anthrax, botulism, brucellosis, cholera, dysentery, hemorrhagic fever, plague, smallpox, syphilis, tick encaphalitis, tsutsugamushi, tularemia, typhoid, and typhus. Other experiments included prolonged exposure of the liver to X rays, freezing body parts to try various methods of thawing, pumping the body full of horse blood, and vivisection.

Although officials of the United States were fully aware of the nature of the experimentation and that American prisoners of war had been used, they concluded that the value of the information obtained far outweighed the value of prosecution because the research greatly augmented scientific knowledge and was believed to be unobtainable anywhere else due to the tight controls on human subject research. The prosecution of the Japanese would have led to admission of this information at trial, which the American officials decided posed a threat to national security because the scientific findings would become available to all countries of the world. The Japanese were offered protection from the Russians in exchange for their full cooperation.

In the period after World War 2, this American complicity with the abuse of subjects by the Japanese was not known. Instead, leaders of biomedical research proclaimed their adherence to the principle of consent. Yet the behavior of American investigators sometimes was otherwise, such as in chemical and biological testing by American military and intelligence agencies from the 1940s to the 1960s.

The original rationale was that such testing was necessary for defensive purposes, on the belief that World War 2 enemies had used such techniques in interrogations, brainwashing, and in attacks designed to harass, disable, or kill Allied personnel and that in the future it would be important to understand how these substances worked and how their effects could be detected. As the potential for offensive use of these substances was recognized, the testing emphasis shifted and included a search for information on how unsuspecting people would respond. Therefore, as part of the testing procedures, unwitting subjects were used in real-life settings.

Two deaths have been directly linked to these experiments. In 1953, Harold Blauer was a patient at New York State Psychiatric Institute. As part of the United States Army Chemical Corps experiments, Blauer was injected with a synthetic mescaline derivative without his knowledge. He died of circulatory collapse and heart failure as a result of the drug. In 1975, the Secretary of the Army announced that Blauer had died while serving as an unwitting subject in Army drug testing. His daughter, Elizabeth Barrett, filed suit charging negligence in the creation and administration of the program and conspiracy to cover up the results (Barrett 1981).[4]

Dr. Frank Olson was an aerobiologist assigned to the Special Operations Division of the United States Army Biological Center at Camp Detrick, Maryland. At a meeting in 1953, five Army and CIA scientists received a dose of LSD in an after-dinner drink. Twenty minutes later they were informed of its presence in the drink. It is unclear whether these scientists ever agreed to be subjects. Olson became seriously depressed and committed suicide nine days later. The CIA provided no information to Olson's family concerning its involvement in his death; this information only emerged years later as a result of an action for damages brought against the government.

Although other allegations of severe harm and even death have not been proven (Nevin 1983), there is no question that many experiments were performed by American investigators between 1946–1965 without the knowledge, much less the consent, of the subjects and otherwise in violation of the existing codes (U.S. Senate 1977; "How U.S. Used Americans" 1986).

RESPECT FOR (INCOMPETENT) PERSONS

The fulcrum on which respect for a person's right to autonomous choice rests is the determination of the person's capacity to make the decision at hand. But how should one apply "respect for persons" when the subject is incapacitated? In the *Belmont Report,* the National Commission (1978, 4) found a second "ethical conviction" embedded in respect for persons: "persons with diminished autonomy are entitled to protection," in other words, respect for their personal well-being.

One situation in which the reach of this principle might be tested arises when parents of a young child with an illness that is usually fatal, such as cancer, refuse to allow an experimental treatment because they believe that the chances for long-term remission are so slim that it would be better to allow the child to die in peace (Holder 1987). Since the child is incapable of making the choice personally, the question is whether the parents' refusal should be binding. On the one hand, the regulations applicable to new drugs make consent a crucial requirement, so that it would not seem reasonable for the physicians simply to treat the child because they are convinced of the wisdom of this course. Moreover, the unproven nature of the treatment makes it unlikely that refusing it would be labelled "neglect" of the child such as to cause a court to transfer care and custody of the child to someone other than the parents. On the other hand, the extreme nature of the situation—when use

---

[4]In May 1987, Mr. Blauer's daughters obtained a $700,000 award against the government in the District Court in Manhattan (Lubasch 1987).

of an unapproved treatment offers the child's only chance of surviving—might lead a court to ignore the niceties of the law.

Plainly, this aspect of "respect for persons" is more difficult to apply than the consent requirement for competent persons. Certain strategies have been developed for minimizing the difficulties, such as relying on the "assent" of subjects who are capable of understanding some or all of the experiment but who are legally too young to give consent, which must be obtained from the child's legal guardian (usually the parents) [National Commission 1977; HHS 1983, §§46.402(b) and 46.408(a)].

When treatment, rather than research, for an incompetent is at issue, the law has generally recognized, and ethicists have generally endorsed, a surrogate decisionmaker (usually the next-of-kin or someone designated before the patient became incompetent) making the decision that the incompetent would have made based on his or her known choices and values. Of course, in many cases such a "substituted judgment" is impossible because the patient was never competent (for example, a young child) or did not express a preference relevant to the medical choice in question. In such circumstances, the surrogate is supposed to make a decision in the person's "best interests," which encompasses treatment choices that the average person would find reasonable under the circumstances. How applicable are such standards to human research? Would the surrogate need to know not only the incompetent person's preferences about treatment but also his or her willingness to take risks and to participate in research when part of the benefit is intended to flow to science and to other patients? In one study designed to examine the side-effects of long-term use of urinary catheters in the elderly, nearly one-third of family members who thought their mentally incompetent relatives (who resided in two nursing homes) would not want to be used for research nevertheless allowed their doctors to include them in the study (Warren et al. 1986). Alternatively, if a surrogate makes a choice according to the best interests standard, what presumption ought the surrogate apply regarding the reasonableness of taking risks in experiments for the benefit of others?

BENEFICENCE

In effect, the second facet of respect for persons—the obligation to protect the personal well-being of those who are incapable of deciding for themselves—might be seen as an aspect of the principle of beneficence, which was said by the National Commission (1978, 6) to give rise to two obligations: "(1) do no harm; and (2) maximize possible benefits and minimize possible harms." Both aspects of beneficence are thus quite compatible with respecting the well-being of the most vulnerable human subjects, those lacking the capacity for autonomous choices.

But when one turns to the first half of the respect for persons principle, the potential for direct conflict with beneficence in human research is enormous. The no-harming or "nonmaleficence" facet of beneficence poses the least risk of trespassing on respect for the choices of autonomous agents. Indeed, the no-harm principle can be derived not only from Hippocrates' Oath and *Epidemics* (Jonsen 1978), but—like respect for persons—also from Kant, since actively to do a person harm is to use him or her as a means to some end (good or perverse) not of his or her own choosing. As the great nineteenth-century researcher Claude Bernard held, one should not injure one person regardless of the benefits that might come to others (Bernard 1865).

Yet Dr. Bernard's oft-quoted "personal code"—among experiments "those that can only do harm are forbidden, those that are harmless are permissible, and those that may do good are obligatory"—illustrates the collision between autonomous choice and the benefit-maximizing aspect of beneficence.[5] After all, this aspect of beneficence goes far beyond the categorical imperative; lacking a common root with respect for persons, it is not surprising that it can easily come into conflict with that principle.

This problem is well illustrated by research conducted between September 1950 and November 1952 among more than 1000 women who received prenatal care at the University of Chicago's Lying-In Hospital. The researchers doubted the then-accepted use of diethylstilbestrol (DES) to prevent miscarriages; with the goal of improving women's health care, but wishing not to upset the pregnant women, they conducted a double-blind study without informing the women of either the study's design or the true nature of the drug they were receiving (Mink 1978). Only when the children of these women began, some twenty years later, to manifest unusually high rates of cancer and other reproductive tract abnormalities did the subjects learn of the experiment's existence. In 1982, a suit brought on behalf of the subjects and their offspring was settled by the University agreeing to provide free lifetime care of adenocarcinoma for any daughter of a subject and to provide other health-related redress for potential victims. In evaluating the tension between beneficence and autonomy in this case, is it relevant that at least some of the women would have received DES anyway (as "standard treatment"), that the study showed DES to be ineffective in preventing miscarriages (thereby benefitting these and many future women), and that the harm that eventually occurred was not anticipated and would not have been included in any statement of risks had the women given "informed consent" at the time of the study?

Quite plainly, the professional goal to search out and try to achieve what is thought to be best for others will sometimes be at odds with the rights of autonomous individuals. If respect for persons is given primacy, as it typically is in contemporary ethical and legal documents on human subjects research, then the principle of beneficence becomes a "side constraint" on the actions of investigators. That is, at a minimum, a researcher should conduct only experiments that have been designed in a manner that minimizes their possible harms; a person's willingness to be a

---

[5]The text analyzes the problems regarding those experiments said by Dr. Bernard to be "obligatory." As Beecher (1970, 226) points out, the rest of Bernard's "splendid sentiments" are equally problematic: he forbids harmful experiments (but such harm is often not known in advance), and he holds harmless ones to be permissible, when in fact they are unethical "unless they are properly organized [including provisions for third-party review and subject-consent?] and give promise of value."

subject is not an adequate sanction for performing an experiment if the investigator could reasonably have reduced the experiment's risks.

This view of the two principles does not remove the tension between them but does permit practical action to occur without abandoning either principle. There is, however, another irony inherent in the two halves of the beneficence principle itself. The nonmaleficence half of the principle emphasizes the paramountcy usually (though perhaps erroneously) given this value in interpreting the Hippocratic tradition: *primum non nocere*. Given the limited understanding and meagre therapeutics of medicine in ancient Greece—and, indeed, up until the middle of this century— the advice "above all, do no harm" was sound. Today, however, intervening despite risks of further harm is often of extreme benefit to patients.

Furthermore, applying the do-no-harm principle to human research (especially nonclinical research unrelated to subjects' well-being) would preclude all experiments; any intervention risks generating some harm. Yet to take this do-nothing posture contradicts the second half of the beneficence principle because the failure to increase biomedical (as well as behavioral and social) knowledge defaults on the obligation to maximize benefits and minimize harms. Certainly, as already remarked, the justification for research as a societal good, which deserves both collective and individual support, is that it not only improves the lot of mankind but also helps to avoid some of the harm that would otherwise be perpetrated because of our present state of ignorance and misguided attachment to practices that are in fact wasteful of resources or actually harmful to individuals. Thus, both a person wishing to carry out a research project and someone who opposes the project could, based upon an agreed set of facts about the risks of the project compared to the risks of the present state of practice, support their positions by reference to opposite halves of the principle of beneficence as articulated by the National Commission and adopted by other commentators (Levine 1986, 16–17).

JUSTICE

As important as the principle of justice is in the Western tradition, it has traditionally played only a minor role in discussions of human research. Failures to respect this principle are, regrettably, legion. One—of which every American needs to be aware—began in 1932 but was not publicly revealed (and halted) until 1972. During those forty years, the U.S. Public Health Service carried out a "study in nature" of untreated syphilis among rural black men near Tuskegee, Alabama, who were kept in ignorance of the experiment and steered away from receiving effective treatment, lest that interfere with the investigators' data (Brandt 1978; Tuskegee Syphilis Study 1973).

While it would generally be agreed that certain gross instances of abuse of research subjects—such as the Tuskegee study and the experiments in the Nazi camps—involved unfair treatment of the subjects, this is simply another way of saying that they manifested a total disrespect for the subjects as persons. The more particular sense of justice as an ethical principle—namely, the comparative use of the concept, which holds that it is unfair to treat like cases differently—is not implicated by these examples, since the experiments conducted by the Nazi physicians would not have been fair even had they selected their victims randomly from among all the inmates, or even from among all Germans.

When this sense of the word justice is employed, the resulting questions—who deserves to bear the burdens of research and to enjoy its benefits?—are interesting and complex. There are many ways of measuring fair distribution. In an egalitarian democracy, these include "(1) to each person an equal share; (2) to each person according to individual need; (3) to each person according to individual effort; (4) to each person according to societal contribution; and (5) to each person according to merit" (National Commission 1978a, 9).

Converting these possible criteria for fairness into operative principles for human research is both conceptually and practically difficult. In many spheres, society gives justice preeminence over other principles. In the collection of taxes, for example, progressive taxation is premised on the idea that it is fair to extract a larger share of income from a wealthy person than from a poor one. However, in human experimentation where respect for the choices of autonomous persons is also a guiding principle, a classic conflict emerges: if autonomy is accorded the primary position it usually enjoys in human-subjects research, then the selection of subjects dictated by justice would only be possible if all the "fairly selected" potential subjects actually agreed to participate. Thus, a just distribution of the burdens of research operates primarily as a side-constraint in the design of experiments, not as justification for enrolling unwilling subjects in attempting to distribute research risks "fairly" in society.

The practical problems in implementing the principle of justice in research are great, even if justice plays a limiting rather than an activating role. Since the connection between many research projects and eventual benefits to people are often remote and difficult to draw even after-the-fact, much less to predict reliably in advance, deciding among research projects with an eye to achieving a fair distribution of their fruits is probably wasted effort and possibly harmful because resources ought to go where they are likely to yield the greatest results, not where determined by a "fairness formula" with dubious predictive power.

The connections between a research project and the burdens it creates are certainly less opaque than its connection to eventual benefits to individuals. Yet even in this aspect, the goal of just distribution is difficult to implement in large measure because of the room for disagreement over defining the groups that ought to be treated "alike." It would seldom if ever be practical or appropriate to hold a lottery that would place every individual in society at equal risk of being recruited into a research project (Capron 1973). Yet if all individuals are not treated as inherently the same, defensible grounds need to be found for dividing them into groups.

Again, the principle of justice may be most serviceable as a constraint rather than a goal: some groupings already exist in society and result in rankings (from the least powerful to the most, from the least well-educated to the best, from the sickest to the healthiest, etc.) to which a researcher selecting subjects can pay attention.

The principle of fairness might be taken to require, for example, that subjects for a study of various birth methods ought to be recruited from among the well-insured patients of obstetricians in private practice as well as from the nonpaying patients in the charity wards.

Certain behaviors are plainly inconsistent with an egalitarian view of justice. As American physician Myron Prinzmetal later wrote, describing his training in the United States (as well as Europe) between the World Wars:

> New drugs, new experimental surgical procedures were commonly tested on charity patients, who rarely understood what was being done to them. Often they were maimed or killed—experimental "animals" sacrificed in the interests of medical progress. . . . In a word—some patients were not treated like animals, but often worse than animals—for some of them understood (Prinzmetal 1965).

A more stringent interpretation would insist on recruiting well-off and well-educated subjects before turning to those who fall lower on the socio-economic scale, based either on John Rawls' argument that justice favors steps that make the least well-off relatively better off (Rawls 1971), or on the conclusion that Jonas draws from his contention that progress is an optional goal, namely that the appeal to participate in the search for progress ought first to be addressed to those who most "identify" with the research enterprise. In this view, one has "an inversion of the normal 'market' behavior . . . namely, to accept the lowest quotation last (and excused only by the greatest pressure of need); to pay the highest price first" (Jonas 1969, 235). Jonas thus ties the notion of a just distribution of research risks back into respect for persons by recruiting first those subjects (such as the researchers themselves) whose "service is not just permitted by [them], but willed. That sovereign will of his which embraces the end as his own restores his personhood to the otherwise depersonalizing context" (Jonas 1969, 236).

> [F]or the scientific community to honor [this idea] will mean that it will have to fight a strong temptation to go by routine to the readiest sources of supply—the suggestible, the ignorant, the dependent, the "captive" in various senses. I do not believe that heightened resistance here must cripple research, which cannot be permitted; but it may indeed slow it down by the smaller numbers fed into experimentation in consequences. This price—a possibly slower rate of progress—may have to be paid for the preservation of the most precious capital of higher communal life (Jonas 1969, 237).

Societal decisions to limit or preclude certain types of research subjects (such as prisoners) show that definitions of justifiable research such as Jonas' can affect policy, but in general the principle of justice seems seldom to be implemented in deciding which research projects to undertake or in selecting the subjects among those legally permitted to participate (such as all adult persons capable of giving informed consent).

Justice also has a role in the design of research. In experiments involving the seriously ill or other "least well-off" groups, Professor Robert Veatch urged "a subject-centered review strategy in which a key question . . . is whether the research design will maximize benefit to the subject (rather than to the researcher, the researcher's institution, or even the pool of knowledge)" (Veatch 1983, 18), indeed, even if it compromises the quality of the research. Veatch argues that justice demands that researchers do not further burden already-burdened patient-subjects by requiring stressful tests or denying access to experimental treatments without randomization.

A timely illustration of this dilemma is the current federal research with AIDS patients to discover an effective therapy. Thousands of desperate AIDS patients are enrolling in drug trials despite unknown risks and the fact that the experiments are blind and randomized; half the subjects receive placebos (inert substances), without knowing in which arm of the protocol they are participating. Many other AIDS victims have complained that it was unfair to exclude them from access to these experimental drugs simply because more subjects were not needed according to the design of the clinical trials.

This situation raises two justice issues in the terms raised by Veatch. First, even when use of placebos is preferable in scientific terms (which is not always the case) should a less conclusive design be used—such as comparing groups using different experimental regimens or utilizing data from a matched group of untreated patients as "historical controls?" Second, should experimental drugs be available outside of formal research programs when they offer the only hope for halting a fatal illness? The government initially justified its policies on the ground that careful research is needed to find an effective therapy; therefore, "the current approach will help the greatest number in the shortest time" (Eckholm 1986), but the Food and Drug Administration (FDA) subsequently revised its rules to permit perscription outside of formal research protocols of certain drugs that have been approved for investigational use. Is sufficient fairness assured if access to an experiment is randomly available to all? Who should bear the burden here—society (in failing to have research that is scientifically adequate) or fatally ill patients (in either being unable to get into a research program where an unproven drug is being dispensed or in being enrolled in a research program with a 50 percent chance of getting an inert placebo)?

ETHICAL REVIEW PROCEDURES

Ethical and legal guidance for experimentation has tended to evolve from one document to the next, sometimes in surprising ways. For example, the Nuremberg Code declared by the American judges in the process of passing judgment on the Nazi camp physicians in 1946 was itself influenced by the 1931 German government regulations, because Boston psychiatrist Leo Alexander, one of the two American medical advisors to the prosecutors of the Nazi physicians, relied on the German standards as well as on those formulated by the American Medical Association after the war in the influential expert testimony that he and Dr. A. C. Ivy provided to the Nuremberg tribunal (Alexander 1966, 15; Conference 1976, 6).

The Nuremberg Code in some ways amounted to a retreat from the German regulations which had emphasized institutional and not merely individual responsibility. The assumption that adequate protection for subject lay in the conscience of the investigator, professional codes (such as the World Medical Association's *Declaration of Helsinki*), and the basic requirement of consent predominated in the first twenty years after the War. Indeed, the only piece of national legislation on the subject during this period—the requirement for "informed consent" from participants in drug trials added to the Food and Drug Act as a minor part of the sweeping 1962 amendments to that statute (Food and Drug Amendments 1962)—also relied primarily on physicians' consciences and subjects' consent.

The changes in the FDA requirements stimulated its sister agency, the Public Health Service, to examine more closely some concerns about a small percentage of research proposals that the PHS was asked to fund (principally through the National Institutes of Health) that seemed to involve ethical problems, such as undue risk to subjects. This led in turn to a system of peer review in the Clinical Center at NIH and then to the guidelines for PHS grantees issued by Dr. Shannon in 1966 which marked a return to collective responsibility for the propriety of research projects. The new federal requirements were not quickly or gladly accepted by the research community (Barber et al. 1973), but their necessity was soon borne out for the larger community, as well as for many researchers, first by Dr. Beecher's revelations and then by the Tuskegee scandal and other studies involving prisoners, aborted fetuses, and mentally retarded persons, among others. Following the recitation of such problems during extensive hearings before a Senate subcommittee in 1973, Congress in the National Research Act (1974) (1) directed the Secretary of HEW to require all recipients of departmental research funds to establish Institutional Review Boards (IRBs), and (2) created the National Commission for the Protection of Human Subjects of Biomedical and Behavioral Research, whose duties included recommending changes in the federal rules on human research. The Commission issued a series of reports between 1974 and 1978, as a consequence of which the Department of Health and Human Services (HHS) promulgated a revised set of regulations on January 26, 1981, which provide the basic framework for oversight of research in the United States (HHS 1983; see also Appendix 2).

The HHS "Institutional Assurance" System

Despite the dominance of the HHS model, the federal government actually uses two systems to protect human subjects. The first applies to situations in which a government agency (most notably HHS, through the extramural programs of the NIH) sponsors research with human subjects. HHS regulations stipulate that an institution receiving funds for research provide "written assurance satisfactory to the Secretary that it will comply with the requirements" of 45 C.F.R. Part 46. The heart of these regulations is the existence of an IRB to determine that each research proposal meets federal requirements. In effect, having set the standards for approval of projects (including minimal requirements for diversity of IRB membership), the government delegates the execution of its rules to research institutions based on their assurance that they will comply.

It seems widely agreed that the process of prospective review of research protocols in general, and the IRB as the means of accomplishing this review in particular, are effective in improving the quality of subjects' consent and in avoiding excessively risky research. Yet few data are actually available to support these conclusions. The National Commission's study (1978b) of IRBs occurred before most institutions had much experience with IRBs as constituted under the present rules, and the present methods by which federal agencies monitor research do not provide much information about the actual operation of IRBs, except when a complaint of abuse is raised against a research project (President's Commission 1981, 35–60; 1983, 53–126).

Nevertheless, an outline can be given for the regulatory process. First, a researcher devises a plan for testing a hypothesis or otherwise developing generalizable knowledge; before carrying out the investigation with human subjects, the researcher will typically have performed theoretical, laboratory and animal studies. In addition to the scientific protocol that describes the research plan and objectives in technical terms from which other scientists can judge the proposal's worth, researchers at many institutions must also prepare a second document for the IRB. This plan explains the population to be studied and how and why the human subjects were chosen, salient aspects of research design (with particular attention to the risks and inconveniences for the subjects) and data interpretation (including provisions for monitoring the accumulating data to allow appropriate adjustments or termination if adverse consequences begin to occur), and the potential significance of the research (Cowan 1975, 537–46). Furthermore, this document includes a copy of the informed consent form that will be read and given to prospective subjects. IRBs devote particular attention to consent forms and frequently request revisions in them (National Commission 1978b, 60–72; President's Commission 1983, 67–97).

Once approved by the IRB and other institutional officials, the research proposal is sent to the federal agency from which funding is being sought—or to another sponsor, since many private sponsors now expect institutions to use the same review methods for protocols involving human subjects, and many institutional "assurances" provide for IRB review for research that will not be federally funded, even though such uniformity of process and standards is not actually a regulatory requirement. There it is appraised (typically on a comparative basis against competing proposals) by a group of the investigator's scientific peers (called "study sections" at the NIH). The IRB's approval is a requirement before the study section may consider funding the proposal. Tension sometimes occurs, however, when the scientific reviewers disagree with an IRB's assessment (for example, if they find the design unduly risky) and want a proposal to be modified for ethical reasons before they will approve it for funding (President's Commission 1983, 37–38). The Office for Protection from Research Risks (OPRR), which negotiates the institutional assurances on behalf of the NIH, does not actually review each protocol and consent form, but is available to provide information for IRBs and study sections and to investigate cases as needed.

The FDA's Retrospective System

Since their revision in 1981, the substance of the FDA's regulations accords with the basic HHS requirements. However, despite the essentially identical process of prior review that will be undergone by a research project subject to FDA jurisdiction, the relationship of the agency to the research institution differs from that of the PHS and the two dozen other federal agencies that fund research with human subjects.

Because the FDA does not usually sponsor research, its oversight of the research institution is indirect. The FDA's protection of human subjects rests on its authority to refuse to approve a new drug or device for general use when the data submitted by the sponsor of the drug or device in support of its approval has been produced through improper research, including research that is unacceptable on ethical grounds. Thus, rather than negotiate "assurances" with institutions and give IRBs prospective approval based on their design and plans as OPRR does, the FDA reviews the adequacy of human subjects protection retrospectively, during its approval process. It is therefore the responsibility of the sponsor to ensure that the protocol complies with the regulations and has been properly reviewed by a legitimate IRB (FDA 1981). When FDA inspectors visit the places where research has been conducted in support of drug applications, they check on the composition and functioning of the IRB and the adequacy of its decisionmaking as part of their review of the "paper trail" that a research protocol leaves in the files of the research institution. The FDA is now taking steps to remedy the gap in its knowledge about what research is being conducted at which institutions with which subjects at any given time but will continue to rely on the sponsor of the drug or device to keep such records as part of the sponsor's responsibility to monitor testing.

State Regulation of Research with Human Subjects

Several states have adopted statutes that establish policies and procedures for medical and psychological research. New York's law, which applies only to research that is not subject to and in compliance with federal regulations, was enacted in 1975 and draws heavily from the federal rules existing at that time. The statute limits the carrying out of research to licensed physicians or persons "deemed appropriately competent and qualified by a human research review committee" [N.Y. 1985, §§2441(6) and 2443]. The requirements for informed consent and for the membership and functioning of the review committee are substantially similar to current HHS rules, except that the reporting and approval requirements tie the institution to the Commissioner of Health in Albany rather than to federal officials (N.Y. 1985, §2444).

California's statute, enacted in 1978, is premised on the *Nuremberg Code* and *Declaration of Helsinki* being legally unenforceable standards and hence incapable of meeting "a growing need for protection for citizens of the state from unauthorized, needless, hazardous, or negligently performed medical experiments on human beings" (Calif. 1984, §24171). Research conducted at an institution with a valid HHS assurance and in conformance with the federal requirements is exempted from most of the procedural provisions of the California law, but the statute's detailed "experimental subject's bill of rights" and its civil and criminal penalties for negligent or willful failure to obtain informed consent still apply (Calif. 1984, §24178).

Nevertheless, the New Jersey Supreme Court recognized the enforceability of professional codes of ethics (Pierce 1980). Although the court denied Dr. Pierce's suit for damages for the termination of her employment that resulted from her refusal to carry-out research she regarded as unethical, the court held that "[e]mployees who are professionals owe a special duty to abide not only by federal and state law, but also by the recognized codes of ethics of their professions" (Pierce 1980, 512).

Overall, the states have legislated little on the subject of human research. What legislation exists is consistent, both in the approach (prior review by an IRB of risks and of informed consent) and in the standards applied standards with the prevailing federal requirements. Of course, like the possibility of a damage action brought by a subject under state tort law, the very existence of state statutory provisions does add an element of uncertainty and procedural complexity to a field in which legal advice could otherwise be largely based on construing a fairly straightforward set of federal regulations that have not been complicated by numerous or divergent judicial interpretations.

CURRENT ISSUES

Having reviewed the history and principles behind the present structure of decision-making about research with human subjects, we turn now to examine some topics that remain as current issues. There are many ways to analyze these issues; the one used here emphasizes the interplay of two central factors—risk and consent—which figure in various combinations in what follows.

Highly Risky Research

UTILITARIANISM VERSUS NONMALEFICENCE

An interesting illustration of the unresolved nature of the interplay of risk and consent is provided by research on the artificial heart. One of the major results of the movement after 1966 away from the investigator's conscience/subject's consent model of acceptable research has been to constrict the range of risks to those that appear acceptable to reasonable members of an IRB (Patullo 1982). Although an

IRB might permit an heroic investigator to engage in some highly risky self-experimentation, many modern studies would not lend themselves to the sort of self-experimentation in which the pioneers in physiology and infectious diseases engaged during an earlier era (Forssmann 1964).

Dr. William DeVries could hardly have implanted an artificial heart into his own chest, rather than that of Barney Clark. Yet healthy people did volunteer themselves to the University of Utah team to have artificial hearts implanted (Grady 1984, 49). From a utilitarian viewpoint, it would be ethical to use such subjects (provided that they really give voluntary, informed consent) because so much more could be learned about the artificial heart (and by extension, also about the functioning of other organs once it is possible to observe a "normal" body in which heart function is totally subject to external manipulation) if it were implanted in a healthy person than in the very sick people who are permitted to be selected as patient-subjects under the existing protocol (Jonsen 1984, 6–8). Yet the obvious excess of risk over benefit *to the subject* makes it highly unlikely that any IRB (or the FDA) would approve such a research design, even though the HHS regulations state that the IRB should be satisfied that "risks to subjects are reasonable in relation to . . . the importance of the knowledge that may reasonably be expected to result" [HHS 1983, §46.111(a)(2)].

It is interesting to note that the conflict between utility and nonmaleficence is customarily resolved in the opposite fashion—that is, in favor of utility—when it comes to vaccine trials, even when it is not possible to leave the weighing of risks and benefits directly to the prospective subjects, who often are young children. (These subjects are selected both because they are the potential victims of the diseases that the vaccines are intended to prevent and because as a group they have a much lower rate of acquired immunity, which would interfere with the scientific measurements in a vaccine trial.)

The reason for the special concern about vaccine trials is that they expose otherwise healthy subjects to harm. Although the same is true with proven vaccines, vaccination programs are justified on the grounds (a) that since all members of society benefit from immunization, it would be unfair to allow an individual to freeload off the risk taken by others in being vaccinated, and (b) that in being vaccinated individuals confer benefits (in immunity to disease) upon themselves as well as upon the community. In an experimental vaccination program, however, the existence of a benefit remains to be proven nor has the degree of risk yet been determined—indeed, these are among the purposes of the trial. Thus, the justification for a vaccine trial is more utilitarian than for ordinary biomedical research with patient-subjects.

The prevailing strategy is to reduce the risks as much as possible (through studies in animals and in adult volunteers) and then, in effect, to take the plunge by using the experimental vaccine on a small number of children. It may be possible to identify characteristics that would make some children better subjects than others: those who do not experience adverse reactions to other vaccines, or those who are most likely to be exposed to the infectious agent and thus stand the most to gain from the discovery of a vaccine. Finally, compensation to subjects injured in the trial as in any experiment would help to overcome the remaining sense of a communal benefit being purchased at a high price to a few individuals (Congress 1980; President's Commission 1982).

RISKY BEHAVIOR AND BENEFICENCE

What compromises should be made in research design because of investigators' obligations to act beneficently toward subjects? Research in the area of preventing Acquired Immune Deficiency Syndrome (AIDS) illustrates the complexity of this ethical issue in several ways.

First, there is a tension between the urgent need to reduce the spread of AIDS and the scientific imperative to develop the most effective means of doing so. The best way to gauge the effectiveness of various programs to prevent the spread of AIDS is to measure the rate of conversion of the population to Human Immunedeficiency Virus (HIV) seropositivity. To avoid biasing the results, the test for the HIV antibody in the blood should be administered unobtrusively, so as not to alter the experimental conditions. "Ethical considerations, however, require the antibody test to be used 'obtrusively' so as to maximize the test's effectiveness as a spur to risk reduction" (Des Jarlais and Friedman 1987, 6).

A second problem will arise once an AIDS vaccine is ready for testing. The vaccine's effectiveness can only be measured if those who are vaccinated are then exposed to the virus. Yet the virus does not spread randomly through the population; exposure requires direct conduct through sexual activities, the sharing of drug paraphernalia, or from pregnant or nursing mother to child. Given the fatal nature of the disease, is it a failure of beneficence for a researcher to test a vaccine on a subject with the expectation—indeed, even the hope—that the subject (who is eligible to be included in the study because he or she has managed to escape HIV infection) will then engage in behavior that risks his or her becoming infected? Is it enough that the subject would have engaged in this behavior anyway, or does the fact of the vaccine research implicate the investigator in the subject's behavior through the failure to do everything in his power ethically and legally to protect the subject from his or her own self-risking activities?

Randomization

At the heart of all concern over human experimentation is the fact that a person in an experiment is being treated differently and exposed to risk that he or she would not encounter absent the experiment. As has already been shown, the two responses to the ethical dilemma that arises once it is decided to go ahead with an experiment anyway are (a) to reduce the actual risk as much as possible through IRB review and the like, and (b) to make the encountering of the risk a matter of the subject's free and informed choice.

A fundamental requisite for ethical experimentation, and hence for IRB approval of a protocol, is appropriate research design because a project that is not scientifically sound is not only wasteful of resources but unnecessarily exposes human beings to risks and inconvenience. Sometimes, however, the attempt to use a scientifically attractive design raises other ethical problems, especially the problem of less than full consent. The use of a randomized design illustrates the difficulties.

In order to measure the effect of the intervention being investigated, it is usually (though not always) necessary to have a "control group" whose members do not receive the intervention. Sometimes it is possible to construct such a group from patients who have received, or are receiving, other forms of treatment or who are untreated; if these control subjects can be "matched" by relevant characteristics with the subjects receiving the experimental intervention, the effects of the latter can be isolated. Such a method is arduous and also fraught with the risk that if all relevant criteria for matching have not been identified, the selection of the control group will be biased in some unrecognized way. For this reason, it is usual to divide potential subjects into at least two groups (i.e., those receiving the experimental intervention and the controls who receive some other treatment or no treatment) for concurrent observation by the investigator.

To avoid conscious or unconscious bias in the assignment of potential subjects to the experimental and control groups, it has become preferred practice to adopt various means of random assignment, particularly in conducting research with patients as subjects. In that case, the design is known as a Randomized Clinical Trial, or RCT.

DISCLOSURE OF RESEARCH DESIGN

The major issues that arise with a RCT are whether and how subjects will be informed of the randomization. The fact of random assignment is plainly an important aspect of research design and is therefore an essential fact to communicate to prospective subjects. It can be argued that it ought not to be material to the decision-making of the subject, because the subject should be able to rely on the physician-investigator to watch out for the subject's interests, and once the null hypothesis has been met (see below) it is, as a matter of definition, in each subject's interests to be randomized (Chalmers 1982). Yet a person entering into research (or treatment, for that matter) is not required to make decisions that are objectively welfare-maximizing. Because potential research subjects who have greater (though misguided) faith in their physicians than in the null hypothesis would want to know that the intervention they are undergoing will be determined by a randomizing procedure than by their physicians' individualized judgments, the randomization procedures should be included in the informed consent process (Fost 1979).

Beyond this, Charles Fried has argued "that there is a continuing duty on the part of the patient's physician . . . to inform his patient about any significant new information coming out of the experiment that might bear on the patient's choice to remain in the study or to seek other types of therapy" (Fried 1974, 35). The word "significant" can also be problematic. Asking a patient to be randomized can be asking her to sacrifice her self-interest, since data which is not significant to the researcher might very well be significant to the subject. Of course, the investigator should also educate subjects about the danger in drawing conclusions from incomplete data; dissuading a patient from withdrawing prematurely is not just a selfish act (to protect the validity of the research) but also a beneficent act toward the patient-subject. Furthermore, in certain cases, a "cross-over" design (in which subjects are switched from one group to the other during the course of the study) can be employed to minimize the ethical problems; likewise, a data review process can be established in order to determine whether statistically significant results have been obtained earlier than expected, allowing the research to be terminated and the better treatment offered to all patients (Chalmers, Block, and Lee, 1972).

THE NULL HYPOTHESIS

Because an RCT involves patients in need of diagnosis and/or treatment, it becomes especially important that a priori one can reasonably maintain that the treatment and control groups will show no difference as a result of the intervention. This position—known as the "null hypothesis"—may seem an odd proposition (why would one test an intervention believed to have no effect compared to a control group?), but its ethical roots are more apparent if the concept is restated as the proposition that a rational person would not prefer a priori to be in one group rather than the other.

It is important to remember that the null hypothesis is a description of an objective state of affairs and not of the subjective sense of the participants. The personal prejudices of physicians and patients (to believe, for example, that a newly developed treatment will be better than any existing treatment) are not enough to deny the null hypothesis when it rests on valid grounds as it usually does in the absence of actual proof one way or the other; nonetheless, such views would, of course, be good reason for particular patients (or even particular physicians) to decline to participate in a randomized experiment. For example, a patient might have a preference for one arm of the research protocol over the other (e.g., in a comparison of surgery and radiation to treat cancer) or might, as a risk-taker in life generally, want to be assigned to the new intervention rather than to the accepted one that is being used as the control.

A current issue involving the null hypothesis arises in the context of studies aimed not at discovering new treatments but at measuring the cost-effectiveness of alternative methods. A prevalent complaint today is that many medical interventions have never been shown to be effective and that even among those that are clinically efficacious, data are often missing by which physicians (and their patients) could compare the relative benefits and costs of alternative forms of preventing, diagnosing, and treating a condition. Although such research was initially promoted as a form of technology assessment that might result in better patient care (Congress 1978), increasingly its objective is to conserve resources.[6] Of course, patients collectively have an interest in avoiding waste in the health-care system; yet

---

[6]With the advent of new forms of third-party payment, especially payments provided on a per capita or prospective basis, the medical community is more interested in researching in this field.

this interest, which is comparable to the collective interest in the advance of knowledge, is not, as Jonas pointed out, sufficient to justify the imposition of burdens or risks on individuals without their consent.

Since the design of a research project on the cost-benefit of various treatments aims to find ways of achieving basically equivalent outcomes for patients while trimming costs to the system, not necessarily to find ways to improve the patients' individual outcomes, these studies are an exception to the general rule that the null hypothesis must be reasonable before randomization is justifiable. One arm may be clearly better than the other; therefore, it becomes very important to ensure that patients participating in such research understand the purpose of the study—to discover just how much better the particular intervention is when compared with an alternative and either justify or discontinue the intervention. One method for avoiding the potential exploitation of patients is to make use of the "natural experiments" that occur as different health providers and insurers adapt to the cost pressures in different ways; however, the uncontrolled variables among the groups often preclude deriving unambiguous or statistically significant results.

Other Features of Research Design

BLIND AND DOUBLE-BLIND STUDIES

It is sometimes impossible to disguise the "arm" of an experiment to which a subject has been assigned, even though knowledge of this fact may affect the subject's responses and perceptions and the investigator's observations and interpretations. Whenever possible, however, it is preferable to conceal the assignment—that is, making it "blind" to the subject or the observer, or "double-blind" to both. Again, this is a fact which must be disclosed to subjects (Curran 1979). While an investigator can do nothing to prevent subjects who are anxious to know whether they are in the active or control group from finding this out, acceptance of the blind condition is a valid basis for accepting, or continuing, a subject in a research project.

PLACEBOS

In some research, the control group is given a placebo: an inactive substance, usually compounded to resemble the size, shape, and so forth, of the substance being tested. (Likewise, outside of drug trials, a sham intervention may be used in place of the true intervention.) The purpose is two-fold: first, to duplicate for the control group the physical experience of the group receiving the experimental intervention, and second, by leading all subjects to believe that they have an equal chance of actually taking the experimental drug or other intervention, to expose all subjects to the elusive but sometimes very powerful effects (both favorable and unfavorable) that patients' beliefs about an intervention can have on their responses.

Two sets of questions arise about placebos. The first involves the information given to subjects. Plainly, if a subject were told whether or not he or she was receiving a placebo, the whole point of this design would be lost; on the other hand, failure to disclose is a form of deception. Would an acceptable solution be to disclose the fact that a placebo will be used but to keep secret the type of intervention actually used? Subjects who find the possibility of receiving a placebo unacceptable could then decline to participate in the experiment. But is it still deceptive not to tell subjects about the possible side-effects of the placebo itself (Connelly 1987)?

The second set of issues around placebos is one of risk more than consent; it concerns the circumstances under which a placebo should not be used. When an effective treatment already exists, the use of a placebo is unacceptable. Ethically, it is justifiable to test a new therapy that promises some advantage (in efficacy, side-effects, cost, etc.) over the existing treatment, but not at the cost of withholding the existing treatment from the control group. In practical terms, the reason for testing a procedure, whether to seek approval of a new drug or to demonstrate a new form of psychological diagnosis, is not to show that it is "better than nothing" (i.e., has more than a placebo effect), but to find something that is preferable to existing treatments. For both these reasons, when a study is being done with patients, it is usually ethically required to assign the control group to the best available form of treatment rather than to a placebo, although there are factors that can outweigh this presumption (such as when the failure to use any treatment would create at worst a small or transient risk to subjects and when the existing treatment differs too much from the intervention being tested to allow a blind or double-blind study).

It would also be unacceptable to use a placebo when doing so would itself create undue risk for subjects. This is why placebo-controlled studies are much rarer in surgery than in medicine and pharmacology: the danger to subjects from sham operations (including the risks of anesthesia and infection) usually preclude their use, despite their obvious value in avoiding the use of unnecessary or worse surgical procedures which will then potentially expose many people to harm or waste over many years (Beecher 1961).

Special Problems of (Non)Consent

Although risk never totally disappears as a topic in human experimentation, some unresolved issues focus more on problems with informed consent as such. These fall into several groups; first, those that arise when investigators are permitted to waive the usual consent requirements for reasons of research design, and second, those that arise because the subjects lack the capacity to give consent.

WAIVER

Several instances (e.g., the use of placebos) have already been mentioned in which subjects may not be fully informed about what is being done to them. A desire to deceive is not, of course, limited to scientific investigators. Columnist Bob Greene relates the story of a young woman who, before going to the beach for her summer vacation, made up business cards in a fictious name, claiming to be "vice president for talent of *Gentlemen's Quarterly*." She found that the handsomest men, who would otherwise not have paid her any attention, not only posed for her but treated her like a celebrity in the hopes they would be selected to appear in the magazine. Would the men's feelings be hurt for having been deceived? "I don't think so," she concluded (Greene 1987). Is there a difference between a "civilian" and a scientist practicing deception of this type?[7]

In some research, investigators have what they regard as more serious reasons to keep subjects uninformed or actively misinformed about the nature, purpose, or even the existence of the research. Largely in response to complaints from social and behavioral scientists that official consent requirements preclude conducting studies in which subjects would alter their behavior if they knew they were being studied or knew the true methods and purposes of the research, the major federal regulations on human subjects research now permit an IRB to alter or even to waive the usual consent rules when (a) the risk to subjects will be minimal; (b) the "rights and welfare" of the subject will not be adversely affected; (c) the project "could not practicably be carried out without the waiver or alteration;" and (d) debriefing of the subjects will occur whenever appropriate [HHS 1983, §46.116(d)].[8]

Several objections can be raised to waiving consent requirements. First, the existence of a waiver provision—like the existence of the exemption for certain research[9]—may encourage a general disregard of the rules to protect human subjects (Leskovac and Delgado 1987, 1155).

More importantly, the waiver provision undermines the very core of the HHS regulations which are premised on the respect for persons. The waiver provision, in contrast, is baldly utilitarian because it shifts the IRB's "focus from the essence of research ethics—protection of human autonomy—to the important, but secondary, consideration of protecting research subjects from physical or emotional harm" (Leskovac and Delgado 1987, 1154). Assuming that direct risk to the subject is "minimal," almost any advance in knowledge will probably be found on utilitarian grounds to justify proceeding with the deception.

For some commentators, any deception of misinformation violates the "rights and welfare" of subjects and thus the waiver provision could never be applied. Others would differentiate between types of waivers: a waiver to permit an epidemiologist to review existing, and personally identifiable, medical records (where the harm would be a small intrusion on privacy); a waiver to permit the epidemiologist then to contact the persons identified in such records, to link prior data

---

[7]Interestingly, Bob Greene writes that the young woman "told herself that there was a valid reason for what she was doing:" 'I've always been interested in the psychology of what goes on in men's minds,' she said. 'What makes them tick. So part of me was thinking that this was a legitimate way to find out' (Greene 1987). Apparently she believed that behaving like a scientist made her conduct less problematic.

[8]The Food and Drug Administration regulations do not provide for deception waivers, though they do permit use of an unapproved drug or device without consent if that is the best way of dealing with a life-threatening emergency (FDA 1981, §50.23).

[9]Investigators are not required to seek IRB approval of certain activities, such as research on normal educational practices in "commonly accepted educational settings," or surveys or interview procedures, or observation of public behavior, except when the information recorded could link identifiable persons to sensitive actions (such as illegal drug use) that could have adverse criminal, civil or social consequences [HHS 1983, §46.101 (b)].

to consequences in their lives (clearly, a more substantial intrusion, not only on private records but on privacy in the sense of personal repose and one's sense of well-being); and a waiver to permit a behavioral scientist to lie to subjects about the purposes of a research project (where the very right of autonomous choice would be denied to the subjects).

One's evaluation of the acceptability of waiver may also turn on the value one finds in the steps that can be taken to mitigate the nondisclosure or deception. Some strategies seek to respect the values behind autonomy by developing substitutes for subjects' prior consent, such as "peer consultants," members of the same group as the potential subjects who can participate with the investigator in design of the research (Baumrind 1978), or debriefing and after-the-fact veto, including an offer to destroy the data generated by their personal involvement (Capron 1982, 221–222). Alternatively, to improve research design (another goal to which the usual requirement of informed consent would contribute) investigators could engage the public in discussion of the need for deception to carry out valuable research; public review and approval would not only provide feedback on the particular project but, perhaps even more important, would lessen the risk that deceptive research would weaken public confidence in science or endanger human interactions (Bok 1978, 194–195). Or, instead of involving the entire public, a group of people who were willing to participate in such research could be used as a "deception pool" from whom subjects could be drawn (Leskovac and Delgado 1987, 1156).

FETUSES AND ABORTUSES

Sometimes the problem with consent lies not in the design of the project but in the inability of the subjects to decide on their own behalf. HHS has recognized the need for extra circumspection in these cases by placing special requirements on researchers. For example, they must obtain approval from a national Ethics Advisory Board or similar group of experts appointed by the Secretary of HHS before the research may be funded [1983, §§46.204 and 46.407(b)(ii)].

Perhaps the most troubled area of special protection is that afforded by the federal regulations and the laws of a number of states to fetuses as possible research subjects. Because of its link to the abortion controversy, this area of research has aroused a great deal of public concern, going back at least to the National Research Act of 1974, which made a study of the subject the first assignment for the National Commission.

The simplest provisions are that any research with a dead aborted fetus be performed only with the consent of its mother, as directly required by statute in a number of states [Arkansas 1985, §82–438; Massachusetts 1983, ch. 112 §12J(a)(II)], and by implication in all states under the Uniform Anatomical Gift Act (UAGA). Furthermore, the federal regulations prohibit use of a fetus ex utero as a subject "until it has been ascertained whether or not" it is viable; vital functions of a nonviable fetus may neither be artificially maintained nor exposed to the risk of more rapid termination, and a viable fetus is to be treated as an infant and not exposed to anything more than minimal experimental risks that are not necessary for treatment (HHS 1983, §46.209). Statutes in several states forbid any research with a fetus ex utero [Arizona 1986, §36–2302(A); Arkansas 1985, §82–438; Massachusetts 1986, ch. 112, §12J(a)(I)].

The direct intersection of the experimentation and abortion issues arises when an investigator wishes to study the fetus in utero. The HHS rules limit such research to activities intended "to meet the health needs of the particular fetus" and involving the minimal increase in risk necessary to meet these needs, or to activities that generate minimal risk, the purpose of which "is the development of important biomedical knowledge which cannot be obtained by other means" [HHS 1983, §46.208(a)]. Similarly, laws in several states limit experimental interventions to those designed to benefit the fetus (Massachusetts 1986, ch. 112, §12J(a)(I); South Dakota 1977, §34–23A–17; Utah 1977, §76–7–310). Does research on prenatal diagnosis fall within the "benefit" or "needs of the fetus" category (when the diagnosis may lead to the decision to abort the fetus)? In interpreting a Louisiana statute that prohibits experimentation upon an unborn child unless it is therapeutic to the fetus (Louisiana 1986, §40:1299.35.13), the federal district court simply side-stepped the plaintiff's claim that the statute was so vague that it would inhibit experimentation and held that prenatal diagnosis is not experimental (Margaret S. 1980). It seems doubtful that a researcher developing new means of antenatal diagnosis, much less new means of abortion, could take much comfort from this decision if prosecuted for violating one of the state laws prohibiting nonbeneficial research involving the fetus.

DEAD OR NEARLY DEAD SUBJECTS

Besides permitting the donation of dead fetuses or their parts for research, the UAGA has general application to dead persons of any age. Unless expressly limited by the donor (i.e., the decedent prior to death or specified family members after the decedent's death), a body donated under the UAGA may be used for education, research, therapy, and/or transplantation. Although an institution could insist that research using dead bodies be reviewed, IRB review is not required by federal regulations, which apply only to living human subjects.

In the context of organ transplantation, a declaration of death is usually based upon the complete cessation of brain functions in bodies whose respiratory and circulatory functions are artificially maintained (Capron 1986; Guidelines 1981). It has been suggested that such brain-dead bodies would be good subjects for research (Carson, Frias, and Melker 1981; Martyn 1986, 8). Despite the potential benefits of, and the apparent authority for, such research, the same ethical concerns involved in fetal research arise in research on dead bodies in which the signs of life are being maintained.

Specifically, research regulations and the UAGA fail to protect against two dangers of research on the brain-dead: the disturbing effect such research could have on family members and the violation of "commonly held convictions about respect for the dead" (President's Commission 1983, 40). The President's Commission recommended that those concerns be addressed by expanding the use of IRBs to all research on the deceased, including the brain-dead (1983, 41). The application to the brain-dead of federal research regulations would require full disclosure of the nature, purpose, and duration of the research as well as the benefits and risks, as well as requiring the research protocol to establish the need of the experiment (Martyn 1986, 25–27). This would give the final right to determine how and whether the body is used to the donors while protecting against infringement of respect for the dead, especially those who in some ways still appear alive (Gaylin 1974, 25).

Beyond potential subjects for research who have lost all brain functions are those who are permanently comatose or anencephalic: both of the latter have intact brainstems (and hence respire spontaneously) but have lost their higher brain functions or, in the case of the anencephalic newborn, never had such capability. Questions may arise about the involvement of such persons in therapeutic research (aimed at finding a means to improve their condition). The difficulties of obtaining consent for research with incompetent subjects are compounded here because the procedures often must be applied on a rapid basis in an emergency room (President's Commission 1983, 39).

The greatest difficulties, however, come with proposals that would involve using persons without higher brain functions as pure subjects (rather than as patient-subjects who might benefit personally from the research). For example, it has been suggested that anencephalic newborns could be useful in physiologic research or as a source of organs for transplantation into other infants and children (Harrison 1986). Approval for the use of this category of subject could be distinguished from using other persons who lack higher brain functions, because an anencephalic infant never had such functions (and will usually die rapidly, even with good support), unlike a fetus (who, if allowed to gestate, will normally develop higher brain functions) or a comatose adult (who may survive for a very long time even after losing all cognitive functions); thus, a foothold may exist against sliding down the "slippery slope." Nevertheless, the removal of organs from—or experimentation with—"a living human being, though one born dying" (Meilander 1986, 22) would violate not only generally accepted medical obligations to patients but also homicide statutes, which protect the lives of all live-born persons. Indeed, even steps to prolong the dying of an anencephalic infant in order to facilitate organ removal after death has occurred would go against the spirit of a conclusion of the National Commission that steps not be taken to "alter the duration of life of the nonviable fetus ex utero" (National Commission 1975, 68).

A FINAL WORD

Needless to say, this list of issues has barely skimmed the surface of the interesting problems that are raised by research with human subjects. One whole complicated area—whether, and if so how, to compensate injured research subjects (President's Commission 1982)—has hardly been touched on here, though the resolution of that issue could have profound consequences for the resolution of other issues, such as the use of subjects (e.g., children) without their consent. Moreover, the analysis has been primarily in ethical terms, with historical illustrations. Different features might have emerged, or sunk into the shadows, had another analytic light been cast on the topic—such as a sociological analysis emphasizing the role and power relationships of the participants in the research process, or a legal analysis focusing on the ways in which the law is capable or incapable of responding to the interests of various parties and how that, in turn, effects their behavior.

REFERENCES

Books and Articles

Alexander, L. "Limitations in Experimental Research on Human Beings." *Lex et Scienta* 3 (1966): 8–15.

Barber, B., J. Lally, J. Makarushka, and D. Sullivan. *Research on Human Subjects.* New York: Russell Sage Foundation, 1973.

Baumrind, D. "Nature and Definition of Informed Consent in Research Involving Deception." In *The Belmont Report,* Vol. 2 (Appendix) (National Commission for the Protection of Human Subjects of Biomedical and Behavioral Research). Washington, D.C.: Government Printing Office, 1978 23–42.

Beecher, H. K. "Surgery as Placebo." *JAMA* 176 (1961): 1102–1107.

———. "Ethics and Clinical Research." *New Engl J Med* 274 (1966): 1354–1360.

———. *Research and the Individual: Human Studies.* Boston: Little, Brown, 1970.

Bernard, C. *An Introduction to the Study of Experimental Medicine* (H. C. Greene, trans.). New York: Macmillan, 1927 (original edition 1865).

Blumgart, J. "The Medical Framework for Viewing the Problem of Human Experimentation." *Daedalus* 98 (1969): 248–274.

Bok, S. *Lying: Moral Choice in Public and Private Life.* New York: Pantheon Books, 1978.

Brandt, A. M. "Racism and Research: The Case of the Tuskegee Syphilis Study." *Hastings Cent Rep* 8, no. 6 (1978): 21–29.

Capron, A. M. "The Law of Genetic Therapy." In *The New Genetics and the Future of Man,* edited by M. Hamilton, 133–156. Grand Rapids, Mich.: Eerdmans Publishing, 1972.

———. "Legal Considerations Affecting Clinical Pharmacological Studies in Children." *Clin Res* 21 (1973): 141–150.

———. "Is Consent Always Necessary in Social Science Research?" In *Ethical Issues in Social Science Research,* edited by T. L. Beauchamp, R. R. Faden, R. J. Wallace, Jr., and L. Walters, 215–231. Baltimore: Johns Hopkins University Press, 1982.

———. "Determination of Death." In *Medicolegal Aspects of Critical Care,* edited by K. Benesch, N. S. Abramson, A. Grenvik, and A. Meisel, 109–132. Rockville, Md.: Aspen, 1986.

Cardon, P. V., F. W. Dommel, Jr., and R. Trumble. "Injuries to Research Subjects: A Survey of Investigators." *New Engl J Med* 295 (1976): 650–654.

Carson, R., J. Frias, and R. Melker. "Case Study: Research with Brain-Dead Children." *IRB* 3, no. 1 (1981): 5–6.

Chalmers, T. C. "The Ethics of Randomization as a Decision-Making Technique, and the Problem of Informed Consent." In *Contemporary Issues in Bioethics,* 2d ed., edited by T. Beauchamp and L. Walters, 538–541. Belmont, Calif.: Wadsworth, 1982.

Chalmers, T. C., J. B. Block, and S. Lee. "Controlled Studies in Clinical Cancer Research." *New Engl J Med* 287 (1972): 75–78.

Conference on the Proper Use of the Nazi Analogy in Ethical Debate. "Biomedical Ethics and the Shadow of Nazism." *Hastings Cent Rep* 6, no. 4 (Supp.) (1976): 1–16.

Congress of the United States, Office of Technology Assessment. 1978. *Assessing the Efficacy and Safety of Medical Technologies*. Washington, D.C.: Government Printing Office.

———. 1980. *Compensation for Vaccine-Related Injuries*. Washington, D.C.: Government Printing Office.

Connelly, R. J. "Deception and the Placebo Effect in Biomedical Research." *IRB* 9, no. 4 (1987): 5–7.

Cowan, D. "Human Experimentation: The Review Process in Practice." *Case W Res L Rev* 25 (1975): 533–564.

Curran, W. J. "Governmental Regulation of the Use of Human Subjects in Medical Research: The Approach of Two Federal Agencies." *Daedalus* 98 (1969): 542–594.

———. "Reasonableness and Randomization in Clinical Trials: Fundamental Law and Governmental Regulations." *New Engl J Med* 300 (1979): 1273–1275.

Des Jarlais, D. C., and S. R. Friedman. "AIDS Prevention Among IV Drug Users: Potential Conflicts between Research Design and Ethics." *IRB* 9, no. 1 (1987): 6–8.

Deutsch, E. *Das Recht der Klinischen Forschung am Menschen: Zulassigkeit und Folgen der Versuche am Menschen Dargest. Im Vergleich zu den amerikan. Beispiel und die internat. Regelungen*. Frankfurt-am-Main: Lang, 1979.

Eckholm, E. "Should the Rules Be Bent in an Epidemic?" *New York Times*, 13 July 1986, §IV, 30.

Eisenberg, L. "The Social Imperatives of Medical Research." *Science* 198 (1977): 1105–1110.

Fost, N. "Consent as a Barrier to Research." *New Engl J Med* 300 (1979): 1271–1273.

Fox, R. C. *The Courage to Fail*. Chicago: University of Chicago Press, 1974.

Forssmann, W. "The Role of Heart Catheterization and Angiocardiography in the Development of Modern Medicine." In *Nobel Lectures, Physiology or Medicine 1942–1962*. Amsterdam: Elsevier, 1964, 506–512.

Frankel, M. *The Public Health Service Guidelines Governing Research Involving Human Subjects: An Analysis of the Policy-Making Process*. Washington, D.C.: George Washington University, 1972.

Fried, C. *Medical Experimentation: Personal Integrity and Social Policy*. New York: American Elsevier, 1974.

Gaylin, W. "Harvesting the Dead." *Harpers* 249 (Sept. 1974): 23–26.

Gomer, R., J. Powell, and B. Roling. "Japan's Biological Weapons: 1930–1945." *Bull Atomic Sci* 37, no. 8 (1981): 43.

Grady, D. "Summary of Discussion on Ethical Perspectives." In *After Barney Clark*, edited by M. Shaw, 42–52. Austin: University of Texas Press, 1984.

Greene, B. "A Beach Party with the Delaware Hunks." *Chicago Tribune* 10 Feb. 1987, §5, 1.

Harrison, M. "The Anencephalic Newborn as Organ Donor." *Hastings Cent Rep* 16, no. 2 (1986): 21–22.

Holder, A. R. "Can a Court Order Participation in Research?" *IRB* 9, no. 4 (1987): 8–9.

"How U.S. Used Americans in Radiation Experiments." *San Francisco Chronicle*, 25 Oct. 1986, 2.

Ivy, A. C. "The History and Ethics of the Use of Human Subjects in Medical Experiments." *Science* 108 (1948): 1–8.

Jonas, H. "Philosophical Reflections on Experimenting with Human Subjects." *Daedalus* 98 (1969): 219–247.

Jonsen, A. R. "Do No Harm." *Ann Intern Med* 88 (1978): 827–832.

———. "The Selection of Patients." In *After Barney Clark*, edited by M. Shaw, 5–10. Austin: University of Texas Press, 1984.

Katz, J. "The Regulation of Human Experimentation in the United States—A Personal Odyssey." *IRB* 9, no. 1, (1987): 1–6.

Leskovac, H., and R. Delgado. "Protecting Autonomy and Personhood in Human Subjects Research." *S Ill Univ L J* 11 (1987): 1147–1158.

Levine, R. J. *Ethics and Regulation of Clinical Research.* Baltimore: Urban & Schwarzenberg, 1986.

Lubasch, A. H. "$700,000 Award Is Made in '53 Secret Test Death." *New York Times,* 6 May 1987, B–3.

Martyn, S. "Using the Brain Dead for Medical Research." *Utah L Rev* (1986): 1–28.

Medical Consultants on the Diagnosis of Death. "Guidelines for the Determination of Death: Report to the President's Commission for the Study of Ethical Problems in Medicine and Biomedical and Behavioral Research." *JAMA* 246 (1981): 2184–2187.

Meilander, G. "The Anencephalic Newborn as Organ Donor." *Hastings Cent Rep* 16, no. 2 (1986): 22–23.

National Advisory Health Council. Stenographic Transcript of the Sept. 28, 1965, Meeting. *Quoted in* Frankel, 1972.

National Commission for the Protection of Human Subjects of Biomedical and Behavioral Research. *Report and Recommendations: Research on the Fetus.* Washington, D.C.: Government Printing Office, 1975.

———. *Report and Recommendations: Research Involving Children.* Washington, D.C.: Government Printing Office, 1977.

———. *The Belmont Report.* Washington, D.C.: Government Printing Office, 1978a.

———. *Report and Recommendations: Institutional Review Boards.* Washington, D.C.: Government Printing Office, 1978b.

Pappworth, M. H. *Human Guinea Pigs: Experimentation on Man.* Boston: Beacon Press, 1968.

Pattullo, E. L. "Institutional Review Boards and the Freedom to Take Risks." *New Engl J Med* 307 (1982): 1156–1159.

Powell, J. "A Hidden Chapter in History." *Bull Atomic Sci* 37, no. 8 (1981): 44–52.

President's Commission for the Study of Ethical Problems in Medicine and Biomedical and Behavioral Research. *Protecting Human Subjects: The Adequacy and Uniformity of Federal Rules and Their Implementation.* Washington, D.C.: Government Printing Office, 1981.

———. *Compensating for Research Injuries.* Washington, D.C.: Government Printing Office, 1982.

———. *Implementing Human Research Regulations.* Washington, D.C.: Government Printing Office, 1983.

Prinzmetal, M. "On the Humane Treatment of Charity Patients." *Med Trib,* 22 Sept. 1965, 15.

Rawls, J. *A Theory of Justice.* Cambridge, Mass.: Harvard University Press, 1971.

Sass, H-M. "Reichsundschreiben 1931: Pre-Nuremberg German Regulations Concerning New Therapy and Human Experimentation." *J Med and Phil* 8 (1983): 99–111.

Tuskegee Syphilis Study Ad Hoc Panel to the Department of Health, Education, and Welfare. *Final Report.* Washington, D.C.: Public Health Service, 1973.

U.S. Senate. *Project MK-ULTRA, The CIA's Program of Research in Behavioral Modification, Joint Hearings Before the Senate Select Comm. on Intelligence and the Subcomm. on Health and Scientific Research of the Senate Comm. on Human Resources.* 95th Cong., 1st Sess. 75, 1977.

Veatch, R. M. "Justice and Research Design: The Case for a Semi-Randomization Clinical Trial." *Clinical Research* 31 (1983): 12–22.

Veressayev, V. *The Memoirs of a Physician* (S. Linden, trans.). New York: Knopf, 1916 (original edition 1901).

Warren, J. W., J. Sobal, J. H. Tenney, J. M. Hoopes, D. Damron, S. Levenson, B. R. DeForge, and H. L. Muncie, Jr. "Informed Consent by Proxy: An Issue in Research with Elderly Patients." *New Engl J Med* 315 (1986): 1124–1128.

World Medical Association. *Declaration of Helsinki*, 1975.

Statutes, Regulations, and Cases

Arizona. *Revised Statutes Annotated*. St. Paul, Minn.: West Publishing, 1986.

Arkansas. *Statutes Annotated* (Supp.). Charlottesville, Va.: Michie, 1985.

Barrett v. Hoffman. 1981. 521 F.Supp. 307 (S.D.N.Y.).

California. *Health and Safety Code*. St. Paul, Minn.: West Publishing, 1984.

Der Minister der geistlichen. Anweisung an die Vorsteher der Kliniken, Polikliniken under sinstigen Krankenanstakten. *Centralblatt der gesamten Unterrichtsverwaltung in Preussen*. Berlin: Prussian Government, 1901, 188–189.

FDA (U.S. Food and Drug Administration). Protection of Human Subjects; Standards for Institutional Review Boards for Clinical Investigations. *Code of Federal Regulations*. Title 21: Part 56, issued in *Fed. Register* 46 (27 Jan. 1981): 8958–8979.

Food and Drug Amendments. Act of 10 Oct. 1962, Pub. Law No. 87–781, *amending* 21 U.S.C. §355, 1962.

HHS (U.S. Dept. of Health and Human Services). "Protection of Human Subjects." *Code of Federal Regulations* 45, Part 46, issued in *Fed. Register* 46 (26 Jan. 1981): 8386–8391 and 48 (4 March 1983): 9269–9270.

Louisiana. *Revised Statutes Annotated* (Supp.). St. Paul, Minn.: West Publishing, 1986.

Margaret S. v. Edwards 1980 488 F. Supp. 181 (E.D.La.).

Massachusetts. *General Laws Annotated*. St. Paul, Minn.: West Publishing, 1986.

Mink v. University of Chicago. 1978. 460 F. Supp. 713 (N.D. Ill.).

National Research Act. 1974. Pub. Law 93–348, 42 USC 289L–3(a).

Nevin v. United States. 1983. 696 F.2d 1229 (9th Cir.).

New York. *Public Health Law*. Albany, N.Y.: McKinney, 1985.

Pierce v. Ortho Pharmaceutical Corp. 1980. 417 A.2d 505 (N.J.).

South Dakota. *Codified Laws Annotated*. Indianapolis: Allen Smith, 1978.

U.S. Public Health Service. *Clinical Research and Investigation Involving Human Beings*, Policy and Procedure Order No. 129, 8 Feb. 1966a.

U.S. Public Health Service. *Clinical Research and Investigation Involving Human Beings*, Policy and Procedure Order No. 129, Revised Supplement No. 2, 12 Dec. 1966b.

Utah. *Criminal Code Annotated*. Indianapolis: Allen Smith, 1982.

APPENDIX 1

THE NUREMBERG CODE

Source: Nuremberg Military Tribunals (1949, 181–82).

The great weight of evidence before us is to the effect that certain types of medical experiments on human beings, when kept within reasonable well-defined bounds, conform to the ethics of the medical profession generally. The protagonists of the practice of human experimentation justify their views on the basis that such experiments yield results for the good of society that are unprocurable by other methods or means of study. All agree, however, that certain basic principles must be observed in order to satisfy moral, ethical and legal concepts:

1. The voluntary consent of the human subject is absolutely essential.

This means that the person involved should have legal capacity to give consent; should be so situated as to be able to exercise free power of choice, without the intervention of any element of force, fraud, deceit, duress, overreaching, or other ulterior form of constraint or coercion; and should have sufficient knowledge and comprehension of the elements of the subject matter involved as to enable him to make an understanding and enlightened decision. This latter element requires that before the acceptance of an affirmative decision by the experimental subject there should be made known to him the nature, duration, and purpose of the experiment; the method and means by which it is to be conducted; all inconveniences and hazards reasonably to be expected; and the effects upon his health or person which may possibly come from his participation in the experiment.

The duty and responsibility for ascertaining the quality of the consent rests upon each individual who initiates, directs or engages in the experiment. It is a personal duty and responsibility which may not be delegated to another with impunity.

2. The experiment should be such as to yield fruitful results for the good of society, unprocurable by other methods or means of study, and not random and unnecessary in nature.

3. The experiment should be designed and based on the results of animal experimentation and a knowledge of the natural history of the disease or other problem under study that the anticipated results will justify the performance of the experiment.

4. The experiment should be so conducted as to avoid all unnecessary physical and mental suffering and injury.

5. The experiment should be conducted where there is an a priori reason to believe that death or disabling injury will occur except, perhaps, in those experiments where the experimental physicians also serve as subjects.

6. The degree of risk to be taken should never exceed that determined by the humanitarian importance of the problem to be solved by the experiment.

7. Proper preparations should be made and adequate facilities provided to protect the experimental subject against even remote possibilities of injury, disability, or death.

8. The experiment should be conducted only by scientifically qualified persons. The highest degree of skill and care should be required through all stages of the experiment of those who conduct or engage in the experiment.

9. During the course of the experiment the human subject should be at liberty to bring the experiment to an end if he has reached the physical or mental state where continuation of the experiment seems to him to be impossible.

10. During the course of the experiment the scientist in charge must be prepared to terminate the experiment at any stage, if he has probable cause to believe, in the exercise of the good faith, superior skill and careful judgment required of him that a continuation of the experiment is likely to result in injury, disability, or death to the experimental subject. . . .

APPENDIX 2

DEPARTMENT OF HEALTH AND HUMAN SERVICES, BASIC HHS POLICY FOR PROTECTION OF HUMAN RESEARCH SUBJECTS

Source: 46 FR 8386, January 26, 1981, 48 FR 9269, March 4, 1983.

§46.101 To what do these regulations apply?

(a) Except as provided in paragraph (b) of this section, this subpart applies to all research involving human subjects conducted by the Department of Health and Human Services or funded in whole or in part by a Department grant, contract, cooperative agreement or fellowship.

(1) This includes research conducted by Department employees, except each Principal Operating Component head may adopt such nonsubstantive, procedural modifications as may be appropriate from an administrative standpoint.

(2) It also includes research conducted or funded by the Department of Health and Human Services outside the United States, but in appropriate circumstances, the Secretary may, under paragraph (e) of this section waive the applicability of some or all of the requirements of these regulations for research of this type.

(b) Research activities in which the only involvement of human subjects will be in one or more of the following categories are exempt from these regulations unless the research is covered by other subparts of this part:

(1) Research conducted in established or commonly accepted educational settings, involving normal educational practices, such as (i) research on regular and special education instructional strategies, or (ii) research on the effectiveness of or the comparison among instructional techniques, curricula, or classroom management methods.

(2) Research involving the use of educational tests (cognitive, diagnostic, aptitude, achievement), if information taken from these sources is recorded in such a manner that subjects cannot be identified, directly or through identifiers linked to the subjects.

(3) Research involving survey or interview procedures, except where all of the following conditions exist: (i) responses are recorded in such a manner that the human subjects can be identified, directly or through identifiers linked to the subjects, (ii) the subject's responses, if they became known outside the research, could reasonably place the subject at risk of criminal or civil liability or be damaging to the subject's financial standing or employability, and (iii) the research deals with sensitive aspects of the subject's own behavior, such as illegal conduct, drug use, sexual behavior, or use of alcohol. All research involving survey or interview procedures is exempt, without exception, when the respondents are elected or appointed public officials or candidates for public office.

(4) Research involving the observation (including observation by participants) of public behavior, except where all of the following conditions exist: (i) observations are recorded in such a manner that the human subjects can be identified, directly or through identifiers linked to the subjects, (ii) the observations recorded about the individual, if they became known outside the research, could reasonably place the subject at risk of criminal or civil liability or be damaging to the subject's financial standing or employability, and (iii) the research deals with sensitive aspects of the subject's own behavior such as illegal conduct, drug use, sexual behavior, or use of alcohol.

(5) Research involving the collection or study of existing data, documents, records, pathological specimens, or diagnostic specimens, if these sources are publicly available or if the information is recorded by the investigator in such a manner that subjects cannot be identified, directly or through identifiers linked to the subjects.

(6) Unless specifically required by statute (and except to the extent specified in paragraph (i)), research and demonstration projects which are conducted by or subject to the approval of the Department of Health and Human Services, and which are designed to study, evaluate, or otherwise examine: (i) programs under the Social Security Act, or other public benefit or service programs; (ii) procedures for obtaining benefits or services under those programs; (iii) possible changes in or alternatives to those programs or procedures; or (iv) possible changes in methods or levels of payment for benefits or services under those programs.

(c) The Secretary has final authority to determine whether a particular activity is covered by these regulations.

(d) The Secretary may require specific research activities or classes of research activities conducted or funded by the Department, but not otherwise covered by these regulations, comply with some or all of these regulations.

(e) The Secretary may also waive applicability of these regulations to specific research activities or classes of research activities, otherwise covered by these regulations. Notices of these actions will be published in the *Federal Register* as they occur.

(f) No individual may receive Department funding for research covered by these regulations unless the individual is affiliated with or sponsored by an institution which assumes responsibility for the research under an assurance satisfying the requirements of this part, or the individual makes other arrangements with the Department.

(g) Compliance with these regulations will in no way render inapplicable pertinent federal, state, or local laws or regulations.

(h) Each subpart of these regulations contains a separate section describing to what the subpart applies. Research which is covered by more than one subpart shall comply with all applicable subparts.

(i) If, following review of proposed research activities that are exempt from these regulations under paragraph (b)(6), the Secretary determines that a research or demonstration project presents a danger to the physical, mental, or emotional well-being of a participant or subject of the research or demonstration project, then federal funds may not be expended for such a project without the written, informed consent of each participant or subject.

§46.102 DEFINITIONS

(e) "Research" means a systematic investigation designed to develop or contribute to generalizable knowledge. Activities which meet this definition constitute "research" for purposes of these regulations, whether or not they are supported or funded under a program which is considered research for other purposes. For example, some "demonstration" and "service" programs may include research activities.

(f) "Human subject" means a living individual about whom an investigator (whether professional or student) conducting research obtains (1) data through intervention or interaction with the individual, or (2) identifiable private information. "Intervention" includes both physical procedures by which data are gathered (for example, venipuncture) and manipulations of the subject or the subject's environment that are performed for research purposes. "Interaction" includes communication or interpersonal contact between investigator and subject. "Private information" includes information about behavior that occurs in a context in which an individual can reasonably expect that no observation or recording is taking place, and information which has been provided for specific purposes by an individual and which the individual can reasonably expect will not be made public (for example, a medical record). Private information must be individually identifiable (i.e., the identity of the subject is or may readily be ascertained by the investigator or associated with the information) in order for obtaining the information to constitute research involving human subjects.

(g) "Minimal risk" means that the risks of harm anticipated in the proposed research are not greater, considering probability and magnitude, than those ordinarily encountered in daily life or during the performance of routine physical or psychological examinations or tests.

§46.103 ASSURANCES

(a) Each institution engaged in research covered by these regulations shall provide written assurance satisfactory to the Secretary that it will comply with the requirements set forth in these regulations.

(b) The Department will conduct or fund research covered by these regulations only if the institution has an assurance approved as provided in this section, and only if the institution has certified to the Secretary that the research has been reviewed and approved by an IRB provided for in the assurance, and will be subject to continuing review by the IRB. This assurance shall at a minimum include:

(1) A statement of principles governing the institution in the discharge of its responsibilities for protecting the rights and welfare of human subjects of research conducted at or sponsored by the institution, regardless of source of funding. This may include an appropriate existing code, declaration, or statement of ethical principles, or a statement formulated by the institution itself. This requirement does not preempt provisions of these regulations applicable to department-funded research and is not applicable to any research in an exempt category listed in §46.101.

(2) Designation of one or more IRBs established in accordance with the requirements of this subpart, and for which provisions are made for meeting space and sufficient staff to support the IRB's review and recordkeeping duties.

(3) A list of the IRB members identified by name; earned degrees; representative capacity; indications of experience such as board certifications, licenses, etc., sufficient to describe each member's chief anticipated contributions to IRB deliberations; and any employment or other relationship between each member and the institution; for example: full-time employee, part-time employee, member of governing panel or board, stockholder, paid or unpaid consultant. Changes in IRB membership shall be reported to the Secretary.

(4) Written procedures which the IRB will follow (i) for conducting its initial and continuing review of research and for reporting its findings and actions to the investigator and the institution; (ii) for determining which projects require review more often than annually and which projects need verification from sources other than the investigators that no material changes have occurred since previous IRB review; (iii) for insuring prompt reporting to the IRB of proposed changes in a research activity, and for insuring that changes in approved research, during the period for which IRB approval has already been given, may not be initiated without IRB review and approval except where necessary to eliminate apparent immediate hazards to the subject; and (iv) for insuring prompt reporting to the IRB and to the Secretary of unanticipated problems involving risks to subjects or others.

§46.107 IRB MEMBERSHIP

(a) Each IRB shall have at least five members, with varying backgrounds to promote complete and adequate review of research activities commonly conducted by the institution. The IRB shall be sufficiently qualified through the experience and expertise of its members, and the diversity of the members' backgrounds including consideration of the racial and cultural backgrounds of members and sensitivity to such issues as community attitudes, to promote respect for its advice and counsel in safeguarding the rights and welfare of human subjects. In addition to possessing the professional competence necessary to review specific research activities, the IRB shall be able to ascertain the acceptability of proposed research in terms of institutional commitments and regulations, applicable law, and standards of professional conduct and practice. The IRB shall therefore include persons knowledgeable in these areas. If an IRB regularly reviews research that involves a vulnerable category of subjects, including but not limited to subjects covered by other subparts of this part, the IRB shall include one or more individuals who are primarily concerned with the welfare of these subjects.

(b) No IRB may consist entirely of men or entirely of women, or entirely of members of one profession.

(c) Each IRB shall include at least one member whose primary concerns are in nonscientific areas; for example: lawyers, ethicists, members of the clergy.

(d) Each IRB shall include at least one member who is not otherwise affiliated with the institution and who is not part of the immediate family of a person who is affiliated with the institution.

(e) No IRB may have a member participating in the IRB's initial or continuing review of any project in which the member has a conflicting interest, except to provide information requested by the IRB.

(f) An IRB may, in its discretion, invite individuals with competence in special areas to assist in the review of complex issues which require expertise beyond or in addition to that available on the IRB. These individuals may not vote with the IRB.

§46.111 CRITERIA FOR IRB APPROVAL OF RESEARCH

(a) In order to approve research covered by these regulations the IRB shall determine that all of the following requirements are satisfied:

(1) Risks to subjects are minimized: (i) By using procedures which are consistent with sound research design and which do not unnecessarily expose subjects to risk, and (ii) whenever appropriate, by using procedures already being performed on the subjects for diagnostic or treatment purposes.

(2) Risks to subjects are reasonable in relation to anticipated benefits, if any, to subjects, and the importance of the knowledge that may reasonably be expected to result. In evaluating risks and benefits, the IRB should consider only those risks and benefits that may result from the research (as distinguished from risks and benefits of therapies subjects would receive even if not participating in the research). The IRB should not consider possible long-range effects of applying knowledge gained in the research (for example, the possible effects of the research on public policy) as among those research risks that fall within the purview of its responsibility.

(3) Selection of subjects is equitable. In making this assessment the IRB should take into account the purposes of the research and the setting in which the research will be conducted.

(4) Informed consent will be sought from each prospective subject or the subject's legally authorized representative, in accordance with, and to the extent required by §46.116.

(5) Informed consent will be appropriately documented, in accordance with, and to the extent required by §46.117.

(6) Where appropriate, the research plan makes adequate provision for monitoring the data collected to insure the safety of subjects.

(7) Where appropriate, there are adequate provisions to protect the privacy of subjects and to maintain the confidentiality of data.

(b) Where some or all of the subjects are likely to be vulnerable to coercion or undue influence, such as persons with acute or severe physical or mental illness, or persons who are economically or educationally disadvantaged, appropriate additional safeguards have been included in the study to protect the rights and welfare of these subjects.

§46.116 GENERAL REQUIREMENTS FOR INFORMED CONSENT

Except as provided elsewhere in this or other subparts, no investigator may involve a human being as a subject in research covered by these regulations unless the investigator has obtained the legally effective informed consent of the subject or the subject's legally authorized representative. An investigator shall seek such consent only under circumstances that provide the prospective subject or the representative sufficient opportunity to consider whether or not to participate and that minimize the possibility of coercion or undue influence. The information that is given to the subject or the representative shall be in language understandable to the subject or the representative. No informed consent, whether oral or written, may include any exculpatory language through which the subject or the representative is made to waive or appear to waive any of the subject's legal rights, or releases or appears to release the investigator, the sponsor, the institution or its agents from liability for negligence.

(a) Basic elements of informed consent. Except as provided in paragraph (c) or (d) of this section, in seeking informed consent the following information shall be provided to each subject:

(1) A statement that the study involves research, an explanation of the purposes of the research and the expected duration of the subject's participation, a description of the procedures to be followed, and identification of any procedures which are experimental;

(2) A description of any reasonably foreseeable risks or discomforts to the subject;

(3) A description of any benefits to the subject or to others which may reasonably be expected from the research;

(4) A disclosure of appropriate alternative procedures or courses of treatment, if any, that might be advantageous to the subject;

(5) A statement describing the extent, if any, to which confidentiality of records identifying the subject will be maintained;

(6) For research involving more than minimal risk, an explanation as to whether any compensation and an explanation as to whether any medical treatments are available if injury occurs and, if so, what they consist of, or where further information may be obtained;

(7) An explanation of whom to contact for answers to pertinent questions about the research and research subjects' rights, and whom to contact in the event of a research-related injury to the subject; and

(8) A statement that participation is voluntary, refusal to participate will involve no penalty or loss of benefits to which the subject is otherwise entitled, and the subject may discontinue participation at any time without penalty or loss of benefits to which the subject is otherwise entitled.

(b) Additional elements of informed consent. When appropriate, one or more of the following elements of information shall also be provided to each subject:

(1) A statement that the particular treatment or procedure may involve risks to the subject (or to the embryo or fetus, if the subject is or may become pregnant) which are currently unforeseeable;

(2) Anticipated circumstances under which the subject's participation may be terminated by the investigator without regard to the subject's consent;

(3) Any additional costs to the subject that may result from participation in the research;

(4) The consequences of a subject's decision to withdraw from the research and procedures for orderly termination of participation by the subject;

(5) A statement that significant new findings developed during the course of the research which may relate to the subject's willingness to continue participation will be provided to the subject; and

(6) The approximate number of subjects involved in the study.

(c) An IRB may approve a consent procedure which does not include, or which alters, some or all of the elements of informed consent set forth above, or waive the requirement to obtain informed consent provided the IRB finds and documents that:

(1) The research or demonstration project is to be conducted by or subject to the approval of state or local government officials and is designed to study, evaluate, or otherwise examine: (i) programs under the Social Security Act, or other public benefit or service programs; (ii) procedures for obtaining benefits or services under those programs; (iii) possible changes in or alternatives to those programs or procedures; or (iv) possible changes in methods or levels of payment for benefits or services under those programs; and

(2) The research could not practicably be carried out without the waiver or alteration.

(d) an IRB may approve a consent procedure which does not include, or which alters, some or all of the elements of informed consent set forth above, or waive the requirements to obtain informed consent provided the IRB finds and documents that:

(1) The research involves no more than minimal risk to the subjects;

(2) The waiver or alteration will not adversely affect the rights and welfare of the subjects;

(3) The research could not practicably be carried out without the waiver or alteration; and

(4) whenever appropriate, the subjects will be provided with additional pertinent information after participation.

(e) The informed consent requirements in these regulations are not intended to preempt any applicable federal, state, or local laws which require additional information to be disclosed in order for informed consent to be legally effective.

(f) Nothing in these regulations is intended to limit the authority of a physician to provide emergency medical care, to the extent the physician is permitted to do so under applicable federal, state, or local law.

§46.117 DOCUMENTATION OF INFORMED CONSENT

(a) Except as provided in paragraph (c) of this section, informed consent shall be documented by the use of a written consent form approved by the IRB and signed by the subject or the subject's legally authorized representative. A copy shall be given to the person signing the form.

(c) An IRB may waive the requirement for the investigator to obtain a signed consent form for some or all subjects if it finds either:

(1) That the only record linking the subject and the research would be the consent document and the principal risk would be potential harm resulting from a breach of confidentiality. Each subject will be asked whether the subject wants documentation linking the subject with the research, and the subject's wishes will govern; or

(2) That the research presents no more than minimal risk of harm to subjects and involves no procedures for which written consent is normally required outside of the research context.

In cases where the documentation requirement is waived, the IRB may require the investigator to provide subjects with a written statement regarding the research.

DISCUSSION QUESTIONS

1. If a physician decides to withold information from a patient about the dangers of the medication the patient is taking in order to protect the patient from harm, what moral principle underlies the decision? Is such a practice justified? What moral principles would justify opposing such a practice?

2. When a physician decides to try an innovative therapy outside of a research protocol, what moral principle would justify such a practice? Should such a practice ever be acceptable outside of a protocol? If so, ought it to be governed by standard rules governing human subjects' research including review by an IRB?

3. In what ways does the principle of justice govern research subject recruitment and research design? Is it ever justified to compromise research design in order to select subjects more fairly or give subjects opportunities to be better off? If so, when?

4. If the ethics of research requires that subjects give a reasonably informed consent, on what grounds, if any, can the following types of information be withheld from subjects: the fact that subjects are randomized? The presence of a placebo in the research design? The presence of deception in the research? The existence of trivial risks that subjects can be expected to know about (such as the pain of an injection)? The fact that medical records will be searched in order to gain research information?

5. Under what circumstances, if any, is it acceptable to conduct research on fetuses: when the pregnant woman is likely to gain? When the fetus has a chance to benefit? When the fetus will not be carried to term? When the fetus has already been aborted?

7

Informed Consent

Tom L. Beauchamp

SUMMARY

This chapter commences with a discussion of the history of informed consent in medical ethics and research ethics. Even in the early writings of the Hippocratic period, the view was held that monitoring medical information in encounters with patients was a basic moral responsibility of physicians. However, these writings had virtually nothing to say about informed consent and thus have contributed little to our understanding of this concept. Informed consent obligations and requirements have emerged from influential cases, potential developments, regulatory interventions, government-appointed ethics commissions, and the occurrence of intra-professional events since the end of World War II to date.

The second section of the chapter discusses the concept and elements of informed consent. It presents several assumptions regarding the notion of informed consent which are commonly held by patients, physicians, and other health-care professionals. Five key elements are fundamental to the concept of informed consent: disclosure, comprehension, voluntariness, competence, and consent. Based on these elements a definition of informed consent is discussed. One can confidently presume that an act is an informed consent if a patient or subject agrees to an intervention based on an understanding of relevant information, the consent is not controlled by influences that engineer the outcome, and the consent given was intended to be a consent and therefore qualified as a permission for an intervention.

The mere listing of these elements and their subsequent transformation into a definition of informed consent may be problematic and confusing. Formulating a definition of informed consent is complicated primarily because there exists at least two common, entrenched and irreducibly different meanings of informed consent. Broadly, these meanings can be categorized as autonomous choice and institutional consent.

The next topic of discussion in this chapter involves the doctrine of informed consent that is derived from the common law. Here the focus is primarily on disclosure and liability for injury. This doctrine has been more influential as an authoritative statement and source of reflection than any other body of thought on the subject.

Next the chapter turns to the quality of the consent obtained. Questions include: How well is the information delivered? How well does the patient/subject understand? And how freely is consent given? The author examines the even more difficult issue of obtaining consent from an incompetent or otherwise vulnerable subject.

Finally, various justifications that are made for not obtaining consent are examined. These might include patient incompetence and therapeutic privilege (the notion that consent be foregone to protect the patient or subject from harm).

The practice of obtaining informed consent has its history predominantly in medicine and medical research, where the disclosure of information as well as the withholding of information are aspects of daily encounters between patient and physician. Although discussions of disclosure and justified nondisclosure have played a role in the history of medical ethics since the Hippocratic writings, the history of informed consent is not ancient. The term "informed consent" never appeared in any literature until 1957, and discussions of the concept as it is used today began only around 1972. Concomitantly a revolution has occurred in the last two decades in the discussion of the patient-physician interaction—a revolution that has increasingly moved from a narrow focus on the physician's obligation to disclose information to the quality of a patient's or subject's understanding and consent.

The forces creating this revolution have been largely, but not entirely, external to medicine and biomedical research and have occurred in the last half of the twentieth century. As long as the "beneficence model" remained the unchallenged model for medical ethics, physicians were able to rely almost exclusively on their own judgment about their patients' needs for information and consultation. Gradually, external forces began in the mid-twentieth century to challenge various assumptions in this model. These forces worked in tandem with widespread social developments. Thus, for example, the Patient's Bill of Rights was connected to various consumer and civil-rights movements that were demanding increased rights to make free and informed decisions.

On the one hand, we cannot hope to understand the arrival of the issue of informed consent in the United States without an awareness of the historical and conceptual background of controversy and its attempted or actual resolution. Accordingly, this text makes historical explanations of how specific controversies, as we know them today, emerged and developed in the United States. On the other hand, one result of these developments has been to introduce both confusion and constructive change in American medicine as that profession struggles to meet unprecedented challenges to traditional medical ethics, and there is thus an increased need for innovative moral thinking that will revise our traditional understanding of informed consent obligations.

In recent years interest in and contributions to the analysis of the concept of informed consent have emerged from many disciplines besides medicine, including other health professions, law, the social and behavioral sciences, and moral philosophy. Law and philosophy have played an especially prominent role in the analysis and revision of more traditional understandings and practices, especially through the opinions of courts and the subsequent analysis of those opinions. Nevertheless, despite its prominent role, the legal vision of informed consent has such severe limitations for medical ethics that it will play only a small part in the analysis below.

We have a strong tendency in the United States to look to legal and regulatory approaches to informed consent for the relevant standards, but it has become progressively clear that the focus of statutory law, case law, and regulatory guideline has been on disclosure and that this focus is misguided. Problems about the quality and adequacy of consent probably cannot be resolved unless conventional disclosure standards are abandoned and a shift occurs toward quality of understanding in the subject, patient, and representative. From this perspective, the central problems about informed consent are issues of communication rather than the abstract and disembodied issues about proper legal standards of disclosure that have so long dominated the subject literature.

MEDICAL ETHICS AND RESEARCH ETHICS

There have been many pioneers of the idea that monitoring medical information in encounters with patients is a basic moral responsibility of physicians. These pioneering ventures are found in the classic historical documents in the history of medicine such as the Hippocratic writings (fifth to fourth century, B.C.), Percival's *Medical Ethics* (1803), the first *Code of Ethics* (1846–1947) of the American Medical Association, as well as in the historically significant didactic writings on medical ethics in the eighteenth and nineteenth centuries, sometimes referred to as the "learned" tradition, comprising discursive study of medical ethics through treatises and books.

Unfortunately these codes and writings have virtually nothing to say about informed consent, and thus have contributed far less to our understanding of this notion than the law. Most of the well known codes and writings are fashioned for clinical medicine, but informed consent has never taken root in medicine by finding its way into the routines of clinical practice. Although codes, regulations, and professional rules in recent years have been extensively used to govern research involving human subjects, even this history never focused on problems of informed consent.

Initial developments in the history of protections for human subjects were directed at eliminating dangerous research that took unfair advantage of subjects' confidence in the physician-patient relationship. Moral requirements were thus adopted to protect individual subjects from harm, exploitation, and injustice. It was only after problems involving the autonomy of subjects gradually grew more insistent, and the idea of respecting autonomy gained equal recognition, that informed consent began to play a central role in research ethics.

Informed consent obligations and requirements, as they have developed in the United States, have emerged and developed through influential cases, political developments, regulatory interventions, government-appointed ethics commissions, and intraprofessional developments extending from the end of World War II to date. It seems likely that this history is still in its early stages and that there is vast room for new developments and synthesis of prior developments. The histories of informed consent in research and in clinical medicine have developed largely as separate threads in a larger fabric of medical ethics, and these threads have never been carefully interwoven.

In therapeutic research the benefits and harms presented to subjects parallel those in medicine—the cure, removal, or prevention of pain, suffering, disability, and disease for the persons involved in the research. In nontherapeutic research, the subjects' interests are less critical because the positive benefit sought by the scientist is new knowledge. Often (but not necessarily) this knowledge is desired because it is expected to contribute to the resolution of important medical or social problems. Therapeutic and nontherapeutic research thus differ in the kinds of benefits each hopes to achieve, and it has been rightly assumed that protections both of consent and of peer review must be more stringent in the research setting than in the clinical context.

Although in both medical ethics and research ethics there is an equally strong imperative to avoid harming the subject, therapeutic research may legitimately present increased potential for harms if they are balanced by a commensurate possibility of benefits to the subject. Here a subject might be permitted to consent to a level of risk that would be impermissible (even if consented to) in the nontherapeutic research context. But in research it has been generally agreed since the late 1960s that standards should be more stringent because there is an increased danger of exploiting subjects in research to gain the investigator's own ends.

This cautious premise should not be understood as denying that risks of harm presented by interventions must constantly be weighed against possible benefits for patients, subjects, or the public interest in both medical practice and research. The physician who professes to "do no harm" is not pledging never to cause harm but rather to strive to create a positive balance of goods over inflicted harms. Not surprisingly, there are dimensions of this balancing that pertain directly to informed consent requirements. In clinical contexts, for example, this balancing can also present situations in which health-care professionals and patients differ in their assessments of the professional's obligations.

THE CONCEPT AND ELEMENTS OF INFORMED CONSENT

Both the concept of informed consent and the practice of obtaining consent are social phenomena that cannot be adequately appreciated or evaluated independent of knowledge of the historical forces that have produced them. No analysis of the concept of informed consent can be distanced from the contexts in which practices of informed consent arose and flourished. However, these contexts often leave considerable vagueness around the term "informed consent," and there is therefore a need to sharpen the concept so that its meaning is clear and faithful to the central meaning of the concept.

Some recent commentators on informed consent in clinical medicine (notably Katz 1984, 86–87; President's Commission 1983, I, 15) tend to equate the idea of informed consent with a model of "shared decisionmaking" between doctor and patient, so that "informed consent" and "mutual decisionmaking" are treated as virtually synonymous terms. Although there is, of course, an historical relationship in clinical medicine between medical decisionmaking and informed consent, it is inaccurate to treat informed consent and shared decisionmaking as synonymous concepts. Informed consent is not restricted to clinical medicine. The term is used no less frequently for research contexts where a model of shared decisionmaking is frequently inappropriate. But even in clinical contexts the personal dynamics and informational interactions through which medical interventions are selected should be distinguished from a subject's or patient's act of autonomously authorizing the intervention.

Presumptions About the Concept

The claim that something is an informed consent or that an informed consent was obtained cannot always be taken at face value. Before we can confidently infer that what appears to be or is called an informed consent is a bona fide instance of informed consent, we need to know what we are seeking. This inquiry requires criteria of what will qualify for the label "informed consent," given the many different criteria that might be proposed.

This task is more difficult than is generally appreciated. If overdemanding criteria of either the nature of information or the nature of consent were employed, it would be impossible to find any practice of informed consent at any time. To avoid this problem this text uses criteria that are neither unreasonably demanding nor so weak as to encompass all discussions and arrangements between professional and patient or subject. Thus, prior to offering any tightened or revisionary analysis of informed consent, presume that an act is an informed consent if a patient or subject agrees to an intervention based on an understanding of relevant information, if the consent is not controlled by influences that engineer the outcome, and if the consent given is intended to be a consent and therefore qualifies as a permission for an intervention.

Many exchanges between a physician and a patient that are often *called* informed consents would be excluded by even this simple conception. For example, truthfulness in disclosure where a patient does not object to anything the physician says has often been taken to be the central matter in informed consent, as if the patient's silence were an implicit authorization to proceed. But a truthful disclosure does not permit any inference whatever about the existence of consent solicitations or practices. Similarly, much of the data available about what are labelled "consent" practices in hospitals or in earlier periods of history are not sufficient to provide adequate evidence about the actual nature and quality of "consents" obtained, and therefore we cannot claim without further evidence that these events involved acts, practices, or policies of consent. Perhaps what some physicians mean by "informed consent" in particular cases is that the patient's signature is obtained on a consent form, or that some kind of disclosure was made. Under the tentative definition above, the mere act of signing a form cannot qualify as an informed consent.

Contemporary Presumptions in Medicine

Interesting data about the meaning of informed consent is found in a survey of physicians conducted by Louis Harris (Harris 1982, 302), which asked physicians "What does the term informed consent mean to you?" Only 26 percent of physicians indicated that informed consent had anything to do with patients' giving permission, consenting, or agreeing to treatment; only 9 percent indicated that it involved patients' making a choice or stating a preference about his or her treatment. Like lawyers and courts, the overwhelming majority of the doctors surveyed appeared to recognize only the *information-providing* dimension of informed consent as the criterion of informed consent. That is, they view informed consent as the explanation given to a patient about the nature of his or her condition and treatment, and recognition by the patient of what is taking place.

If informed consent means only telling things to an attentive patient, and not asking anything (such as questions or permission) of the patient, how are we to interpret claims by physicians that they regularly "obtain consents" from patients before medical procedures? The answer is that such claims are entirely unreliable unless we know the actual procedures involved in some detail. Matters may be even worse than they appear: perhaps all physicians understand by informed consent is that the patient's signature was obtained, or perhaps they mean only that some kind of disclosure was made. This interpretation fits better with the results of studies of informed consent that proved more negative. Some studies failed to find any sizeable evidence of informed consent in clinical medicine; other studies found little evidence that the consents obtained are meaningful exercises of informed choice by patients (Lidz and Meisel 1982, 333–340; Faden and Beauchamp 1986, 98–100).

The Authority of Oaths, Codes, and Treatises

There are numerous related problems regarding what can be reasonably inferred from oaths, prayers, codes of ethics, published lectures, and general pamphlets and treatises on medical conduct, usually written by individual physicians or medical societies for their colleagues. In the absence of more direct data about actual consent practices, these documents have been relied on heavily in numerous historical writings on informed consent as sources that provide information about related matters of clinical medical ethics.

However, it is often difficult to determine whether the statements that appear in these documents were primarily exhortatory, descriptive, or self-protective. Some writings describe, for educational purposes, conduct that was in accordance with prevailing professional standards. Other documents aim at reforming professional conduct by prescribing what should become established practice. Still others seem constructed to protect the physician from suspicions of misconduct or from legal liability. Moreover, informed consent has never been mentioned in any of these classic sources of medical tradition. Thus, historical and conceptual distortions may be introduced by accepting at face value prescriptions in various writings to the effect that consent must be obtained. Informed consent is a creature of a broad range of social practices and institutions in the twentieth century. To remove the notion from contemporary cultural and historical contexts in which it was nourished in order to test retrospectively for its presence in other cultures is a dangerous undertaking requiring special precautions.

The Elements of Informed Consent

Legal, philosophical, regulatory, medical, and psychological literatures have generally tried to define or analyze informed consent in terms of its "elements." The following elements have been identified as fundamental to the concept: 1) Disclosure, 2) Comprehension, 3) Voluntariness, 4) Competence, and 5) Consent (Levine 1978, 3–9; Meisel and Roth 1981; National Commission 1978, 10). There is a surprising amount of agreement over the acceptability of this analysis in the literature, where these conditions are treated as defining informed consent—or, as some prefer to say, as providing a definition of valid consent (Culver and Gert 1982, 42–63). On either formulation, the idea is that something is an informed consent if and only if some of the elements 1–5 above (and maybe all, depending on the particular analysis) are conditions that are satisfied in the circumstances. That is, one gives an informed consent to an intervention if and only if one receives a thorough disclosure about it, one comprehends the disclosure, one acts voluntarily, one is competent to act, and one consents to the intervention.

At first glance this definition of informed consent seems both attractive and faithful to the uses of the term in such practical contexts as clinical medicine and law. Nevertheless, the list of conditions in this analysis is distorted by the specific orientations of medical convention and malpractice law. Conditions 1–5 are less suitable as conditions in a conceptual analysis of the *meaning* of informed consent than as a list of the elements of informed consent as they have emerged in institutional or regulatory settings in which consent requirements appear in policies. We shall later see why this approach is too narrow to grasp the basic meaning of informed consent.

To take but one instance of the kind of bias at work in this form of definition, the US Supreme Court in *Planned Parenthood of Central Missouri v. Danforth* found cause to reflect on the meaning of informed consent: "One might well won-der . . . what 'informed consent' of a patient is. . . . We are content to accept, as the meaning, the giving of information to the patient as to just what would be done and as to its consequences" (67, *n*.8). This definition is strikingly similar to the assump-tions made by physicians in the national survey discussed previously, because both have an almost exclusive focus on disclosure. But the definition is profoundly inade-quate as a treatment of the general meaning of informed consent. It is tainted by an implicit assumption of medical authority and by an unrelieved legal focus on the theory of liability, which delineates not a meaning of informed consent but rather a duty to make disclosures.

There is nothing about the nature of an informed consent per se that requires disclosure as part of its meaning (or that makes disclosure a necessary element in the analysis), and to require disclosure as the central element is to misunderstand the concept. A patient or subject—already knowledgeable about a proposed inter-vention—could give a thoroughly informed consent without having received any disclosure from a second party. Similarly, other conditions in the above list of conditions are not necessary. For example, some persons who are legally incompe-tent (see element 4) may give informed consents, and in some instances even psychologically incompetent persons (also often the referent of element 4) may be able to give an informed consent.

The transformation of the above five-fold set of elements into a definition of informed consent thus raises as many problems and confusions as it offers insights. The meaning of informed consent is simply not found by listing these elements. That is, there is no necessary connection between listing the hallmark characteristics of informed consent in its literature and the conditions of informed consent that govern its meaning. However, there is a reason why so much confusion has pervaded the analysis of informed consent, as we shall now see.

Two Meanings of Informed Consent

The question "What is an informed consent?" is complicated because there are at least two common, entrenched, and irreducibly different meanings of informed consent. That is, the term is analyzable in different ways because different concep-tions of informed consent have emerged from the history of struggles with the concept. In one sense an informed consent is analyzable as an autonomous autho-rization by individual patients or subjects. In the second sense, informed consent is analyzable in terms of cultural and policy rules of consent that collectively form the social practice of informed consent in institutional contexts where groups of patients or subjects must be treated in accordance with the rules. Here, informed consents are not always autonomous acts, nor are they necessarily meaningful authorizations (Faden and Beauchamp 1986, 276–287).

This text refers to the second kind of consent as "institutional consent" because informed consent in this second sense does not refer to autonomous authorization, but to a legally or institutionally effective (sometimes misleadingly called valid) authorization from a patient or a subject. Such an authorization is effective if obtained through procedures that satisfy the rules that govern specific institutional practices of consent. Any consent is informed if it satisfies whatever operative rules apply to the practice in the context.

Whenever federal regulations and hospital policies govern whether an act of authorizing is effective, a patient or subject can autonomously authorize an intervention, and so give an informed consent in the first sense, and yet not effectively authorize that intervention and thus not given an informed consent in the second sense. For example, if the person consenting is a minor and therefore not a legally authorized agent, the person may autonomously authorize without giving an effective consent. All of this should come as no surprise in light of the fact that the legal system and health-care institutions need a generally applicable informed consent mechanism by which injury and responsibility can be readily and fairly assessed in court.

The definition of informed consent as institutional consent expresses the present-day mainstream conception in the regulatory rules of federal agencies as well as in health-care institutions. The documents governing consent in these contexts derive from some conception about what the rules must be in order to enable effective authorizations in these institutions, but these rules are premised only rarely on a conception of autonomous authorization that has more than a superficial quality. However, if a court, institution, or physician obtains an institutional consent under the prevailing rules, it does not follow that the best or even acceptable standards were used in light of a stricter autonomy-based model requiring autonomous authorization.

In principle, although less clearly in practice, the conditions of informed consent as autonomous authorization can function as model standards for fashioning the institutional and policy requirements of informed consent—a model of autonomous choice thus serving as the benchmark against which the moral adequacy of prevailing rules and practices might be evaluated. But this proposal only leads to further questions about what such a model of autonomous choice entails.

Autonomous Choice

Because of the close associations between the concept of autonomy and the concept of informed consent, we need to examine the meaning of autonomy in conjunction with the meaning of informed consent. The reason is that informed consent is rooted in concerns about protecting and enabling autonomous or self-determining choice by patients and subjects. In the literature on informed consent, "autonomy" and "respect for autonomy" are terms loosely associated with several ideas, such as privacy, voluntariness, self-mastery, choosing freely, the freedom to choose, choosing one's own moral position, and accepting responsibility for one's choices. Because of this conceptual uncertainty, the concept of autonomy and its connection to informed consent need careful analysis.

In moral philosophy personal autonomy has come to refer to personal self-governance: personal rule of the self by adequate understanding while remaining free from controlling interferences by others and from personal limitations that prevent choice. Many issues about consent concern failures to respect autonomy, ranging from manipulative underdisclosure of pertinent information to nonrecognition of a refusal of medical interventions. To respect an autonomous agent is to recognize with due appreciation that person's capacities and perspective, including his or her right to hold certain views and to take certain actions based on personal values and beliefs.

The idea of an informed consent in the sense of autonomous authorization suggests that a patient or subject does more than yield to, express agreement with, acquiesce in, or comply with an arrangement or a proposal. He or she actively authorizes the proposal in the act of consent, and does not merely assent to a treatment plan through submission to a doctor's authoritative order. Any such submission would not incorporate the person's own authority in order to give permission. The act is more like that of an embarrassed citizen who submits, yields, or assents to an officer's order to produce a driver's license. Just as citizens sometimes simply submit to an authority, in a system where the lines of authority are clear, so often do patients.

In sum, in contrast to informed consent as institutional consent, an informed consent based on an autonomous authorization entails that a subject or a patient substantially understands the circumstances, decides in substantial absence of control by others, and intentionally authorizes a professional to proceed with a medical or research intervention (Faden and Beauchamp 1986, Chs. 7–8).

THE LIMITS OF THE LAW

The law of informed consent has almost certainly been more influential as an authoritative set of statements and source of reflection than any other body of thought on the subject. "The doctrine of informed consent," as it is sometimes called, is the legal doctrine; and informed consent is often treated as synonymous with this "legal doctrine." The doctrine derives from common law and includes the entire body of law dealing with the obligation to obtain informed consent and valid exceptions to the obligation.

The legal doctrine derives in American case law almost exclusively from the physician-patient relationship in therapy, not from the researcher-subject relationship in research. A physician has a duty both to inform patients and to obtain their consent. If a patient is injured as a result of a failure on the part of a physician to disclose information about a procedure, then the patient may collect money damages from the physician for causing the injury. This legal vision has been fashioned for an adversarial court setting and is almost entirely focused on *disclosure* and on *liability for injury*. There are good reasons, as we shall now see,

; on such a narrow basis and also why it is ill-equipped to stray
ndaries.

lity

The primary basis for the legal doctrine is tort law. A tort is a civil injury to one's
person or property that is inflicted by another and that is measured in terms of, and
compensated by, money damages. This law imposes duties on members of society,
and one who fails to fulfill a legal duty is liable to compensation for the misdeed (in
the civil law). The theory of liability under which a case is tried determines the duty
that must be fulfilled. In recent informed consent cases, negligence is the theory of
liability almost always applied. However, the informed consent doctrine originally
developed and flourished under battery, which is a different theory of liability.
Currently no unified legal theory underlies all informed consent cases.

Under battery theory the defendant is held liable for any intended (i.e., not
careless or accidental) action that results in physical contact for which the plaintiff
has given no permission. A defendant need not have an evil intent, nor must injury
result; the unpermitted contact is itself considered wrongful. The battery theory of
liability protects the right to choose whether to permit others to invade one's physical integrity, and thus is based on the general right of self-determination in the law.

A physician who performs an invasive procedure without the patient's permission may be found guilty of a battery even if a reasonable person would have
authorized the procedure if asked. The physician may be found to have committed
battery if no consent at all was obtained, if consent was obtained for a procedure
different in scope or kind from the one actually performed, or if the physician failed
to inform the patient adequately about potential consequences of the procedure. In
general, if the physician performs a particular procedure without proper permission then any apparent consent is rendered invalid (Berkey 1969; Meisel 1977, 80;
Schloendorff 1914).

Under negligence theory, by contrast, unintentional, "careless" action or omission is the source of liability. The carelessness occurs in regard to some activity in
which the defendant has a duty to take care or to behave reasonably toward others,
and an injury measurable in monetary terms is caused by failure to discharge the
duty. Medical malpractice is but one type of professional negligence, where the
physician is held liable for violation of a duty to exercise proper skill and care.

Duty of Disclosure

Two competing disclosure standards have evolved as attempts to resolve problems
regarding the nature and amount of the information that must be disclosed: the
professional practice standard and the reasonable person standard. (A third standard, the subjective standard, is also discussed in legal commentary.) The professional practice standard holds that both the range of the duty to disclose and the
criteria of adequate disclosure are properly determined by the customary practices
of a professional community. These practices establish the standards of care for

disclosure and care alike. The patient, subject, or reasonable person lacking expert knowledge is considered unqualified to decide what should be disclosed.

Although the professional practice standard remains the primary standard in informed consent law, it contains serious inadequacies and it may even be doubted whether a customary standard of disclosure actually exists for much of medical practice. A basic problem is that negligent care might be perpetuated if relevant professionals throughout the profession offer inferior information, and another doubtful premise is that physicians have sufficient expertise to be able to judge in many cases what information their patients need. However, the principal objection to this standard is its failure to promote decisional autonomy, the protection of which is generally accepted as the primary function and moral justification of informed consent requirements.

By contrast to the professional practice standard, the reasonable person standard focuses on the information a "reasonable person" needs to know about procedures, risks, alternatives, and consequences. The legal test of an adequate disclosure is the "materiality," or significance, of information to the decisionmaking of the patient. Thus, the right to decide what information is material and due is shifted away from the physician to the reasonable patient. The reasonable person standard requires a physician to divulge any fact that is material to a reasonable person's decision, but there is no requirement to meet the unreasonable demand of a patient.

This reasonable person standard is as vulnerable to criticism as the professional-based standard. It can be doubted whether the reasonable person standard serves the interests of those patients who know little about either their informational needs or the medical system. The interpretation of the standard for clinical practice is also difficult, because it specifies no precise duty for physicians; and both the concept of material information and the central concept of the reasonable person are left at an intuitive level. It can therefore be doubted whether the reasonable person standard more adequately protects the patient's right to choose than does the professional practice standard.

These arguments are not intended to eliminate standards of professional disclosure. In the absence of a disclosure initiated by the professional, patients or subjects often cannot formulate their concerns and ask meaningful questions. A patient or subject needs to understand what an informed professional judges to be of value for most patients or subjects as material information, and what it means for consent to be an authorization to proceed. The problem is not whether we need adequate disclosures but rather whether a legal vehicle can be expected to provide an adequate standard of disclosure for clinical practice. This issue is reconsidered below under the discussion of "the quality of consent."

The larger problem with disclosure standards, for our purposes, is that they will not much help us formulate a conception of informed consent for clinical medicine and research. Because courts are captivated by the context of after-the-fact resolution of narrow and concrete questions of duty, responsibility, blame, injury, and damages in specific cases, the law has no systematic way of affecting contemporary medical practice other than by a somewhat muted threat of prosecution for legal wrongdoing. For all of these reasons, the heart of issues about informed consent is not legal but moral, because informed consent has less to do with the liability of professionals as agents of disclosure, and more to do with the autonomous choices of patients and subjects.

Giving the Law Its Due

This assessment is not meant as a criticism of law. Case law is extremely influential, not directly upon medical practice but rather on many disciplines in the intellectual history of informed consent—probably more influential than the writings emanating from any other discipline. The law contributed the term "informed consent" and set others on the road to conception of the social institution of consent rules as a mechanism for the protection of autonomous decisionmaking. As a just tribute, the courts must be acknowledged as the pioneers of today's concerns about informed consent.

THE QUALITY OF CONSENT

In discussing both autonomous choice and the limits of law, we may note that problems about the quality and adequacy of consent probably cannot be resolved unless conventional disclosure rules are abandoned and a shift occurs toward the quality of understanding present in a consent. This approach focuses on the need for communication, and a dispensing with liability-oriented discussions about proper legal standards of disclosure. The key to effective communication is to invite participation by patients or subjects in an exchange of information and dialogue. Asking questions, eliciting the concerns and interests of the patient or subject, and establishing a climate that encourages the patient or subject to ask questions may be more important than the full corpus of disclosed information.

A question-and-answer approach recognizes that an informed consent includes many of the features of a valid contract, chief of which is that the parties share an understanding and agree with the essential elements of the arrangement. Absent such agreement, there can be no assurance that an informed consent is a bona fide informed consent to the proposed intervention. If investigator and subject have different conceptions of the proposed intervention, and the differences have implications for what is to be implemented, generally only the investigator's conception will be effected.

Without introduction of the proper climate into the consent context, a request from a professional that the patient or subject ask for information is as likely to result in silence as to elicit the desired result of a meaningful informational exchange and consent. Patients find it difficult to approach physicians with questions or concerns, and even when they do not understand their physicians, many still do not ask questions. The extent to which this passive attitude characterizes research subjects is less clear. Although still understudied, it is a good guess that relatively little educating of this quality occurs at present in either clinical practice or research in the United States. There are also many unresolved issues about how to handle these problems in the case of special populations, such as children.

VULNERABLE SUBJECTS, COMPLIANT PATIENTS, AND COERCIVE SITUATIONS

A necessary condition of autonomy is that a person be free. Patients and subjects are entitled to expect that those who are in a position to influence them such as physicians and research investigators will do so through a fair presentation of accurate information and without undue influence in the form of coercion and manipulation. To understand what would be required to approach the ideal of free choice in practice we need to examine the broad concept of influence.

Control is always exerted through some form of influence, but not all influences are controlling. Influences come in a multiplicity of forms including threats of physical harm, promises of love and affection, economic incentives, reasoned argument, lies, press releases, gossip, etc. The degree of influence actually exerted can vary dramatically, and many forms of influence are easily resistible. Some types of influence have a major effect on an individual's ability to do things, while others make no difference. It is important, therefore, to recognize the kind and degree of influence at work.

Problems of influence have their place in both clinical ethics and research ethics, but they have played an especially prominent role in research ethics, where much discussion about the morality of involving subjects in research centers not on how informed the subjects are, but rather on how free they are. For example, this topic consumed a great deal of time in the deliberations of the National Commission for the Protection of Human Subjects over the involvement of prisoners in drug research. The Commission raised the question "Whether prisoners are, in the words of the Nuremberg Code, 'so situated as to be able to exercise free power of choice.'" The Commission answered that "although prisoners who participate in research affirm that they do so freely, the conditions of social and economic deprivation in which they live compromise their freedom. The Commission believes, therefore, that the appropriate expression of respect consists in protection from exploitation" (National Commission 1976, 5–7).

The Commission went on to recommend a ban on drug research involving prisoners, on grounds that in such coercive institutions free choice would be too often compromised. Six years later this argument still raged on: Robert Levine, who had been on the staff of the Commission, argued—as had a minority of Commissioners—that prisoners are actually better off, not worse off, by their involvement in research, and that exclusion from research was a far worse restriction of free choice (Levine 1982, 6). Many were dubious, however, that such abstract statements take account of the realities of coercion in the prison (Dubler 1982, 10).

Much the same controversy was extended into 1982 and 1983 by Dr. Mortimer Lipsett at NIH (NICHD) and by respondents to an article he published dealing with the question whether Phase I clinical trials of cancer chemotherapies involve a special class of subjects deserving special protections. He presented the problem as follows:

> The President's Commission for the Study of Ethical Problems in Medicine and Biomedical and Behavioral Research developed and extended the concept of the vulnerable subject in medical research. Children, prisoners, and the mentally disabled were defined as vulnerable because a variety of constraints and inducements effectively removed their capacity to function autonomously. Similarly, patients with advanced cancer are faced with inducements that may sway their judgment of the risk-benefit ratio. Should such patients be treated as vulnerable research subjects necessitating extraordinary supervision by third parties? (Lipsett 1982, 941–942)

He answered that every patient entering such a therapeutic trial is vulnerable by virtue of the disease state and the unique opportunity to receive a promising drug, but he maintained that the problem could be and was being overcome by "painstaking consultation and preparation" involving families, IRBs, third-party consultation, etc. He concluded that, as conducted, the phase I clinical trials of "cancer chemotherapies are ethical and necessary" (Lipsett 1982, 941–942).

Some published responses to Lipsett were less sanguine. Alexander Capron, who had been staff director of the President's Commission, as well as Terrence Ackerman and Carson Strong, argued that the notion of therapeutic intent in the trials is easily subject to misunderstanding by patients, who may be misled to the hope of a favorable effect, especially when the prospect for therapeutic efficacy is as exceedingly remote as it often is at the dosage level offered. They maintained that patients should be given a realistic picture of how they are contributing to medical knowledge. They noted the dangers of "manipulating" subjects and of subjecting them to "affective" factors that impair understanding and judgment. In general, they challenged the view that present safeguards are sufficient to preclude exploitation (Ackerman and Strong 1983, 883; Capron 1983, 882–883).

Underlying these discussions—which are perennial issues about many populations used in research—is a theoretically difficult and partially unresolved set of problems about free choice, coercion, and manipulation. Certain forms of withholding information, playing on emotion, or presenting constraints can rob a person of the capacity of free choice by manipulation or coercion. Deceptive and misleading statements limit freedom by restricting the range of choice and by prompting a person to do what the person otherwise would not do. The National Commission was worried about coercion in the case of prisoners; by contrast, those engaged in the discussion of Phase I trials and cancer chemotherapies were interested in manipulation.

There is a continuum of controlling influences in our daily lives, running from coercion, which is at the most controlling end of the continuum (compare the

National Commission's model of prisoners), to persuasion and education, which are not controlling at all, even though they are influences (compare Lipsett's model of drug patients). Influence thus does not necessarily imply constraint, governance, force, or compulsion, although these concepts are essential to certain kinds of influence. Important decisions are usually made in contexts replete with influences in the form of competing claims and interests, social demands and expectations, and straightforward or devious attempts by others to bring about the outcome they desire. Some of these influences are unavoidable, and some may even be desirable. Clearly not all of them interfere with or deprive persons of autonomous belief and action, as when patients are persuaded by sound reasons to do something.

Coercion—which involves a threat of harm so severe that a person is unable to resist acting to avoid it—is always completely controlling. It entirely negates freedom because it entirely controls action. Persuasion, by contrast, is the intentional and successful attempt to induce a person, through appeals to reason, to freely accept the beliefs, attitudes, values, intentions, or actions advocated by the persuader. Like informing, persuading is entirely compatible with free choice, even though both are forms of influence.

The most sweeping and difficult area of influence is manipulation, a broad, general category that runs from highly controlling to altogether noncontrolling influences. The essence of manipulation is getting people to do what the manipulator intends without resort to coercion or to reasoned argument. In a paradigm case of manipulation in contexts of informed consent, information is managed so that the person does not know what the manipulator intends. Whether such uses of information necessarily compromise or restrict free choice is an unresolved and untidy issue, but one plausible view is that some manipulations (e.g., the use of rewards such as reduced medical fees for being involved in research) are compatible with free choice, whereas others (such as deceptive offers of hope where there is none) are not compatible with free choice.

Manipulation in this sense also may not be immoral (e.g., a criminal might be tricked into surrendering), but the use of manipulative techniques almost always requires justification. Manipulation is often characterized as necessarily immoral because it uses another person to one's ends without the other's consent (DeGeorge 1982, 182). However, this argument is unpersuasive; the moral character of offering an incentive that noncoercively alters a person's choices (e.g., a retirement-bonus incentive program intended to make early retirement attractive to employees) differs markedly from the moral character of an act of deception that tricks a person into doing that which he or she otherwise would not do. Yet both are manipulative.

In informed consent contexts, the central issues turn on how to differentiate proposals that are compatible with substantial autonomy from those that are not. The central question is not whether we are entirely free of even manipulative influences, but whether we are sufficiently free to remain autonomous—free to perform our own actions—as opposed to controlled by the actions of another. The thorniest of all problems about autonomy and manipulation is not that of punishment and threat but the effect of rewards and offers. This category refers to the intentional use of offers of rewards to bring about a desired response. For example, during the Tuskegee Syphilis experiments various methods were used to stimulate and sustain the interest of subjects in continued participation. They were offered free burial assistance and insurance, free transportation, and a free stop in town on the return trip. They were also rewarded with free medicines and free hot meals on the days of the examination. The deprived socioeconomic condition of these subjects made them easily manipulable by those means.

This general range of problems is compounded still further by what is sometimes called the problem of "coercive situations." Normal definitions of coercion require that coercion be intentional by the coercer, but the problem of coercive situations is that of whether there can be nonintentional coercion where the person is controlled by the situation, not by the design of another person. Sometimes people unintentionally make other persons feel threatened, and sometimes situations such as illness and economic necessity prevent threats of serious harm that a person feels compelled to prevent at all costs. The earlier example of using prisoners in experimentation is again applicable in this context, if we assume that a prisoner is left without any viable alternative to participation in research because of the awfulness of the alternatives in the circumstance or because of what may appear to be threats presented by prison officials. As Alvin Bronstein, Director of the National Prison Project, puts the problem for informed consent, "You cannot create . . . [a prison] institution in which informed consent without coercion is feasible" (Bronstein 1975, 130–131).

Beyond the prison, in circumstances of severe physical or health deprivation, a person might accept an offer or sign a contract that the person would refuse under less stringent circumstances. Cancer patients are good examples: The prospect of death if an otherwise objectionable offer of a toxic drug is rejected seems to "coerce" a choice of the drug no less than an intentional threat. The psychological effect on the person forced to choose may be identical, and the person can appropriately say in both cases, "There was no real choice; I would have been crazy to refuse." But if, as we usually believe, a contract signed under another person's threat is invalid (and the consent behind the signing an invalid consent), can we not say that a person who agrees to drug experimentation in a coercive situation has made an invalid contract (and given an invalid consent)?

However, it is a mistake to suppose that persons in such coercive situations cannot act freely. Many consenting patients of all types are persons left without meaningful choices in just this respect: to survive they have no meaningful choice but to elect the procedure. This loss of alternatives cannot be equated with coercion. Many of these patients have carefully deliberated about their situations and may have reached a decision under noncoercive circumstances. It is, then, a confusion to move from a correct claim about a deprivation or loss of freedom caused by desperate circumstances to a (fallaciously drawn) conclusion that there has been a loss of autonomy because of a coercive situation.

Nevertheless, even if knowledgeable intent to threaten is not present, one may feel just as forced to a choice and may just as heartily wish to avoid it, and this is why the worry is often presented in the language of "vulnerable subjects." Their situation does make them vulnerable, even desperately vulnerable, and may subject them to control by their emotions and anxieties to an abnormal degree. Again, the paradigm is the presumptively dying patient. The principle of therapeutic benefit will, as Lipsett correctly argues, generally enjoin the clinician to offer an intervention with lifesaving potential, even if the person is incapable of resisting the offer of the proposed intervention because of the threat of death. Despite the horribly tense and pressured nature of such circumstances, patients can, if properly managed, consent freely. What may be doubted is how often a free informed consent does in fact occur.

RIGHTFUL AUTHORITY

The law is a form of authority, but perhaps the central problem of authority in contexts of informed consent is that of decisionmaking authority. The problem of whether health providers ever have rightful authority to override the decisions of patients in order to benefit them or prevent harm to them is one dimension of the problem of medical paternalism, in which a parental-like decision by a professional overrides an autonomous decision of a patient. Much of the literature about consent focuses on such moral problems as when consent need not be obtained and when refusals need not be honored.

In law, philosophy, and health-care literatures the prevailing view now seems to be that competent persons are always entitled to make their own decisions, but a premise to the effect that decisions about health care must finally rest with competent and informed patients can lead to some disquieting consequences from the perspective of a health provider. For example, the premise entails that the right to autonomous choice includes the choice to forego life-sustaining treatment, thus defeating normal presumptions in the medical community in favor of providing care and even sustaining life. Recognition of a strong patient's-rights premise as authoritative could have a pervasive and unsettling effect on hospitals, where such behavior as foregoing treatment is still generally viewed as suspect and disruptive despite pronouncements about patients' rights (President's Commission 1983, Chs. 1–2).

The central problem of authority in these discussions is whether an autonomy model of medical practice that gives premier decisionmaking authority to patients should be allowed to gain practical priority over a beneficence model that gives authority to providers to implement sound principles of health care. The "autonomy model" here refers to the view that the physician's responsibilities to the patient of disclosure and consent-seeking are established primarily (perhaps exclusively) by the principle of respect for autonomy. The "beneficence model" depicts the physician's responsibilities of disclosure and consent-seeking as established by the principle of beneficence, in particular through the idea that the physician's primary obligation (surpassing obligations of respect for autonomy) is to provide medical benefits. The management of information is understood, on the latter model, in terms of the management of patients (due care) generally. That is, the physician's primary obligation is to handle information so as to maximize the patient's medical benefits. (Beauchamp and McCullough 1984, Ch. 2).

Atypical handling of the problem of conflict between these two models is found in the following statement by the President's Commission:

> The primary goal of health care in general is to maximize each patient's well-being. However, merely acting in a patient's best interests without recognizing the individual as the pivotal decisionmaker would fail to respect each person's interest in self-determination. . . .
>
> When the conflicts that arise between a competent patient's self-determination and his or her apparent well-being remain unresolved after adequate deliberation, a competent patient's self-determination is and usually should be given greater weight than other people's views on that individual's well-being. . . .
>
> Respect for the self-determination of competent patients is of special importance. . . . The patient [should have] the final authority to decide. (1983, 26–27, 44.)

Professionals and patients alike tend to see the authority for some decisions as properly the patient's and authority for other decisions as primarily the professional's. It is widely agreed, for example, that elective surgery involving significant risk is properly the patient's but that decisions about whether and under what conditions to administer a sedative to a frightened patient screaming in an emergency room is properly the physician's. However, many cases are far more ambiguous as to proper decisionmaking authority—for instance, who should decide which aggressive therapy, if any, to administer to a cancer victim or whether to prolong the lives of severely handicapped newborns.

Judgments that the patient ought to serve as the primary decisionmaking authority are not always justified by a principle of respect for autonomy, because these judgments may rest on the principle that the patients' welfare is maximized by allowing them to be decisionmakers. The idea that authority should rest with the patients or subjects is justified, from this perspective, by arguments from beneficence to the effect that decisional autonomy by patients enables them to survive, heal, or otherwise improve their own health. These arguments range from the simple contention that making one's own decisions promotes one's psychological well-being to the more controversial observation that patients generally know themselves well enough to be the best judges, ultimately, of what is most beneficial for them.

In research settings a similar argument holds that requiring the informed consent of subjects will serve as a curb on research risks presented to subjects. For example, the earliest and premier moral and legal concern in the history of research ethics was to control the risks presented to subjects by research, and not to enable autonomous choice about participation. Consent requirements first appeared in research codes and guidelines with the intent of protecting subjects' welfare.

In each of these arguments autonomous choice for patients and subjects is valued only extrinsically for the sake of health or welfare rather than intrinsically for its own sake. Those who maintain that respect for autonomy is the sole justification of requirements to obtain informed consent generally stand entirely opposed to these views of the justification for decisionmaking authority, although not opposed to the authority given to patients and subjects. As autonomy-based justifications for the consent provision have flourished, so has the view that an autonomy model of decisionmaking authority should replace a beneficence model in medicine.

Unfortunately, this goal of enabling autonomous choice has often been only vaguely formulated in the quest for satisfactory medical and research ethics, with little general agreement about how respect for autonomy is to be understood or implemented in the obtaining of consent. There has also been sparse agreement about the contexts in which respect for a subject's or patient's decision ought to extend. Historically and sociologically, we can claim little beyond the almost indisputable fact that there has developed a general, inchoate societal demand for the protection of patients' and subjects' rights, most conspicuously their autonomy rights.

Autonomy is almost certainly the most important value discovered in medical and research ethics in the last two decades, and it is the single most important moral value for informed consent. However, the concern in contemporary medical ethics should not be whether the principle of respect for autonomy is lexically ordered so as to trump the principle of beneficence and restore the proper lines of authority to patients. In any approach to medical decisionmaking, it is important that autonomy not be either overvalued or undervalued. Although the burden of moral proof will generally be on those who seek to intervene in another's choice with a claim of rightful authority, it is still a reasonable view that as the need to protect persons from harm becomes more compelling, thereby increasing the "weight" of moral considerations of beneficence in the circumstances, it becomes more likely that these considerations will constitute a sufficient reason for overriding competing moral demands to respect autonomy.

COMPETENCE TO CONSENT

We noticed earlier in discussing the elements of consent that competence is often listed as a necessary condition of informed consent. In legal and policy contexts, reference to competent persons is more common than reference to autonomous persons. In these contexts competence functions as a gatekeeping concept for informed consent (Faden and Beauchamp 1986, 288). That is, competence judgments function to distinguish persons from whom consent should be solicited from those from whom consent need not or should not be solicited.

The incompetent person is one who, for one or more of a number of reasons, is unable to given an informed consent. Competence can be either a factual or a presumptive, categorical determination. Minors, for example, are presumed incompetent in law, whereas adults can generally be declared legally incompetent only on the basis of some "factual" determination. The issue of legal capacity is more complex for adult patients, for whom an individualized determination normally must be made. If a person is incompetent, the physician is usually required, absent an emergency, to secure some form of third-party consent from a guardian or other representative legally empowered to give it. There is no widely agreed-upon standard, test, or definition of incompetence—a set of issues surrounded by considerable ambiguity and confusion.

Judgments of competence and incompetence determine from whom consent rightly should be solicited and are therefore normative. Often there is an underlying moral appeal to respect for autonomous persons. If a person is autonomous and situated in a context in which consent is appropriate, it is a prima facie moral principle that informed consent should be sought from the person. By contrast, if a person is nonautonomous and situated in a context in which some form of consent is required, it is a prima facie moral principle (not derived from the principle of respect for autonomy, but rather from beneficence) that some mechanism for the authorization of procedures or decisions other than obtaining the person's consent should be instituted.

Thus, gatekeeping by allowing autonomous persons—competent persons—to give informed consent and not allowing nonautonomus persons—incompetent persons—to give informed consent is accomplished by an appeal to the moral principle that autonomous persons are rightfully the decisionmakers. Gatekeeping of this description is not the only framework for determining who is competent and who incompetent, and therefore who should and should not be solicited to give an informed consent. But classically this perspective has been a deeply embedded model governing the "element" of competence, as that element appears in treatments of informed consent in policy and legal contexts.

The special commitments of medicine, law, psychiatry, philosophy, psychology, and other professions have led to competing perspectives on competence that are in many instances incompatible. The definition and criteria of competence are not waters into which we can here wade, but it is important to note how placement of the label "incompetent" on a patient or subject can almost automatically introduce the possibility of coercive treatment and the presumption that there is no need to obtain consent. Competence commonly functions to denote persons whose consents, refusals, and statements of preference will be accepted as binding, while incompetence denotes those who are to be placed under the guidance and control of another.

The competent person, then, is treated as one who must be dealt with as his or her own person; that person's will, and not the will of another, must prevail as the source of authorization or refusal. If such a competent person cannot make an informed choice merely because of eliminable ignorance, it seems morally imperative that the information required to remove ignorance must be supplied. Similarly, if the competent person is in danger of control by the exertion of family pressures, then steps should be taken to ease the family pressures. But in the case of the incompetent person, matters are starkly different because information will be provided to a third party authorized to decide on the incompetent's behalf, and the decision will be reached by that party.

Where the cut-off line should be situated on the continuum of decisionmaking ability that divides competence from incompetence is a normative question with several levels. Establishing the requisite abilities is a first level of evaluation; then thresholds for each of those abilities must be fixed. Still a third normative dimension is present if a test of competence is used to determine who passes and who fails. The inherently ethical aspect of such decisions has not always been duly appreciated in medical contexts, where there has been a tendency to think of such decisions as medical rather than moral.

JUSTIFICATIONS FOR NOT OBTAINING CONSENT

The claim that a patient is incompetent is one way to justify overriding the normal presumption that consent must be obtained, but there are other prominent justifications as well. In clinical settings the so-called "therapeutic privilege" has long been used to justify not obtaining consent and has elicited a particularly furious exchange over whether autonomy rights can be validly overridden for paternalistic reasons.

If framed broadly, the therapeutic privilege can permit physicians to withhold information if disclosure would cause any countertherapeutic deterioration, however slight, in the physical, psychological, or emotional condition of the patient. If framed narrowly, it can permit the physician to withhold information if and only if the patient's knowledge of the information would have serious health-related consequences—for example, by jeopardizing the success of the treatment or harming the patient psychologically by critically impairing relevant decisionmaking processes.

The narrowest formulation is that the therapeutic privilege can be validly invoked only if the physician has good reason to believe that disclosure would render the patient incompetent to consent to or refuse the treatment, that is, would render the decision nonautonomous. To invoke the therapeutic privilege under such circumstances does not conflict with respect for autonomy, because an autonomous decision could not be made in any event. However, broader formulations of the privilege that require only "medical contraindication" of some sort do operate at the expense of autonomy. These formulations may unjustifiably endanger autonomous choice altogether, as when the invocation of the privilege is based on the belief that an autonomous patient, if informed, would refuse an indicated therapy for what the medical community views as incorrect or inappropriate reasons.

Such paternalism is sometimes resolutely and properly contested, because it threatens the basic values underlying the informed consent obligation. There are also many problems in formulating an acceptable standard for determining what information may be withheld, and there has been confusion regarding appropriate measures of rationality, psychological damage, and emotional stability under the standard. Unless the therapeutic privilege is tightly and operationally formulated, the medical profession can use it to deprive the unreasonable but competent patient of the right to make decisions, especially if the physician sees his or her commitment to the patient's best interest as the overriding consideration. Loose standards can permit physicians to climb to safety over a straw bridge of speculation about the psychological consequences of information. In short, there is a significant potential for abuse of the privilege because of its inconsistency with the patient's right to know and to decline treatment (Faden and Beauchamp 1986, 38).

In research settings some quite different reasons have been put forward for not disclosing information and thereby not receiving informed consents. One argument is that if full disclosure is made, some subjects will withdraw and therefore will bias the results; others will be made unnecessarily anxious by disclosure of randomization. In many cases anything like full disclosure will destroy or threaten the trial, because patients will not knowingly submit to what might be a therapeutically disadvantaging situation. Participating physicians may also intrude bias. Because the overall research situation has therapeutic intent, it seems justified, according to this line of argument, to withhold information that would bias the results (Chalmers 1979; Lasagna 1970; Meier 1979; Shaw and Chalmers 1970).

This approach, although still defended, is widely regarded as unsatisfactory because it will inevitably lead to avoidable distrust and suspicion, and, more importantly, likely violates the autonomy or therapeutic rights of subjects. Some form of more adequate disclosure therefore is morally required. But an adequate disclosure is sometimes provided even though it is not a complete disclosure, and there may be ways around some of these methodological and moral problems. Subjects may consent to having some information, even data, withheld. For example, subjects are sometimes informed that they cannot be told the purpose or the specific subject of the research, and in some cases they are asked to consent to studies after being informed that the research procedures will be intentionally deceptive.

Is any form of withholding of information along these lines compatible with informed consent? Here the question is whether potential subjects who understand that they are being kept partially ignorant about a particular intervention or research project can given informed consents to that project or intervention. The answer depends on the subject's ability to judge the materiality of the information being withheld, but subjects are not always in a good position to make such a determination, and it is sometimes difficult to assess whether various events and bits of information are likely to be important or trivial. Generally, this depends on the kind and amount of information being withheld.

The resolution of these problems depends at least in part on an analysis of the intervention or arrangement to which the subject is consenting. If the subject cannot confidently evaluate the materiality of withheld information, and it remains doubtful whether the subject has a substantial understanding of the proposed research project, the subject may not be able to give an informed consent to participation in that particular research project. The subject may nonetheless be able to give an informed consent to participate in research being conducted by the investigator, under the guarantees and terms of ignorance that have been discussed, provided the subject has an understanding of that which is material to her or his decision to authorize the professional to proceed under the specified conditions.

It is often dilemmatic whether informed consents can be given under the condition of an open withholding of information, but it would be precipitous to maintain that patients and subjects can never give informed consents merely because they lack some relevant descriptions. They may, in the end, have every material description needed. In other cases, they may not have adequate information, and we may need to shift to other expedients such as the following: retaining subjects in a trial who refuse to be randomized; then distributing subjects into four groups—two nonrandomized and two randomized, with an experimental treatment and a standard treatment operation in each pair (Veatch 1983). Such a procedure may, in some cases, be the most acceptable balance between ethical requirements and the canons of research design.

CONCLUSION

Jay Katz argues that the history of the physician-patient relationship from ancient times to the present reveals how inattentive physicians have been to their patients' rights and needs to make their own decisions. Little appreciation of disclosure and consent can be discerned in this history, except negatively, in the emphasis on patients' incapacities to understand the mysteries of medicine:

> It is the history of silence with respect to patient participation in decision making. . . .
> When I speak of silence I do not mean to suggest that physicians have not talked to their patients at all. Of course, they have conversed with patients about all kinds of matters, but they have not, except inadvertently, employed words to invite patients' participation in sharing the burden of making joint decisions. (Katz 1984, 3–4, 28)

Katz is equally unrelenting in his criticisms of court decisions and legal scholarship. He regards the declarations of courts as filled with overly optimistic rhetoric. The problem, in his view, is that the law has little to do with fostering real communication in the clinic and tends to line up with the professional judgments of physicians in the crucial test cases. In Katz's view, judges have only "toyed briefly" with the idea of informed consent since 1957, "bowing" in its direction largely to set it aside. Like physicians, judges always defer to a model of medical care rather than a model of the right to make one's own informed decisions, and thus both have failed to appreciate that "autonomous decisionmaking requires two-way conversation" (Katz 1984, 2, 49–50, 79).

There is much to be said for Katz's indictments of law and medicine, although every relevant discipline, including ethics, deserves no less stern criticism for the failure to develop an adequate conception of informed consent. But in reaching to condemn these efforts we should place them in an historical and contemporary context. Until recently—roughly the 1957 date mentioned by Katz as the birthdate of informed consent—the justification of practices of disclosure and consent-seeking were largely governed by a beneficence model rather than an autonomy model of the physician's responsibility for the patient.

Because these two models embrace distinct perspectives on responsibilities to patients, they can and often do emerge in conflict in decisions about the management of information for patients. The beneficence model not only traditionally dwarfed any nascent autonomy model in medical practice but led to an environment in which autonomy figured insignificantly or not at all in reflections about disclosure. The consent practices emerging from this consent were not meaningful exercises of autonomous decisionmaking, despite the bows in the direction of respectfulness and truthtelling found in a few codes, treatises, and practices.

Certainly Katz is correct in judging that informed consent has always been an alien notion in the history of medicine and medical ethics and that informed consent has not changed the fundamental character of the physician-patient relationship. The lines of authority today seem roughly to be what they were in Percival's time: the beneficence model is overwhelmingly predominant. Many patients therefore routinely acquiesce to medical interventions rather than autonomously authorizing them.

At the same time, however, the scene in American medicine is slowly undergoing what may prove to be an extensive transformation through the implementation of the idea of informed consent. In hospitals and clinics all over the United States, patients are giving more and more "informed consents" and more and more attention is being paid in institutions to the quality of those consents. While these consents may be less than substantially autonomous decisions, the practice of medicine seems profoundly altered. It also seems indisputable that something dramatic has occurred to affect research ethics and policies.

Accordingly, before we reach to condemn the writings and practices of the past, it is well to remember that informed consent is still under development and that our own failures may be no less apparent to future generations than are the failures that we find with the past. The autonomy model is, in the light of history, still a novel and provocative idea and perhaps a model that must always compete with the beneficence model in the care of patients. It is also well to remember that although the autonomy model underlies the twentieth century movement to informed consent, the autonomy model is not the whole of medical ethics.

REFERENCES

Ackerman, Terrence F. and Carson M. Strong. In "Letters." *JAMA* 249 (18 Feb. 1983): 882-83.

American Medical Association. *Proceedings of the National Medical Conventions.* Held in New York, May 1846, and in Philadelphia, May 1847. Adopted May 6, 1847 and submitted for publication in Philadelphia, 1847.

Beauchamp, Tom L., and Laurence McCullough. *Medical Ethics: The Moral Responsibilities of Physicians.* Englewood Cliffs, N.J.: Prentice-Hall, 1984.

Berkey v. Anderson. 1 Cal. App. 3d 790, 82 Cal. Rptr. 67 (1969).

Bronstein, Alvin. "Remarks." In *National Academy of Sciences, Experiments and Research with Humans: Values in Conflict.* Washington, D.C.: National Academy, 1975, 130–131.

Capron, Alexander M. In "Letters." *JAMA* 249 (18 Feb. 1983): 882–883.

Chalmers, Thomas. "Invited Remarks." *Clin Pharmacol Ther* 25 (May 1979): 649–650.

Culver, Charles, and Bernard Gert. *Philosophy in Medicine: Conceptual and Ethical Issues in Medicine and Psychiatry.* New York: Oxford University Press, 1982.

"Declaration of Helsinki: Recommendations Guiding Medical Doctors in Biomedical Research Involving Human Subjects." Adopted by the 18th World Medical Assembly, Helsinki, Finland, 1964. Published in *N Engl J Med* 271 (1964): 473; revised by the 29th World Medical Assembly, Tokyo, Japan, 1975. As reprinted in Levine, Robert J. *Ethics and Regulation of Clinical Research.* Baltimore: Urban & Schwarzenberg, 1981, 287–289.

DeGeorge, Richard T. *Business Ethics.* New York: Macmillan, 1982.

Dubler, Nancy. "The Burdens of Research in Prisons." *IRB* 4 (Nov. 1982): 9–10.

Faden, Ruth R., and Tom L. Beauchamp. *A History and Theory of Informed Consent.* New York: Oxford University Press, 1986.

Harris, Louis et al. "Views of Informed Consent and Decisionmaking: Parallel Surveys of Physicians and the Public." In President's Commission for the Study of Ethical Problems in Medicine and Biomedical and Behavioral Research. *Making Health Care Decisions,* Vol. 2 (1982): 17–316.

Hippocrates. In *Hippocrates,* 4 vols. Translated by W. H. S. Jones. Cambridge, Mass.: Harvard University Press, 1923–1931.

Katz, Jay. *The Silent World of Doctor and Patient.* New York: The Free Press, 1984.

Lasagna, Louis. "Drug Evaluation Problems in Academic and Other Contexts." *Ann NY Acad Sci* 169 (1970): 506.

Levine, Robert. "The Nature and Definition of Informed Consent in Various Research Settings," Appendix: Vol. I. In *The Belmont Report* Washington, D.C.: DHEW Publication No. (OS) 78–0013, 1978, (3–1)–(3–91).

Levine, Robert J. "Research Involving Prisoners: Why Not?" *IRB* 4 (May 1982): 6.

Lidz, Charles, and Alan Meisel. "Informed Consent and the Structure of Medical Care." In President's Commission, *Making Health Care Decisions.* Washington, D.C.: Government Printing Office, 1982.

Lipsett, Mortimer B. "On the Nature and Ethics of Phase I Clinical Trials of Cancer Chemotherapies." *JAMA* 248 (27 Aug. 1982): 941–942.

Meier, Paul. "Terminating a Trial—The Ethical Problem." *Clin Pharmacol Ther* 25 (May 1979): 637.

Meisel, Alan. "The Expansion of Liability for Medical Accidents: From Negligence to Strict Liability by Way of Informed Consent." *Nebraska Law Rev* 56 (1977): 51–152.

Meisel, Alan, and Loren Roth. "What We Do and Do Not Know About Informed Consent." *JAMA* 246 (Nov. 1981): 2473–2477.

Meisel, Alan, and Loren H. Roth. "Toward an Informed Discussion on Informed Consent: A Review and Critique of the Empirical Studies." *Arizona Law Rev* 25 (1983): 265–346.

National Commission for the Protection of Human Subjects. *Research Involving Prisoners.* Washington, D.C.: DHEW Publication No. (OS) 76–131, 1976.

National Commission for the Protection of Human Subjects of Biomedical and Behavioral Research. *The Belmont Report.* Washington, D.C.: DHEW Publication No. (OS) 78–0012, 1978.

Percival, Thomas. *Medical Ethics; or a Code of Institutes and Precepts, Adapted to the Professional Conduct of Physicians and Surgeons.* Manchester: S. Russell, 1803. The available edition is Leake, Chauncey D., ed. *Percival's Medical Ethics.* Huntington, N.Y.: Krieger Publishing, 1975.

Planned Parenthood of Central Missouri v. Danforth. 428 U.S. 52, 67 n.8, 1976.

President's Commission. *Deciding to Forego Life-Sustaining Treatment.* Washington, D.C.: Government Printing Office, March 1983.

President's Commission for the Study of Ethical Problems in Medicine and Biomedical and Behavioral Research. *Making Health Care Decisions,* Vol. 1, Chapter 1, 1982.

Salgo v. Leland Stanford Jr. University Board of Trustees. 317 P.2d 170, 1957.

Schloendorff v. Society of New York Hospitals. 211 N.Y. 125, 105 N.E. 92, 1914.

Shaw, L. W., and Thomas Chalmers. "Ethics in Cooperative Clinical Trials." *Ann NY Acad Sci* 169 (1970): 487–495.

United States v. Karl Brandt, Trials of War Criminals Before the Nuremberg Military Tribunals Under Control Council Law No. 10, Vols. 1 and 2, "The Medical Case." Military Tribunal I, 1947. Washington, D.C.: Government Printing Office, 1948–1949.

Veatch, Robert M. "Justice and Research Design." *Clin Research* 31 (Feb. 1983): 12–22.

DISCUSSION QUESTIONS

1. Is the purpose of consent to benefit the individual or to promote autonomous choice? What should happen when providing information may do more harm than good?

2. Is consent more important in research in which the subject cannot benefit or in therapeutic medicine? In which circumstance is consent harder to obtain?

3. Are there any good reasons for obtaining consent for interventions in research or therapy that can do no harm to patients or subjects?

4. If patients want some information about therapy, but clinicians, customarily, tend not to provide it, is there any moral reason for providing it?

5. Should physicians have a duty to provide information that individual patients desire even if most reasonable patients would not desire it? If so, under what circumstances?

8

Genetics and Reproductive Technologies

LeRoy Walters

SUMMARY

This chapter covers three major topics: reproductive technologies, genetic testing and screening, and genetic engineering and therapy. On the issue of reproductive technologies, several key issues are explored. The first section considers the challenges that reproductive technologies present for the traditional notion of the family and genetic lineage, and analyzes what is now meant by the term family. It also examines issues surrounding the appropriate role of government and the effects of new reproductive technologies on the lives of citizens. The chapter discusses metaphysical, legal, and ethical dilemmas presented by artificial insemination, in vitro fertilization, embryo freezing and storage, and the future applications of technology for sex selection, diagnosis of disease, and/or research. The dilemmas and ethical and public-policy questions surrounding surrogate motherhood are also explored.

The discussion of genetic testing and screening begins with an introduction to the technical and legal background of such techniques as neonatal, prenatal, carrier testing and screening, and current efforts to map and sequence the human genome. The discussion that follows consists of an analysis of the major ethical and public-policy issues surrounding genetic testing and screening, including freedom and coercion in genetic testing, the confidentiality or disclosure of test results, access to genetic testing services, and the probable benefits and harms of genetic testing and screening programs.

In the final section, the issues surrounding human gene therapy and genetic engineering are explored. To facilitate this discussion, the author first distinguishes several possible types of genetic intervention. Various ethical and public-policy questions are then discussed in terms of both present and future implications.

Some obstacles and alternatives to genetic intervention are explored, especially the enhancing of human characteristics. The new science of gene mapping and gene sequencing may lead to breathtaking and unanticipated possibilities as well as potentially serious harms. It is therefore prudent to consider these technological possibilities and their potential social impact well before they are upon us.

REPRODUCTIVE TECHNOLOGIES

Before considering specific reproductive technologies such as artificial insemination and in vitro fertilization, we will examine some of the background assumptions that cut across the various technologies.

Background Assumptions

The Naturalness or Artificiality of the New Technologies

If one believes that nothing artificial should intrude into the sexual relations between human beings, that belief will have profound implications for one's attitude toward contraceptive techniques and reproductive technologies. One critic of the new reproductive technologies has formulated his objection as follows:

> Is there possibly some wisdom in that mystery of nature which joins the pleasure of sex, the communication of love, and the desire for children in the very activity by which we continue the chain of human existence? . . .
>
> My point is simply this: there are more and less human ways of bringing a child into the world. I am arguing that the laboratory production of human beings is no longer *human* procreation, that making babies in laboratories—even "perfect" babies—means a degradation of parenthood (Kass 1972, 49).

Diametrically opposed to this anti-technological viewpoint is the perspective of those who regard the rational control of nature as one of the major achievements of human beings. On this view, liberation from some of the unpredictable aspects of human reproduction is a major boon to the human species.

> Should we leave the fruits of human reproduction to take shape at random, keeping our children dependent on the accidents of romance and genetic endowment, of [the] sexual lottery or what one physician calls

"the meiotic roulette of his parents' chromosomes?" Or should we be responsible about it, that is, exercise our rational and human choice, no longer submissively trusting to the blind worship of raw nature? (Fletcher 1974, 36).

A third position tends to mediate between these radically divergent views. In agreement with the first, it accepts reproduction without technological assistance as natural and good. However, this third position also argues that the development and use of new methods of contraception or reproduction can be morally justifiable, depending on the circumstances and on the reasons adduced. On this view, it is natural for human beings to create culture in an effort to cope with some of the uncertainties and inconveniences of the natural world. Technology is an important part of that culture (Callahan 1972, 100–101).

THE MORAL STATUS OF THE EARLY HUMAN EMBRYO

To speak of the moral status of anything is to use a shorthand expression for more complex formulations like "What are our moral obligations to X?" or "What moral rights does X possess?" Analogously, one can speak of the legal status of an adult, a newborn infant, or a human embryo.

There are three principal viewpoints on the moral status of the early human embryo—here defined as the embryo within the first fourteen days post-fertilization. The first viewpoint asserts that human embryos are entitled to protection as human beings from the time of fertilization forward. On this view, any research or other manipulation, such as freezing, that damages an embryo or interferes with its prospects for transfer to a uterus and subsequent development is ethically unacceptable. This perspective on embryonic status is based on two kinds of factual evidence. First, the embryonic genotype is established at the time of fertilization. Second, given the proper environment, early embryos have the potential to become full-term fetuses, children, and adults.

A second viewpoint denies that early human embryos have any moral status. According to this view, we who are adult human beings have no moral obligations to early human embryos. This viewpoint also appeals to scientific evidence, especially the fact that only about 30–40 percent of embryos produced through human sexual intercourse develop to maturity in utero and are delivered as live infants (Leridon 1973). It also notes that the biological individuality of the early embryo is established only toward the end of the first fourteen days of development; before that time one embryo can divide into twins or, more rarely, two embryos with different genotypes can combine into a single hybrid embryo. Finally, this position argues that an undifferentiated entity like the early embryo, which has no organs, no limbs, and no sentience, cannot have moral status.

Again on this issue there is a mediating position. This viewpoint accords some moral status to the early embryo, on grounds of its genotype and its potential. These characteristics differentiate the early embryo from other human tissues or cells.

However, this third view acknowledges that our prima facie moral obligations to early human embryos can be outweighed by other moral duties, for example, the duty to develop new and better methods of providing care to infertile couples.

THE ROLE OF THE FAMILY AND GENETIC LINEAGE

The practice of donating gametes or early embryos has occasioned debate among commentators on the new reproductive technologies. One view is that even though the new reproductive technologies are not unnatural, they should be employed only within the family unit. Proponents of this view argue that if a couple cannot conceive a child by means of their own sperm and egg cells, even with medical assistance, they should accept their infertility and explore other alternatives like the adoption of a child. On this view, adoption is qualitatively different from the deliberate and premeditated introduction of "foreign" gametes or embryos into the family unit because adopting parents rescue an already-existing child from a situation of homelessness. The opposing viewpoint on gamete and embryo donation is that these practices are morally justified when employed by a couple for good reasons, such as untreatable infertility or the presence of a genetic abnormality in one or both partners. The use of the new reproductive technologies is thus seen as a useful adjunct that allows couples to approximate, as closely as possible, the usual experience of reproduction.

Another controversial issue is the meaning of the term "family." The traditional understanding of family was that it included a husband, a wife, and one or more children. This traditional understanding has been called into question not by the new reproductive technologies but by several social developments of the twentieth century—especially divorce rates that are approaching 50 percent in the United States and the increasing number of children born to single women. The general debate about the meaning of family will, however, be carried over into discussions of the new reproductive technologies as members of non-traditional families—unmarried heterosexual couples, single men or women, and members of homosexual couples—request technical assistance in reproduction.

THE APPROPRIATE ROLE OF GOVERNMENT

The classical Western view of the proper role of government, articulated by philosophers like Plato, was that government should promote virtue in the citizens, who were viewed in some sense as parts of an organic whole, the state. In modern times this view has been rejected by most Western political philosophers. The closest modern parallel to the Platonic view is that governments should ensure that citizens act in accordance with the principles of morality. According to this view, governments are justified in intervening to prevent even private immoral behavior, such as illicit sexual activity, because such behavior in the long run undermines the public good (Devlin 1965, 14–15). A second view sees the primary role of government as protecting individual liberties and preventing individuals from inflicting harm on others. This view often includes the "clear and present danger" test often used in debates about freedom of speech—namely, that only serious, imminent harms are of sufficient importance to warrant government intrusion (Feinberg 1973, 41–45). On this view, government would not normally intervene in the private sexual activities or reproductive efforts of consenting adults except, perhaps, to prevent tangible, highly-probable physical harm to potential offspring. A third view would limit individual liberty not only to protect citizens from harm but also to ensure that every citizen enjoys at least a certain minimum of welfare—that is, income, food, clothing, shelter, and health care (Daniels 1985; Rawls 1973). Applied to the new reproductive technologies, this view of government might include infertility treatment within the scope of the minimum health services that every citizen should be guaranteed by society.

Artificial Insemination

Artificial insemination is widely used in animal husbandry, especially in the breeding of cattle. The technique was first demonstrated unequivocally in toads in 1779 by Lazaro Spallanzani, Italian priest and physiologist. The first known successful artificial insemination of a human female occurred in 1790, when John Hunter, Scottish anatomist and surgeon, inseminated the wife of a linen draper, using her husband's sperm (Corea 1985, 35). Almost a century later William Panacost, a medical school professor in Philadelphia, performed artificial insemination with donor sperm. When a wealthy Philadelphia couple requested his help in overcoming their infertility, Panacost asked the best-looking member of his medical school class to volunteer as a semen donor. The insemination was performed in the doctor's office under general anesthesia, and neither the husband nor his wife was informed about the method employed to initiate the pregnancy (Andrews 1985a, 148).

Two types of artificial insemination are usually distinguished, artificial insemination using the husband's semen (AIH) and artificial insemination using a donor's semen (AID). AIH is often considered as a therapeutic intervention when a couple has tried unsuccessfully for several years to conceive a child by means of sexual intercourse. One or more factors may be responsible for the couple's infertility, among them the husband's impotence, a low sperm count, or an immunological incompatibility between the husband's semen and the wife's cervical or vaginal secretions. The freezing of semen samples for possible future AIH is also considered by some couples when the husband is about to undergo surgery, drug treatment, or radiation treatment that may cause sterility or damage the sperm cells.

The technique of AIH is quite straightforward. One or more semen samples are produced by the husband through masturbation. After treatment by various laboratory techniques, the samples, or the sperm from the samples, are placed by a health professional into the vagina, cervical canal, or uterus of the wife (American Fertility Society 1986, 34S). No patterns of handicapped offspring have been observed following the use of AIH.

The major ethical objection raised against AIH by some critics is that it separates the love-making and procreative aspects of human sexual activity (Pius XII 1956). This objection seems to be based on an ideal of natural reproduction and on a rejection of at least some kinds of technological interventions into the reproductive process. Defenders of AIH respond by arguing that it is nature itself, not the husband and wife, that causes the separation of love-making and reproduction for couples who are involuntarily infertile. Proponents of AIH also assert that couples who resort to AIH merely extend the sphere of their love-making to include the physician's office and the technological assistance of a third party (McCormick 1978, 1458; 1985, 399).

AID is usually considered as an option by a couple when the husband has no viable sperm in his semen, when there is a rhesus (abbreviated Rh) incompatibility between husband and wife, or when the husband does not want to transmit a genetic defect to offspring. As noted above, donor semen has been used by some physicians in treating infertile couples since the late nineteenth century. The technique precisely parallels AIH, except that the provider of semen in AID is not the husband.

Because AID involves the introduction of third-party gametes into the marital relationship, the use of this technique is a more complicated matter, both ethically and legally. Some critics of AID have suggested that the practice undermines the family or that it could have negative psychological effects on the husband or the potential child. These are empirical questions and can be systematically studied. The meager data currently available indicate no pattern of such psychological harms if the husband has consented to AID and if resulting children are informed of the circumstances of their conception in a reasonable way (Andrews 1985a, 168).

From the standpoint of safety to the wife and to the potential child, the most important issue of AID is appropriate screening of the semen donor, who is often technically a "vendor" rather than a donor. In several tragic cases fatal genetic diseases in children have resulted from improper screening of the biological father. Communicable diseases, including infection with the human immunodeficiency virus which causes AIDS, have also been transmitted from semen donors to recipient women (Stewart et al. 1985). At a minimum, the prospective donor's family history should be taken, and he should be tested for evidence of infectious disease. Whether his chromosomes should also be examined through karyotyping is currently a matter of debate. Careful, permanent records about the donor's health status should be maintained in a confidential file, to which medical practitioners should have access if later follow-up with the donor becomes necessary (American Fertility Society 1986, 37S).

As currently practiced in the United States, AID often includes a commercial dimension. If fresh semen from a nonrelative is used for AID, the "donor" is usually a student who receives $25–$50 per acceptable specimen. If frozen semen is employed, it is most likely to be purchased from one of approximately 25 commercial sperm banks in the United States. One can debate whether a paid "donor" is being compensated for his time and inconvenience or for the gametes themselves. However, some critics of AID object to what they call the commercialization of the reproductive process when semen donors are paid and sperm banks become profit-making enterprises. They argue that the collection and distribution of sperm should be conducted in the same voluntary, nonprofit way that whole blood and transplantable organs are. France has gone a step further by establishing a centralized, national system for the sperm donors. Fertile males who have already fathered healthy children are urged to consider donating semen to the national sperm banking system, as a fulfillment of a civic duty (United Kingdom, 1984, 27–28).

In Vitro Fertilization

CLINICAL APPLICATIONS

The birth of Louise Brown in Lancashire, England, on July 25, 1978, inaugurated a new era in the history of the reproductive technologies. Louise had been conceived, not inside her mother's body, but rather in a Petri dish, where eggs from her mother were mixed with sperm from her father, and where fertilization took place.

In vitro fertilization (IVF) is most often proposed when the members of a married couple are unable to reproduce because of obstructions in the wife's reproductive tract or because of the husband's low sperm count. Typically, the egg cells used in IVF are surgically removed from the wife's ovaries, and the semen is provided by the husband. In most cases no early embryos are frozen, and one or more developing embryos are transferred to the uterus of the wife.

The possible risks of clinical IVF to offspring were, in the 1970s, the object of rather vigorous debate. By the mid-1980s, however, a series of more than 2000 births following IVF showed no clear evidence of an increased incidence of congenital defects. The longterm consequences of IVF on children conceived by means of this technique have, of course, not yet been assessed.

The major ethical reservation about clinical IVF in cases involving only the reproductive cells of the husband and wife is that this technical procedure separates love-making from procreation. This reservation and the counter-argument to it exactly parallel the discussion in the case of AIH.

There are several emerging and potential future uses of clinical IVF that have occasioned considerable debate. These include the freezing and storage of early human embryos, the donation or sale of human embryos, early gender selection, and early diagnosis of genetic or chromosomal abnormalities (American College of Obstetricians and Gynecologists 1986; American Fertility Society 1986).

The freezing and storage of early human embryos is currently a research procedure. This technique is widely used in animal husbandry, especially in the cattle-breeding industry. There are several reasons why the freezing and storage of early human embryos might be useful to infertile couples. Infertile women are often given hormonal stimulation so that their ovaries produce multiple eggs in a given cycle. After fertilization with the husband's sperm, these multiple eggs may develop into multiple early embryos, perhaps even five or six embryos. The freezing and storage of some of these embryos may help to solve the "surplus-embryo" problem. Rather than transferring all five or six embryos at one time—thus perhaps risking the possibility of a triplet or quadruplet pregnancy—the couples's physician may elect to transfer only two or three and to freeze and store the remaining embryos until a later cycle. Further, the freezing and storage of embryos spares the wife the trauma of another surgical procedure for retrieving eggs in a subsequent ovulatory cycle.

At the same time, however, human embryos freezing may raise metaphysical, ethical, and legal problems. The metaphysical problem is what status to ascribe to an undifferentiated human entity that can be preserved for years in a state of suspended animation. The ethical and legal problems center on the question whether frozen, stored embryos should be regarded as in some sense the "property" of the couple whose reproductive cells combined to produce the embryos. A famous case in Australia, the Rios case, sparked a lively public debate about what should be done with frozen early embryos that were suddenly "orphaned" by the deaths of their future "social parents" in a plane crash (Sellar 1984).

The new techniques for freezing or storing embryos will also facilitate the donation or sale of human embryos to third parties. The question of embryo donation or sale closely parallels the question of semen donation or sale discussed above. In the future human egg freezing and storage may also become technically feasible. The same issues of third-party involvement, donor screening, and public policy on donation or sale that we examined in connection with AID also arise in connection with the freezing and storage of human embryos. In addition, many would argue that the ethical stakes are higher in the case of an embryo that may one day develop into a human adult than with a sperm or egg cell.

Noninvasive techniques for determining whether early human embryos are destined to be males or females are likely to be developed in the future. If these techniques were used to help a couple avoid transmitting a sex-linked genetic disorder to their children, the use of these techniques would seem, in the view of most commentators, to be morally justifiable. They would have the advantage, as compared with prenatal diagnosis and selective abortion, of sparing the woman physical trauma and of intervening when the embryo is relatively undeveloped. The use of gender selection techniques for purely social reasons, such as the desire to "have a boy first" raises subtle, and hotly-debated, questions about sex discrimination and possible longterm effects on the sex ratio.

Another future application of IVF and freezing and storage techniques may be early—that is, preimplantation—diagnosis of genetic or chromosomal abnormalities. The technique likely to be employed will remove one or more cells from the developing embryo for diagnostic purposes, then freeze the remaining cells. Various tests could then be performed on the removed cells. If a particular embryo were found to be free of detectable defects, it would be transferred to the uterus of the woman in a subsequent ovulatory cycle. Any embryo found to be affected by a genetic or chromosomal abnormality would presumably not be transferred but, rather, would be discarded. Again in this case preimplantation intervention would seem morally preferable to intervention on the basis of prenatal diagnosis after a pregnancy is already well established. However, the consequences, for the later development of potential children, of removing embryonic cells will need to be established in careful scientific studies.

RESEARCH

Laboratory research with early human embryos has been proposed as a way to gain important information about fertilization, the prevention of fertilization (that is, contraception), and the causes of birth defects in children. However, critics of laboratory research with early human embryos argue that such research is not compatible with the kind of respect that should be shown to developing entities that may have the potential to become human beings.

Contrasting viewpoints on the ethics of human embryo research are clearly based on differing conceptions of the moral status of the early human embryo (Robertson 1986). The public-policy debate on this question has raged in several countries with no clear resolution. Most public bodies charged with reaching a judgment on human embryo research have found the research to be ethically acceptable, in principle, if the research is intended to develop important knowledge that cannot be gained in any other way (Ontario 1985; United Kingdom 1984; U.S. Ethics Advisory Board 1979; Victoria 1984).

Surrogate Parenthood

Surrogate parenthood arrangements are generally proposed when a wife who wishes to bear and raise a child is medically incapable of carrying a pregnancy. She may, for example, have been born without a uterus. Or she may be afflicted with a medical condition that would make pregnancy a life-threatening condition for her.

The first documented attempt to employ a surrogate motherhood arrangement in the United States occurred in 1976, under the direction of Michigan attorney Noel Keane (Keane and Breo 1981). In the early years of this new social practice the relatively old technology of artificial insemination donor (AID) was employed, using sperm provided by the husband of the future social mother. Thus, the child in the usual or "full" surrogate motherhood arrangement results from the union of the surrogate mother's egg and the social father's sperm. In 1985 the first instance of surrogate motherhood assisted by in vitro fertilization occurred. In this arrangement the future social mother was able to produce fertilizable eggs but medically unable to carry a pregnancy. Her eggs were fertilized in vitro with sperm from her husband, and the resulting embryos were then transferred to the uterus of a surrogate mother (Utian et al. 1985). In this latter arrangement, which is sometimes called "partial surrogacy," the gestational mother is often called a "surrogate carrier" because she makes no genetic contribution to the child.

While surrogate motherhood in the United States has usually involved a professional who formalizes the arrangements between the surrogate and the social parents, as well as arranging for the payment of a fee to the surrogate mother, a formal and commercial relationship is not a necessary part of surrogate motherhood. In some subcultures a fertile wife readily conceives and bears an extra child for her sister if the sister is infertile. Further, there have been anecdotal reports of noncommercial surrogacy arrangements in which a fertile woman bore a child for an infertile friend or coworker. In fact, some commentators on surrogate motherhood have argued that the earliest pretechnological surrogate arrangement occurred in biblical times, for example, when Sarah suggested that Abraham conceive a child with her maid Hagar because Sarah herself was infertile (Genesis 16:1–15).

There are four principal ethical and public-policy questions that have been raised about surrogate motherhood arrangements.

1. If the surrogate mother decides during the pregnancy or at the time of delivery to keep the child that she had agreed to bear for a couple, who should have parental rights?
2. To what extent should the adopting couple be able to control the lifestyle of the surrogate mother during the pregnancy?
3. If the child is born with physical or mental handicaps, are the adopting parents nonetheless obligated to accept the child as their own?
4. If the surrogate mother receives payment, for what is the payment made, and how can exploitative or coercive relationships be avoided?

What all these questions suggest is that the duration and intent of third-party involvement in surrogate motherhood arrangements raise special problems. In the case of semen or egg donation, or even embryo donation, the act of donation can be completed in a few minutes, at most. However, surrogate mothers are pregnant for approximately nine months, interact physically with the fetus, give birth to a child, and perhaps even develop a relationship with the future social parents. This extended period of de facto interdependence among surrogate mother, fetus, and adopting parents plus the uncertainties inherent in any pregnancy probably means that complications will always arise in at least a small fraction of surrogate motherhood arrangements.

Given these likely complications, should surrogate motherhood arrangements be legally prohibited? The answer to this question has varied from country to country. The United Kingdom and the state of Victoria in Australia have banned commercial surrogate motherhood arrangements (King 1986, 131–132). In 1985 the Ontario Law Reform Commission recommended that surrogate motherhood arrangements be permitted only with the active participation of a court in the entire transaction (1985, 242–262). In the United States the two most thorough committee analyses of surrogate motherhood have described potential problems in the practice, but have stopped short of recommending legal prohibition even of commercial surrogacy (American College of Obstetricians and Gynecologists 1983; American Fertility Society 1986). The 1986 report of the American Fertility Society recommended that, if surrogate motherhood is practiced, it should be regarded as a clinical experiment, with formal research protocols and oversight by a research review committee. The same report also urged practitioners and social scientists to publish data about surrogate motherhood programs, so that society will have a better basis on which to reach a well-founded ethical judgment about this practice (American Fertility Society 1986, 67S).

In the future it is possible that an artificial placenta or artificial uterus will be developed that will make extracorporeal gestation possible. Such a device, if demonstrated to be safe and efficacious, might make the current practice of surrogate motherhood obsolete. However, this new technology would raise interesting ethical questions in its own right (Fletcher 1974, 163–165).

GENETIC TESTING AND SCREENING

There can be no doubt that we live in the golden age of medical genetics. Even before the 1950s Gregor Mendel's classic work on various modes of inheritance was available as a theoretical framework for understanding how genetic disease is transmitted. However, Watson and Crick's description of the molecular structure of DNA in 1953 and the rapid advances based on the use of recombinant DNA techniques in the 1960s and 1970s have opened up entirely new possibilities in genetic diagnosis and therapy.

As we shall see, the principal benefits of medical genetics through the mid-1980s have been diagnostic and predictive rather than therapeutic. We now understand much more clearly the genetic dimensions of many human diseases, including conditions that in the past were not thought to have any genetic components—for example, manic-depressive disorders and malignant melanoma. For a minority of genetic diseases some helpful therapy can currently be offered to patients. For the most part, however, the medical treatment of genetic disease is a future goal.

Genetic disorders exact an enormous toll of human suffering. In the latest edition of the standard catalog of Mendelian disorders in humans, 4000 distinguishable genetic or chromosomal conditions are described (McKusick 1986). Genetic disorders are the second leading cause of death among 1- to 4-year-olds in the United States and the third leading cause of death in 15- to 17-year-olds. It is estimated that 25–30 percent of admissions to U.S. acute-care hospitals for persons under eighteen are for genetic conditions; about 13 percent of adult admissions are for genetically-related conditions. In addition, 20–25 percent of persons institutionalized because of mental retardation have genetically-caused diseases (*Antenatal Diagnosis* 1979, I–27 to I–30).

This section of the present chapter will discuss the various types of genetic testing and screening and some of the ethical and public-policy questions currently being raised, or likely to be raised in the future, by genetic screening programs in particular. Genetic testing is here defined as the use of diagnostic procedures for determining the presence or absence of one or more genetic traits or conditions in an individual. Genetic screening refers to the use of such tests in programs that are intended to reach a large percentage of persons who have a particular genetic trait or condition. Thus, genetic screening always involves genetic testing, but genetic testing may not always involve a systematic, organized screening program.

Technical and Legal Background

As currently practiced, genetic testing usually occurs at one of three stages of life: (1) in the neonatal period; (2) prenatally; or (3) when couples are considering marriage or childbearing. In the future the technique of gene mapping and the sequencing of the human genome may significantly extend medicine's current diagnostic capabilities.

NEONATAL SCREENING

Historically, the capacity to test newborns for phenylketonuria (PKU)—a so-called "inborn error of metabolism"—was the first to be used in a mass screening program. In 1962 Massachusetts tried a voluntary screening program for PKU, using a test developed by Dr. Robert Guthrie. The following year Massachusetts adopted the first mandatory PKU newborn screening law in the United States (U.S. President's Commission 1983, 13).

From these modest beginnings, newborn screening has since expanded until forty-eight states and the District of Columbia had statutes governing newborn screening in 1985 (Andrews 1985b, 1). Of these programs, all but three—those in Maryland, the District of Columbia, and North Carolina—were mandatory. The list of genetic conditions screened for has gradually expanded, as well. Many states now attempt to detect hypothyroidism, galactosemia, homocystinuria, and maple-syrup urine disease, as well as PKU (Andrews 1985b, 156–160). In the early 1970s twelve states and the District of Columbia passed statutes authorizing sickle-cell screening. Most of these laws have since been repealed or revised (Andrews 1985b, 147–149).

The principal rationale for newborn screening is that it makes possible the early diagnosis of a disease that can be treated through appropriate medical intervention. In the case of PKU, for example, a special diet can help to prevent much of the damage that PKU would otherwise cause to children's brains. However, at least one city-wide program has screened newborns for hemoglobin disorders not only for the purpose of managing the infants' diseases but also to provide reproductive information to the infants' parents (Townes 1986).

PRENATAL DIAGNOSIS

The second type of genetic testing developed, historically, was prenatal diagnosis. In 1966 a report was published of the first study of chromosomes taken from cultured cells withdrawn from the amniotic sac by amniocentesis. In the following two years successful prenatal diagnosis of a chromosmal disorder and an inborn error of metabolism was reported in scientific publications (U.S. President's Commission 1983, 23). Since the early 1960s other diagnostic methods have also become available for the prenatal detection of genetic or chromosomal abnormalities. These include ultrasonography (which provides echo-like pictures of the developing fetus), the withdrawal of a blood sample from the umbilical cord with the aid of fetoscopy, the testing of blood samples from pregnant women, and the removal of fetal cells from chorionic villi inside the uterus toward the end of the first trimester of pregnancy (U.S. President's Commission 1983, 25–31). The techniques for studying fetal cells have also become more precise and sophisticated in the intervening years.

Prenatal diagnosis has for the most part, been conducted on the basis of physician recommendation or patient request as a part of individualized prenatal care. However, in the late 1970s a large collaborative study of maternal serum alpha-fetoprotein screening was conducted in Great Britain (U.K. Collaborative Study 1977). This study involved testing blood samples taken from pregnant women for an elevated level of the substance alpha-protein (AFP). Elevated levels of AFP are frequently correlated with the presence of fetal brain absence (anencephaly) or a fetal spinal cord defect (spina bifida). MSAFP screening is now made available to all pregnant women in Great Britain through the National Health Service. In the United States several regional MSAFP screening programs have been developed; California has a coordinated prenatal-diagnosis program that offers MSAFP testing to all pregnant women and amniocentesis to all pregnant women who will be 35 years old or older at the time of delivery (Steinbrook 1986).

CARRIER TESTING AND SCREENING

This third type of genetic testing and screening is most frequently employed when couples are considering marriage or reproduction. In the United States the earliest carrier screening programs focused on two diseases, Tay-Sachs disease, which affects primarily people of Ashkenazi Jewish descent, and sickle-cell anemia, which is most prevalent among members of the black population (U.S. President's Commission 1983, 17–23). In the Mediterranean region similar programs have been developed for thalassemia, a hemoglobin disorder that is in some respects similar to sickle-cell disease. In 1986 three hospitals, one each in Massachusetts, New York, and Maryland, also began offering genetic testing to adults who are at risk for carrying the gene that causes Huntington's chorea (Zoler 1986).

In carrier testing a genetic counselor helps couples to understand their relative risk of transmitting a genetic defect to their children. Typically both members of the couple provide cell samples which are then studied in the laboratory. The results of the laboratory tests help the genetic counselor to explain a series of probabilities to the couple. For example, if only one member of the couple carries the gene for a recessive genetic disease, then the couple is not at risk of producing a child afflicted with the disease but has a one in two chance of producing a carrier. However, if both members of a couple carry the gene for a recessive genetic disease that is not sex-linked, the couple has a 25 percent chance of producing an unaffected child, a 50 percent chance of producing a carrier, and a 25 percent chance of producing a child who will have the disease.

In the future "carrier testing and screening" may come to have a more extended definition. New diagnostic techniques will increasingly make it possible to give distant early warning to individuals who are destined to be afflicted with a genetic disease later in life. Huntington's chorea testing is the most striking example of this new capability. This disease usually strikes its victims between the ages of 35 and 45. Until recently no reliable test existed that could determine whether a healthy 20-year-old would or would not be afflicted with the disease in later life. Now a relatively accurate test does exist, and individuals who are at risk are having to make a very difficult decision—whether to be tested or not. Similar tests may one day be available for other genetically-related conditions, such as the tendency to develop serious heart disease in one's thirties or forties.

GENE MAPPING AND THE SEQUENCING OF THE HUMAN GENOME

Human beings usually have twenty-three pairs of chromosomes in the nuclei of every one of their cells. In turn, these chromosomes contain the genes that code for proteins and other products that our bodies need to function, as well as intervening stretches of DNA whose function is not well understood at present. The smallest coding units within the genes and intervening sequences are called bases. It is estimated that our twenty-three pairs of chromosomes contain 50,000 to 100,000 genes and 3 to 3.5 billion base pairs. Scientists are eager to learn more about the structure and function of human genes and chromosomes, which, all taken together, are called the human genome. Thus, researchers plan first to map the genome, then to sequence areas of special interest, and finally to sequence (or decipher the genetic letters contained in) all 3 to 3.5 billion base pairs that comprise our genome (Lewin 1986).

Perhaps a geographical analogy will be helpful for understanding how gene mapping and sequencing work. If you wanted to make a physical map of the United States, you might first use a satellite photograph to get an overview of the whole country. That largest map would correspond to locating the twenty-three pairs of human chromosomes. In mapping the United States you might then divide the country into 1000 regions, each comprised of a certain number of square miles. For this more detailed map you might use photographs taken from airplanes. Similarly, scientists will divide the human genome into major regions, each of which will consist of perhaps 40,000 base pairs. In our geography project, there might be certain regions that required special attention even at this stage of mapping—for example, major metropolitan areas or areas with potentially dangerous geological faults. In a parallel way, scientists have already discovered that certain disease-related genes are located in particular regions of particular chromosomes. They will therefore subject these regions to special scrutiny at this stage of mapping. The final stage in the geography project might be a highly-detailed map that indicates individual streets or even individual buildings on those streets. This fine level of detail would correspond to knowing the sequence in which some or all of the 3 to 3.5 billion base pairs are arranged in human chromosomes.

This massive project of gene mapping and sequencing will initially provide detailed knowledge about where important genes are located and how they function. The first application of this new knowledge will probably be diagnostic: tests will be developed for large numbers of diseases, and these tests will then be able to be used in newborn screening, prenatal diagnosis, and carrier screening. At the same time, however, gene mapping and sequencing may help scientists and clinicians to develop ways to correct, or at least compensate for, at least some genetic defects.

Ethical and Public-Policy Issues

Much has been written about the ethical and public-policy issues surrounding genetic testing and screening. Four issues have been central to this discussion: (1) freedom and coercion in genetic testing and screening; (2) the confidentiality or disclosure of test results; (3) access to genetic testing services; and (4) the probable benefits and harms of genetic testing and screening programs.

Freedom and Coercion

As we noted above, all programs of prenatal diagnosis and nearly all programs of carrier screening have been voluntary. In contrast, virtually all newborn screening programs are mandated by state governments. The major rationale for mandatory newborn screening programs is that such programs protect the helpless from serious, avoidable harm through the use of low-risk, minimally intrusive diagnostic procedures (U.S. President's Commission 1983, 51). The arguments in favor of newborn screening for treatable conditions are so strong, in fact, that the overwhelming majority of parents want such screening to be performed on their newborns. A study of Maryland's voluntary newborn screening program for PKU found, for example, that the parental refusal rate was only .05 percent—one refusal for every 1999 acceptances (Faden et al. 1982). One can view this result in two ways. On the one hand, the result indicates that so-called "mandatory" newborn screening programs are probably not perceived as coercive by a large majority of parents. On the other hand, this high rate of voluntary parental compliance suggests that laws or regulations mandating newborn screening may not be necessary; at the very least, the social costs of initiating any kind of mandatory program need to be weighed against the benefits conferred to a tiny minority of newborns and their families.

There is a second type of mandatory program that can be distinguished from the unconditionally-mandatory screening imposed by a state. We might call such testing "contingently mandatory." For example, an employer might hypothetically require all applicants for employment to undergo a battery of genetic-diagnostic tests. These tests would not be mandatory in the sense that anyone could decide not to apply for work in a company that has adopted such a screening policy. However, the tests would be mandatory for all applicants. Similar questions may arise if health insurance companies begin requiring batteries of genetic tests before writing individual insurance policies. The debates that currently surround drug-testing in the workplace and testing for antibody to the human immunodeficiency (AIDS-causing) virus in a variety of settings suggest that contingently-mandatory genetic testing may become an important public-policy issue in the future.

In its report on genetic counseling and screening the President's Commission on Bioethics reached the following conclusion:

> In sum, the fundamental value of genetic screening and counseling is their ability to enhance the opportunities for individuals to obtain information about their personal health and to make autonomous and noncoerced choices based on that information (U.S. President's Commission 1983, 55).

This conclusion clearly states the autonomy-oriented approach to genetic testing and screening. However, moral freedom is generally accompanied by moral responsibility. Thus, a complementary and balancing thesis is that individuals and couples have a moral duty to learn what they can about the likelihood that they will transmit genetic conditions to their offspring and to take reasonable steps—steps that are compatible with their other ethical convictions—to avoid causing preventable harm to their descendants. This "ethics of genetic duty" (Ramsey 1970, 57) need not, and in the author's view should not, be enacted into law. It does, however, qualify the ethic of autonomy in the genetic and reproductive spheres.

CONFIDENTIALITY AND DISCLOSURE

If a genetic condition is detected through either a mandatory or a voluntary testing or screening program, there remains a further question: who, besides the individual and his or her health provider, should have access to the information about the genetic condition? This question arises primarily in two contexts—an extended-familial context and what might be called a business context. In the extended-family context, individuals or couples who learn that they have a genetic disease or carry a genetic trait may face decisions about whether to inform their parents, their siblings, their children, and even more distant relatives. For example, if an individual discovers that he has the gene for a late-onset genetically-dominant disorder like Huntington's chorea, he will also know that each of his siblings will have a 50 percent chance of having the gene and, if one or more siblings have the gene, a 50 percent chance of transmitting the gene to each of their children. Most individuals in this situation would probably want to warn their siblings voluntarily, especially given the fact that none of us is causally or morally responsible for the genetic conditions with which we are born. However, if an individual refuses to disclose such information voluntarily, and serious harm to others is likely to result from the nondisclosure, then a case can be made for breaching the normal duty to protect the confidentiality of information about a patient's genetic condition (U.S. President's Commission 1983, 44–45).

The business context for questions about confidentiality in medical genetics is likely to involve either employers or insurers. For example, health insurance companies might charge a higher premium for, or even refuse to insure at all, an individual who is afflicted with a certain kind of genetic condition. Similarly, an employer might be reluctant to hire and train an individual if the employer knew that she were at high risk of premature death from a lethal genetic disease. These are highly complicated issues that cannot be solved with simple formulas. On the one hand, employers and insurance companies have a legitimate interest in controlling their costs. On the other hand, there is the possibility that individuals will be unfairly discriminated against because of medical conditions over which they have no control. The result for these individuals may be loss of access to employment or to the health-care system.

The President's Commission on Bioethics argued that, because of "the potential for misuse as well as unintended social or economic injury, information about genetic conditions should be disclosed to insurers or employers only with the explicit consent of the person tested" (1983, 44). This argument may be an important element in an overall public policy about confidentiality and genetic testing, but it should be supplemented by a more thorough analysis of society's responsibility, or lack of responsibility, to provide access to employment and health care to every member of society. Specific mechanisms, at the state or federal level, for spreading the financial risks of caring for members of high-risk groups should also be addressed (National Academy of Sciences 1986, 168–173).

ACCESS TO GENETIC TESTING SERVICES

Problems of access to genetic testing services can arise in at least two ways. First, because health-insurance systems are often oriented toward the performance of procedures, insurance carriers will often reimburse their clients for tests but not for the counseling and interpretation that should accompany the tests. The result may be either the loss of critical information or a major unanticipated expense.

Second, in some cases an individual may not know what further tests may be required if the results of an initial test are positive or suspicious. For example, MSAFP screening usually involves only a single test of a blood sample from a pregnant woman. However, an initial positive test may lead to a repeat blood (serum) test, detailed ultrasonography, amniocentesis, and a decision about selective abortion. Pregnant women who are uninsured or underinsured may be able to afford the initial and repeat serum tests but be unable to bear the expense of the later, more sophisticated tests in the series. The State of California has sought to confront this kind of access problem by providing a statewide and state-run program that charges a nominal flat fee—in 1986 the figure was $40—to every pregnant woman who enrolls for MSAFP testing. The $40 fee guarantees access to all necessary diagnostic tests (Steinbrook 1986).

PROBABLE BENEFITS AND HARMS

We have already considered a series of possible benefits and harms of genetic testing and screening programs. The principal benefits noted are knowledge, the ability to avoid transmitting genetic disease to offspring, and, in some cases, the ability to secure timely treatment for a genetic condition. We have also seen that genetic testing and screening programs can cause harm—through coercion, through leading to exclusion from the work force or the health-care system, and through providing incomplete information or partial services.

Two other dimensions of the benefit-harm question deserve brief consideration. The first is that a positive genetic test, even if it does not lead to economic loss, may result in the stigmatization of the individual tested. Sometimes this stigmatization is based on erroneous information, as was the case in the early 1970s when carriers of the sickle-cell trait, who did not have sickle-cell anemia, were subjected to several baseless restrictions (Andrews 1985b, 147–148). The stigmatization may also result from informing children of their genetic problems or carrier status when they are not yet able to cope with the information.

In a curious way the new techniques of gene mapping and gene sequencing may help to "democratize" genetic disease. We all know, theoretically, that we have certain genetic tendencies and may in fact carry several potentially lethal genes. In addition, our chromosomes include a set of dormant but nonetheless potentially dangerous cancer-causing genes called proto-oncogenes. As more is learned about the human genome, and as diagnostic tests for more genetic diseases and traits become available, it may become clearer that visible and invisible genetic problems are simply an omnipresent aspect of the human condition.

Finally, the technique of prenatal diagnosis and selective abortion raises special ethical questions. Some commentators argue that abortion is always wrong, even if performed for so-called "fetal indications" (Ramsey 1970, 114). Other commentators have raised the question whether it is psychologically possible to advocate the selective abortion of fetuses discovered to have genetic defects while at the same time pressing for nondiscriminatory treatment of the already-born who are handicapped (Hauerwas 1986, 159–181; Motulsky and Murray 1983). This quandary may be resolved, in part, by the development of new and better methods of intrauterine intervention, both medically and surgically (Fletcher 1983a; Walters 1986a). However, some conditions that are detectable prenatally may never be amenable to corrective treatment.

HUMAN GENE THERAPY AND GENETIC ENGINEERING

Types of Genetic Intervention

There are four major kinds of genetic intervention in humans that may one day become technically feasible. These types of possible interventions can be represented schematically as follows:

	cure of disease	enhancement of capabilities
somatic cells	1	3
germ-line cells	2	4

The first type of genetic intervention would aim to cure a condition that is generally acknowledged to be a disease by genetically altering the nonreproductive cells of a patient. For example, the bone-marrow cells of a patient suffering from sickle cell anemia may be able to be treated and the patient cured of his or her disease. However, this cure would not be transmitted to the patient's descendants. In the second type of genetic intervention both somatic (nonreproductive) and reproductive cells would be treated, so that the changes of the genetic "cure" would be passed on to the patient's descendants. (Depending on the type of genetic alteration and the stage of development at which it were performed, it is possible that only some of the patient's descendant's would be cured.)

The distinction between "the cure of disease" and "the enhancement of capabilities" may not always be clear. However, a plausible example of enhancement would be doubling the efficiency of an individual's longterm memory. If this enhancement were based on somatic-cell alterations, one would have the third type of genetic intervention. If this enhancement also affected the reproductive cells of the subject—who would perhaps not be called a "patient"—improved long-term-memory efficiency would also be passed on to at least some of the subject's descendants. This germ-line enhancement of a human capability would be·an example of the fourth type of genetic intervention.

As of 1988, no human patient has been cured of genetic disease by means of gene therapy. However, almost twenty years of experience with the analogous procedure of bone marrow transplantation (Parkman 1986) and the success of laboratory studies (Anderson 1984; Hock and Miller 1986) suggest that somatic-cell gene therapy for the cure of disease may soon be a technical possibility.

The most likely candidates for early type-1 gene therapy are enzyme deficiency single-gene defects. A leading candidate for such treatment is a adenosine deaminase (ADA) deficiency, which causes the total 's immune systems. Because of their immune deficiencies, chil- ADA deficiency inevitably fall prey to bacterial or viral infections the results of such infections by the age of two.

The technique for performing gene therapy on such children might be called "bone marrow transplantation with an extra step." Bone marrow cells will be removed by needle from the upper parts of the patient's own hip bones. The removed bone marrow cells will be taken to the laboratory where an attempt will be made to add a properly-functioning gene to as many of the bone-marrow cells as possible. (The real targets of this procedure are not the bone-marrow cells themselves but the relatively small number of stem cells that later give rise to bone-marrow cells and other kinds of cells.)

The vehicle most likely to be used for delivering properly functioning genes to the cells is a retroviral vector. Scientists have been able to "domesticate" certain kinds of retroviruses, so that they no longer have the capacity to multiply and move from cell to cell. Instead, the viruses are induced to enter a cell and remain there. This domestication is achieved primarily through removing some of the retrovirus's three or four native genes. The removal of the genes, in turn, creates space in the retroviral genome, so that the desired "payload"—the properly functioning gene for the missing enzyme—can be added to what remains of the retrovirus.

If the laboratory procedure works properly, the remaining part of the retrovirus, which is called a vector or vehicle, will carry a copy of the properly functioning gene into the nucleus of each bone marrow cell and especially into the nuclei of stem cells. There the vector and the added gene will be "adopted," so to speak, by one of the chromosomes present in those cells. If all goes well, the added gene will be integrated into one of the native chromosomes and will begin to produce the missing enzyme. As soon as the vectors and genes have been successfully introduced into the patient's bone-marrow and stem cells, the patient will be given a transfusion of his or her own modified cells. Researchers hope that the modified cells containing the properly functioning gene will multiply and will ultimately supplant the patient's own native bone marrow cells. If so, the modified cells with the added gene would produce enough of the missing enzyme to cure the patient's disease (Walters 1986b).

Germ-line gene therapy is likely to take an entirely different tack. Several researchers have been able to introduce genetic changes into the reproductive cells of laboratory animals by adding new DNA to early embryos of the animals. In studies involving mice, for example, genes have been added to one-cell mouse embryos after the sperm had penetrated the egg but before the genetic material from the sperm and egg are joined within the same nucleus. If the experiment is successful, these added genes are then adopted by the embryo. As the embryo grows and the number of embryonic cells increases, the added genes become part of every new embryonic cell. Later, when the sperm or egg cells of the mouse develop, the added genes are included in approximately half of these reproductive cells. Thus, when the mouse reproduces, some of its progeny receive the added genes, and so on through the generations. Genetic defects have been corrected in the germ line in at least three laboratory experiments, one with fruit flies and two with mice (Costantini, Chada, and Magram 1986; Hammer, Palmiter, and Brinster 1984; Rubin and Spradling 1982).

The closest approximation to "enhancement" studies in laboratory animals has been the attempt to produce very large mice by means of genetic intervention. In widely publicized studies a team of researchers introduced the gene for either rat growth hormone or human growth hormone into one-cell mouse embryos. A small fraction of the embryos developed to maturity; some of the mature mice expressed the added gene and, as a result, grew to be significantly larger than their siblings. Several of the offspring of these "supermice" were also abnormally large—thus demonstrating that the genetic change had indeed been passed on through the germ line (Palmiter et al. 1982, 1983).

Ethical and Public-Policy Questions

For the short-term future, only somatic-cell gene therapy for the cure of disease—that is, type-1 gene therapy—will be proposed for use with human patients. Because the changes effected through somatic-cell gene therapy will not be passed on to future generations, many commentators think that this technique will not be qualitatively different from other biomedical innovations, for example, kidney transplants (U.S. Congress Office of Technology Assessment 1984, 1, 7, 28; U.S. President's Commission 1982, 45, 61).

As in the case of other new therapies, the probable benefit/harm ratio for patients or others of somatic-cell gene therapy will be an important consideration. There are clearly some risks and some unknowns associated with even this simplest type of gene therapy. For example, it is not presently possible to control where the retroviral vectors will "touch down" when they reach the nuclei of the patient's bone-marrow and stem cells. In other words, currently-available vectors are unguided missiles. There is some concern among researchers that the vectors may disrupt properly-functioning genes and therefore kill some cells or, more seriously, that the vectors may activate some previously dormant cancer-causing genes. It is also possible that the domesticated retroviral vectors will recombine with other DNA or other viruses and so recapture their native capacity to produce more retroviruses and to infect large numbers of cells. Further, because there are few good animal models of the enzyme-deficiency diseases that afflict humans, laboratory "cures" of such diseases may not be able to be demonstrated. Thus, if gene therapy works as a treatment for, say, ADA deficiency, the first cured subjects are likely to be human beings.

There are other ethical questions, as well, that will be raised by the first attempts to perform gene therapy in human patients. If there are more candidates for gene therapy than can be initially treated, a fair procedure for selecting among candidates will need to be devised. Informed consent will also be an important issue. Patients will deserve a thorough explanation of the potential hazards and benefits of gene therapy. If, as seems likely, the first patients are young children, parents or guardians will need to be well informed before making decisions on behalf of their children or wards. Privacy and confidentiality may also be important questions. The press and the public will be eager to know about the early attempts to perform gene therapy. In the earliest uses of heart transplantation and the artificial heart, this desire to know sometimes created a circus-like atmosphere that posed a risk to the patient's health. With gene therapy a balance will need to be struck between the disclosure of information to the press and the public, on the one hand, and the patient's need for rest and privacy, on the other.

A special public review process for somatic-cell gene therapy has been established in the United States. After a gene-therapy proposal has been reviewed and approved by an institution's local research review committee (often called an "institutional review board"), the proposal will be forwarded to the Recombinant DNA Advisory Committee at the National Institutes of Health. That committee's Human Gene Therapy Subcommittee will perform an initial public review of the proposal and forward its recommendations to the parent committee. If the parent committee, the Recombinant DNA Advisory Committee, also approves, the proposal will be forwarded to the NIH Director for final approval. Thus—for publicly funded research, at least—everyone interested in the topic of gene therapy will be able to know about the researchers, the institution, and the disease to be treated before gene therapy is performed (Walters 1986b, 226).

Type-2 gene therapy, germ-line gene therapy for the cure of disease, may raise qualitatively new kinds of ethical questions, for the genetic alterations performed in this case are likely to be passed on to at least some of the subject's descendants (Fletcher, 1983b). As noted above, the germ-line approach to the treatment and prevention of disease in fruit flies and mice has been modestly successful in a few laboratory experiments. Why would germ-line gene therapy be proposed for the cure or prevention of human disease? One rationale might be that the cells in some parts of the body can only be reached and effectively treated if gene therapy is administered very early, probably at the embryonic stage of development. Certain diseases of the brain, for example, may fall into this category (Office of Technology Assessment, 1984, p. 24). In an experiment aimed at treating otherwise-unreachable brain cells, the researcher's primary intention would no doubt be to prevent the brain-based disease from occurring in the future person; a side-effect of the early intervention would be to effect a genetic alteration in the reproductive cells of the future person, as well.

A second possible rationale for the germ-line approach would be a simple argument from efficiency. It might seem more reasonable to correct a defect once, through germ-line gene therapy, and to have that correction passed on to the subject's descendants than to repeat somatic-cell gene therapy, generation after generation, in a family afflicted by a genetic disease. (Given the current method of gene addition as the likely means of performing gene therapy, it should be noted that only some of the subject's descendants would receive the properly-functioning added gene, while others would receive only the malfunctioning gene. Only if a technique for replacing the malfunctioning genes with properly functioning genes is developed will germ-line gene therapy have the desired effect of eliminating a genetic disease from a particular family line.)

The major current obstacles to germ-line gene therapy through, for example, the treatment of early human embryos, are technical rather than ethical. One technical obstacle is that the large majority of mouse embryos into which added DNA is microinjected either do not survive the injection procedure, do not implant, do not survive because of a new lethal mutation, or do not express the added gene or genes. Further, if one is thinking of therapeutic interventions with human embryos at the time of fertilization, one would not know in most cases whether a particular embryo were destined to be afflicted with a genetic disease. Think, for example, of the case in which both parents are carriers of a recessive genetic trait. Any embryo produced by those parents has a 25 percent chance of being completely unaffected, a 50 percent chance of being a carrier of the genetic trait, and a 25 percent chance of having the genetic disease. In other words, in the situation described any given embryo has a 75 percent chance of not having the genetic disease. Those seem like poor odds for early genetic intervention, especially if the intervention has a moderate or high probability of harming embryos that would otherwise not manifest the disease.

As noted above, a possible alternative to genetic intervention with early human embryos has been suggested by some commentators, namely, preimplantation genetic testing or screening (American College of Obstetricians and Gynecologists, 1986). With this method, a few cells would be removed from an 8-cell embryo, or even a later embryo (a blastocyst) for diagnostic purposes. The remaining cells of the embryo would be frozen and stored. Various genetic tests would then be run on the removed cells. If the results of the test showed an embryo to be free of the genetic disease about which the potential parents were concerned, the remainder of the embryo that had been frozen would be thawed at the appropriate time and transferred to the uterus of the wife. If the diagnostic tests indicated that an embryo would develop genetic disease in the future, it would probably not be transferred but would, rather, be discarded.

It is possible that ways to overcome the current technical obstacles to germ-line therapy will be found and that safe and effective ways to repair either sperm or egg cells or early embryonic cells will be developed. In that case, germ-line genetic intervention for the prevention of genetic disease in some or all of one's descendants will become technically feasible. We will then face the question of deciding whether we ought to do what we now can do. While the action of intervening in a way that intentionally and directly affects multiple future generations will be a momentous one, it is difficult to see why this type of preventive strategy should not at least be considered. Reducing the probability that couples will pass on genetic problems to their descendants—assuming that they freely consent to the intervention—would provide benefits to the couple, their descendants, and perhaps to the wider society, as well.

The question of enhancing human characteristics, whether by somatic-cell or germ-line intervention, is surely controversial. Many commentators on gene therapy and genetic engineering have argued that the negative quest to cure or prevent disease, even through the germ-line, is ethically acceptable but that attempts to improve the capabilities of human beings by genetic means are ethically unacceptable (Anderson, 1985, p. 289–90). These commentators would presumably not be opposed to attempts by an individual to improve him- or herself (or his or her children) through good diet, adequate exercise, and advanced training. It is specifically genetic modes of improvement to which objection is registered.

There are several specific arguments that have been raised against the genetic enhancement of human beings. One is that such an endeavor is a manifestation of hubris, or, in religious language, an attempt to play God. A second objection is that such a program would inevitably lead to eugenics, an attempt by society or the state to coerce everyone to participate in the genetic improvement program. A third objection is that such a program would be utopian; it would attempt to develop a perfect human being or a perfect society. A final objection is that different cultures have different ideals and that therefore human beings would not be able to agree on which traits are better or worse for human beings.

The most provocative and sustained philosophical defense of human enhancement by genetic means is to be found in Jonathan Glover's book, *What Sort of People Should There Be?* Glover proposes a voluntary program of genetic improvement that could be freely accepted or rejected by parents (1984, 29). He argues that such a program need not be utopian; it would simply aim for modest improvements in human capabilities, one family at a time (1984, 185). There are two respects, in particular, in which human beings seem to Glover to be good candidates for improvement—intellectually and ethically. On the intellectual front, Glover believes that enhancement might produce not simply a boost in IQ, but also the capacity to think in new ways (1984, 180). In the ethical sphere, Glover notes our emotional and imaginative limitations, as well as the restricted range of our sympathies. In his view, we have in some respects retained a tribal ethic while achieving great feats technologically, especially in the military sphere (1984, 181–84).

The types of genetic enhancements that Glover envisions may never be technically feasible. If so, we and our descendants will not face momentous choices about the kinds of persons we wish to be, genetically speaking. On the other hand, the new science of gene mapping and gene sequencing may lead to breathtaking and unanticipated possibilities of the kind Glover describes. It may therefore be prudent to consider these technological possibilities and their potential social impact well before they are upon us.

REFERENCES

American College of Obstetricians and Gynecologists, Executive Board. *Ethical Issues in Surrogate Motherhood.* Washington, D.C.: ACOG, May 1983.

American College of Obstetricians and Gynecologists, Committee on Ethics. *Ethical Issues in Human in Vitro Fertilization and Embryo Placement.* Washington, D.C.: ACOG, July 1986.

American Fertility Society, Ethics Committee. 1986. "Ethical Considerations of the New Reproductive Technologies." *Fertil Steril* 46, suppl. 1 (1986): i–94S.

Anderson, W. French. 1984. "Prospects for Human Gene Therapy." *Science* 226 (1984): 401–409.

———. "Human Gene Therapy: Scientific and Ethical Considerations." *J Med Philos* 10 (1985): 275–291.

Andrews, Lori B. *New Conceptions: A Consumer's Guide to the Newest Infertility Treatments.* New York: Ballantine Books, 1985a.

———, comp. *State Laws and Regulations Governing Newborn Screening.* Chicago: American Bar Foundation, 1985b.

Antenatal Diagnosis: Report of a Consensus Development Conference Sponsored by the National Institute of Child Health and Human Development. Bethesda, Md.: National Institutes of Health, December 1979.

Callahan, Daniel. "New Beginnings in Life: A Philosopher's Response." In *The New Genetics and the Future of Man,* edited by Michael Hamilton, 90–106. Grand Rapids, Mich.: Eerdmans, 1972.

Corea, Gena. *The Mother Machine: From Artificial Insemination to Artificial Wombs.* New York: Harper & Row, 1985.

Costantini, Frank, Kiran Chada, and Jeanne Magram. "Correction of Murine Beta-Thalassemia by Gene Transfer into the Germ Line." *Science* 223 (1986): 1192–1194.

Daniels, Norman. *Just Health Care.* New York: Cambridge University Press, 1985.

Devlin, Patrick. *The Enforcement of Morals.* New York: Oxford University Press, 1965.

Faden, Ruth R., et al. "A Survey to Evaluate Parental Consent as Public Policy for Neonatal Screening." *Am J Public Health* 72 (1982): 1347–1352.

Feinberg, Joel. *Social Philosophy.* Englewood Cliffs, N.J.: Prentice-Hall, 1973.

Fletcher, John C. "Emerging Ethical Issues in Fetal Therapy." In *Research Ethics,* edited by Kare Berg and Knut Erik Tranøy, 293–318. New York: Alan R. Liss, 1983.

———. "Moral Problems and Ethical Issues in Prospective Human Gene Therapy." *Virginia Law Rev* 69 (1983b): 515–546.

Fletcher, Joseph. *The Ethics of Genetic Control: Ending Reproductive Roulette.* Garden City, N.Y.: Anchor Press/Doubleday, 1974.

Glover, Jonathan. *What Sort of People Should There Be? Genetic Engineering, Brain Control and Their Impact on our Future World.* New York: Penguin Books, 1984.

Hammer, Robert E., Richard D. Palmiter, and Ralph L. Brinster. "Partial Correction of Murine Hereditary Growth Disorder by Germ-Line Incorporation of a New Gene." *Nature* 311 (1984): 65–67.

Hauerwas, Stanley. *Suffering Presence: Theological Reflections on Medicine, the Mentally Handicapped, and the Church.* Notre Dame, Ind.: University of Notre Dame Press, 1986.

Hock, Randy A., and A. Dusty Miller. "Retrovirus-Mediated Transfer and Expression of Drug Resistance Genes in Human Haematopoietic Progenitor Cells." *Science* 320 (1986): 275–277.

Kass, Leon R. "Making Babies—The New Biology and the 'Old' Morality." *The Public Interest* 26 (1972): 18–56.

Keane, Noel P., and Dennis L. Breo. *The Surrogate Mother.* New York: Dodd, Mead, 1981.

King, Patricia L. "Reproductive Technologies." In *BioLaw: A Legal and Ethical Reporter on Medicine, Health Care, and Bioengineering Resource Manual.* Frederick, Md.: University Publications of America, 113–148.

Leridon, H. "Démographie des éches de la reproduction." In: *Les accidents chromosomiques de la réproduction,* edited by A. Boué, and C. Thibault, pp. 13–27. Paris: Centre International de l'Enfance, 1973.

Lewin, Roger. "Proposal to Sequence the Human Genome Stirs Debate." *Science* 232 (1986): 1598–1600.

McCormick, Richard A. "Reproductive Technologies: Ethical Issues. In *Encyclopedia of Bioethics,* edited by Warren T. Reich, 1454–1464. New York: Free Press/Macmillan, 1978.

———. "Therapy or Tampering? The Ethics of Reproductive Technology." *America* 153 (1985): 396–403.

McKusick, Victor A. *Mendelian Inheritance in Man,* 7th ed. Baltimore: Johns Hopkins University Press, 1986.

Motulsky, Arno G., and Jeffrey Murray. "Will Prenatal Diagnosis with Selective Abortion Affect Society's Attitude Toward the Handicapped?" In: *Research Ethics,* edited by Kare Berg and Knut Erik Tranøy, 277–291. New York: Alan R. Liss, 1983.

National Academy of Sciences and Institute of Medicine. *Confronting AIDS: Directions for Public Health, Health Care, and Research.* Washington, D.C.: National Academy Press, 1986.

Ontario, Law Reform Commission. *Report on Human Artificial Reproduction and Related Matters,* 2 Vols. Toronto: Ministry of the Attorney General, 1985.

Palmiter, Richard D. et al. "Dramatic Growth of Mice That Develop from Eggs Microinjected with Metallothionein-Growth Hormone Fusion Genes." *Nature* 300 (1982): 611–615.

_____. "Metallothionein-Human GH Fusion Genes Stimulate Growth of Mice." *Science* 222 (1983): 809–814.

Parkman, Robertson. "The Application of Bone Marrow Transplantation to the Treatment of Genetic Diseases." *Science* 232 (1986): 1373–1378.

Pius XII. 1956. "Address of His Holiness, Pope Pius XII, to the Second World Congress on Fertility and Sterility." In *Proceedings of the Second World Congress on Fertility and Sterility,* edited by G. Tesauro [Naples, Italy, 18–26 May 1956]. 2 Vols. Naples: Institute of Clinical Obstetrics and Gynecology, University of Naples, 1957–1958.

Ramsey, Paul. *Fabricated Man: The Ethics of Genetic Control.* New Haven, Conn: Yale University Press 1970.

Rawls, John. *A Theory of Justice.* Cambridge, Mass.: Belknap Press of Harvard University Press, 1973.

Robertson, John A. "Embryo Research." *U Western Ontario Law Rev* 24 (1986): 15–37.

Rubin, Gerald M., and Allan C. Spradling. "Genetic Transformation of *Drosophila* with Transposable Element Vectors." *Science* 218 (1982): 348–353.

Sellar, Jeffrey. "Australian IVF: Orphan Embryos." *Nature* 309 (1984): 738.

Steinbrook, Robert. "In California, Voluntary Mass Prenatal Screening." *Hastings Cent Rep* 16 (Oct. 1986): 5–7.

Stewart, G.J., et al. "Transmission of Human T-Cell Lymphotropic Virus Type III (HTLV-III) by Artificial Insemination by Donor." *Lancet* II (1985): 581–584.

Townes, Philip L. "Newborn Screening: A Potpourri of Policies," Editorial. *Am J Public Health* 76 (1986): 1191–1192.

United Kingdom Collaborative Study on Alpha-Fetoprotein in Relation to Neural Tube Defects. "Maternal Serum Alpha-Fetoprotein Measurement in Antenatal Screening for Anencephaly and Spina Bifida in Early Pregnancy." *Lancet* I (1977): 1323–1332.

United Kingdom, Department of Health and Social Security. *Report of the Committee of Inquiry into Human Fertilisation and Embryology.* London: Her Majesty's Stationery Office, July 1984.

United States Congress, Office of Technology Assessment. *Human Gene Therapy: Background Paper.* Washington, D.C.: OTA, December 1984.

U.S. Department of Health, Education, and Welfare, Ethics Advisory Board. *HEW Support of Research Involving Human in Vitro Fertilization and Embryo Transfer,* 2 Vols. Washington, D.C.: HEW, 4 May 1979.

United States President's Commission for the Study of Ethical Problems in Medicine and Biomedical and Behavioral Research. *Screening and Counseling for Genetic Conditions.* Washington, D.C.: Government Printing Office, February 1983.

_____. *Splicing Life: The Social and Ethical Issues of Genetic Engineering with Human Beings.* Washington, D.C.: Government Printing Office, November 1982.

Utian, W.H., et al. "Successful Pregnancy After in Vitro Fertilization and Embryo Transfer from an Infertile Woman to a Surrogate." *N Engl J Med* 313 (1985): 1351–1352.

Victoria, Australia, Committee to Consider the Social, Ethical and Legal Issues Arising from in Vitro Fertilization. *Report on the Disposition of Embryos Produced by in Vitro Fertilization.* Melbourne: F.D. Atkinson Government Printer, August 1984.

Walters, LeRoy. "Ethical Issues in Intrauterine Diagnosis and Therapy." *Fetal Therapy* 1 (1986a): 32–37.

———. "The Ethics of Human Gene Therapy." *Nature* 320 (1986b): 225–227.

Zoler, Mitchel L. "Genetic Tests Creating a Deluge of Dilemmas." *Medical World News* 27 (22 Sept. 1986): 34–52.

DISCUSSION QUESTIONS

1. Should human characteristics be enhanced by genetic means if such a technique becomes possible?

2. Does it make any difference morally whether the genetic changes are made in somatic or germ-line cells?

3. Should couples be free to use prenatal genetic diagnosis and abortion to assess and terminate pregnancy in cases where fetuses have any characteristics of which the couple disapproves? Does this include minor medical problems? Sickle cell trait? XYY Syndrome? A fetus of a sex not desired by the couple?

4. What are the moral differences between the use of reproductive technologies such as artificial insemination and in vitro fertilization within a marriage and outside of marriage? Should persons have the liberty to produce pregnancies involving third parties? What is the moral difference, if any, between artificial insemination by donor and surrogate motherhood? Do these procedures unfairly or coercively force lower-income persons into contributing to reproduction for the sake of other persons?

5. How do the new reproductive technologies challenge the traditional notion of the family? What other social developments are also calling the family into question? What are the advantages and disadvantages of non-traditional families?

g

Ethical Issues in Organ Transplantation

Albert R. Jonsen

SUMMARY

Organ transplantation poses serious moral questions about the intrinsic morality of transplantation, the determination of the death of the source of a cadaveric organ, the right of persons to donate their own organs, the selection of recipients for scarce organs and the procurement and allocation of organs as a scarce social resource.

Some question the intrinsic morality of organ transplantation. Does a person have the right to give up, for any reason, an important bodily part? Is it morally legitimate to remove a vital organ from one person in order to replace it in another's body? Is it morally right for a donor to consent to the deliberate excision of an important bodily part?

Particular features of the Roman Catholic and Judaic faiths are relevant to the morality of organ transplantation including whether there is an ethical duty to risk one's own life or well-being for the benefit of another.

Regarding the procurement of organs, the first issue is the need for free and informed consent. Another is the determination of death. When does death really occur, legally and medically? While death used to be determined based on heart-lung criteria, it now is based on brain-death criteria. The shift has important implications for the supply of organs.

Several factors determine of how large or small the organ pool is. Ethical and policy issues surround each one. This chapter reviews proposals to increase the supply. Given that the number of organs is significantly smaller than the supply, it is often difficult to determine who should receive scarce organs. Approaches for determining the recipients of organs include the utilitarian and egalitarian models are discussed.

On December 3, 1967, in the Schur Groot Hospital, Capetown, South Africa, Dr. Christiaan Barnard transplanted a living heart from the thoracic cavity of a presumably dead person into the chest of a patient suffering from end-stage cardiac disease. That patient lived for eighteen days. Again, on January 2, 1968, Barnard attempted the same procedure to save the life of Dr. Philip Blaiberg who lived eighteen months. These events, heralded as "The Miracle of Capetown" ushered in the Age of Transplantation. It can be said, with only slight exaggeration, that the same events ushered in the Age of Bioethics. Certainly, the transplantation of a major human organ, the kidney, had begun almost two decades before and, by 1967, had achieved considerable success in extending the lives of some 5000 patients with end-stage renal disease. Certainly, discussion of bioethical problems stimulated by the allocation of renal dialysis, by abortion, and by advances in genetics, had taken place with some intensity for several years. But the first transplantation of a human heart focused the attention of the world and of scholars on the science and practice of organ transplant and the ethical problems that leap immediately to mind (Wolstenholme and O'Connor 1968).

The public fascination with the sight of one human being kept alive by the heart of another and the scientific curiosity over the problem of immunological rejection of foreign tissue did much to focus attention on the "Miracle of Capetown." But public and scientific interest are not enough to create an ethical problem. There was something in organ transplantation that seemed to sound the depths of human ethical concern. That depth—the fundamental question of ethics—is the question of the nature and degree of one human person's obligations to another. In all transplantation of major organs between individuals of the same species, a part of one person is useful for the survival of another. Whether the source of the organ be a person who has died, as it always is in heart transplantation, or whether the one who grants an organ is a living donor, as is often the case in renal transplantation, the question can be asked "does one human owe this to another?" This echoes the ancient question, "am I my brother's keeper?" This conjunction between an extraordinary medical technology and a profound ethical question stimulated the questions and answers that make up the new complex discipline of bioethics. In a certain sense, that profound question lies at the heart of all bioethical questions about all forms of technology and medicine.

Organ transplantation has come far from the day in 1954 when doctors at the Peter Bent Brigham Hospital in Boston performed the first successful kidney transplantation. Great strides in the understanding of the immunological system and its medical manipulation have made the transplantation of major organs a common event. The solid organs are kidney, heart, lung, pancreas, liver; bone marrow is also transplanted. The success rates, in terms of survival of grafts, survival of patient and subsequent quality of life, though variable from organ to organ, are reaching the point where these procedures either are, or soon will be, considered "accepted and standard therapy" for diseases that destroy major organ function and lead to death. In 1985, kidney transplant centers report a graft survival rate of 85 percent and a patient survival rate of 95 percent for one year after cadaver transplant; if the organ comes from a living related donor, graft survival and patient survival rates reach 95 percent and 98 percent. By 1985, 1500 heart transplants and 1200 liver transplants were performed worldwide; heart patients show survival rates of 80 percent after one year and 47 percent after six years. All these procedures are expensive: they cost, on the average, between $75,000–150,000.

Thus, it is clear that organ transplantation is well established. Its science will progress and, in all probability, will show even greater prospects for success and will prompt even greater boldness. On November 1, 1985, the Transplant Team at one of the most active centers, Presbyterian-University Hospital in Pittsburgh, announced that it was considering a simultaneous transplantation of a liver, spleen, stomach, pancreas, and small and large intestine into one patient in a single operation. In what sense does this medical-surgical accomplishment give rise to ethical problems more specific than the general question mentioned above? What are the ethical issues usually associated with organ transplantation and what are the opinions of scholars about them? This chapter will review these issues: the intrinsic morality of transplantation, the determination of the death of the source of a cadaveric organ, the right of persons to donate their own organs, the selection of recipients for scarce organs and the procurement and allocation of organs as a scarce social resource.

THE INTRINSIC MORALITY OF ORGAN TRANSPLANTATION

Is it morally legitimate to remove a vital organ from one person in order to place it in another's body? At first sight, this question can be readily answered. Certainly it is moral to do so if the donor consents or if the source of the organ is one who has died. Certainly it is moral if the recipient needs the organ for continued life. However, on closer inspection, these obvious answers are not so obvious: each of them has given rise to much debate. Is it morally right for the donor to consent to the deliberate excision of an important bodily part? What does it mean to say that a person is dead and what can morally be done to a dead body? Does a person in need of an organ have any moral claim on the organs of another? Whose moral claims take priority when there are more needy persons than available organs? The discussion of these questions and their reasonable resolution constitutes the ethics of organ transplantation.

The most fundamental moral question asks whether a person has the right to give up, for any purpose, an important bodily part. This is an ancient question, raised long before organ transplantation was possible: do persons have the authority to mutilate their bodies, that is, to separate from themselves a part or organ that would appear to be a natural constituitive part? Roman Catholicism and Judaism have long forbidden self-mutilation. A person is only steward of his or her body; dominion over the body is God's alone. Any mutilation is morally justified only if it will contribute to the well being of the person whose body is mutilated. Thus, removal of a diseased limb to save one's life was permitted. The advent of successful corneal transplants called for refinement of this traditional position. In both faiths, the predominant opinion at present allows that the removal of an organ for immediate and genuine benefit of another person should not be considered a reprehensible self mutilation; indeed it is an act of charity. However, this position envisages that the removal of the organ will not cause serious detriment to the donor; certainly, it would not be tolerated if the removal of the organ was attended with the donor's certain death. Thus, donation of one's heart while still living would be forbidden and condemned as suicide (Kelly 1956; Rosner 1979).

While Roman Catholicism and Judaism condemn a donation that would be tantamount to suicide, could not an argument in support of such an act be constructed in secular ethics? Contemporary secular ethicists rarely argue against suicide. Further, would not a suicide that benefits another seem praiseworthy? In fact, several cardiac transplant centers have reported such offers. Arguments against such a practice would have to rely on the possibility of coercion and inducement that would undermine the presumption of free consent. Also, the reaction of the living recipient to the fact of being alive as the result of another's deliberate death might be devastating. Thus, donation of an organ that would directly lead to the death of the donor would seem ethically unacceptable.

Thus, the ethics of donation in the Roman Catholic and Jewish traditions seems sound. Persons are morally justified in giving up a bodily part for the benefit of another. They cannot do so, however, if that donation directly leads to their own death. Thus, the donation of a kidney, of a cornea, of bone marrow, is morally acceptable. However, the problem is yet more complicated. The donor should make the donation responsibly, that is, understanding what donation entails and consenting freely to it. The donor should give informed consent to the donation. From the earliest days of organ transplantation, it has been recognized that informed consent posed a particularly difficult ethical problem.

Since the body rejects tissue that its immunological system does not recognize, the most successful transplants are those between persons who are genetically related. Given this biological phenomenon, the social and psychological pressure to donate an organ to a close relative can be extreme, even to the point of coercion. An honest effort must be made to relieve the pressure that may come from a concerned family; but it is difficult to relieve the internal compulsion that arises from a sense of duty to save one's relative. There is of course a difference between a sense of duty and an actual duty. Here a second ethical question, almost the opposite of the problem of mutilation, arises: is there an ethical duty to risk one's own well-being in order to contribute to the well-being of another?

Again, this ethical question antedates transplantation; the Catholic and Jewish traditions have long debated the problem in other contexts. Their answer is a qualified "yes;" such a duty does exist and its stringency depends on the degree of affinity to the one in need, on the seriousness of the need and of the risk one must take, and, finally, on the likelihood that the helping action will really help. This sort of duty has generally been identified as an obligation in charity, rather than a duty in justice: its force is less strict, that is, certain circumstances can exempt from it and the recipient has no right to demand its fulfillment. Thus, donation of bone marrow, which poses little risk to the donor, would impose a greater, but not absolute, obligation on a potential donor. The higher likelihood of failure of this sort of therapy might justify a refusal to undergo even the lesser risk. On the other hand, the greater possibility that a renal transplant might succeed would lay on the potential donor an obligation to undergo the greater risks of contributing a kidney. To many, this traditional approach to the morality of altruistic action seems more reasonable than a utilitarian approach in which one's moral obligation is dictated by "the greater good of the greater number." This would seem to lead to the absurd conclusion that, since the two kidneys of one person could save the lives of two persons in need, the first person has a utilitarian duty to sacrifice both kidneys. Critics of utilitarianism point out that it would oblige persons to extreme sacrifices for the greater good; its defenders have countered that the existence of certain rules favoring one's own welfare and absolving from continual and excessive sacrifice are themselves necessary for the preservation of the greater good.

Even if a qualified moral duty to donate can be established, such a duty has not been recognized by the law. The effort of a person in need of a bone marrow transplantation to force his cousin, who was the most compatible donor, to contribute, was rejected by a court. The court noted that, while it found the cousin's refusal to undergo the minor risks of bone marrow aspiration morally reprehensible, the law's respect for the privacy of persons and their right over the integrity of their bodies could not be overcome by a duty of charity or supererogation (*McFall v. Shimp* 1978).

The free and informed consent of the donor, then, is required, even if the donor has a moral duty, since a moral duty must be carried out—or rejected—by means of responsible decisions. In this respect, the use of minor children as donors for their siblings has posed a difficult problem. The first case that came to public notice actually involved a sibling who was retarded. The court approved the taking of the retarded brother's kidney only through the tortuous reasoning that the retarded child would himself be benefited by the continued life of his brother, to whom he was devoted. In so reasoning, the court upheld, though shakily, the principle that a person should not be put at risk unknowingly and unwillingly, unless a benefit would accrue to the person himself [*Strunk v. Strunk,* Ky 1969]. Still, in recent years, the practice of taking a kidney from a minor sibling has disappeared (fortunately, advances in immunosuppression have made it less necessary). At the same time, there seems to be little hesitation to take bone marrow from a minor. This is justified on the grounds that the risk of so doing is trivial. However, the invasion of the body of an unconsenting person is not justified by the smallness of the risk, but only by the existence of a moral duty to benefit another. Some authors have argued that such a duty exists on the presumption that the child would accept if able to comprehend and choose. This is a controversial position. (McCormick 1974; Ramsey 1976).

THE DETERMINATION OF DEATH

Organs can be removed from the body of a dead person and transplanted into the body of a living one. This can be done for all major organs and must be done in those cases when the organ is essential for life; thus, hearts, livers and lungs must come from cadaver donors; kidneys and bone marrow can come either from living or cadaver donors. However, it is not quite correct to say that an organ can be removed from a dead person and transplanted to a living person. The removed organ must be viable, in the sense that it retains those biological properties that will enable it to function within the recipient. Thus, the body of the donor must still have some sort of vitality at the time of removal. At the same time, removal of the heart renders continued life impossible (unless another organ or artificial prosthesis replaces it). Removal of a heart from a living human would appear to be homicide in the moral and legal understanding of that term. Yet removal of a heart from a cadaver in which the vital functions, particularly the perfusion of organs by oxygenated blood, have totally ceased, provides an organ too damaged for transplantation. Thus, the first attempt to grapple with this problem, "A Definition of Irreversible Coma: Report of the Ad Hoc Committee of Harvard Medical School to Examine the Definition of Brain Death," opens with the remark that their revision is prompted by the belief that "obsolete criteria for definition of death can lead to controversy in obtaining organs for transplantation" (Ad Hoc Committee 1968).

Indeed, there was controversy. The literature of medical ethics is filled with it in the late 1960s and early 1970s. During the several previous decades, it had become possible to maintain vital functions by mechanical support. At the same time, ability to diagnose extensive destruction of the brain had become sharper. Thus, the way out of the impasse appeared to be adoption of a "new" basis for determining death. The "old" basis had relied on clinical perception that heart and lungs had ceased to function because heart beat, pulse and breathing had stopped. The "new" basis would rely on the clinical perception, assisted by the technique of encephalography, that the activity of the brain had ceased. Thus, on this new basis, an individual might still have heart beat and respiration supported mechanically and, at the same time, be declared dead because no brain activity was detectable. From this point of view, partial death seemed possible; an individual was dead in the brain but still living in the rest of the body. If medical practice would adopt this approach and if the law could be brought to sanction it, vital organs could be removed from dead bodies.

This approach was filled with ambiguities. Yet, under pressure to clarify the legal status of cadaveric transplantation, states began to enact "brain-death" statutes to replace or supplement their "obsolete" cardio-respiratory statutes. Peculiar cases began to appear in the courts. Trauma services hesitated to cooperate with transplant services. The philosophers argued about the meaning of death. Medical practitioners were uncertain of the differences between total brain death and permanent coma or vegetative state. The media reflected the doctors' confusion. In 1978 the Congress of the United States created the President's Commission for the Study of Ethical Problems in Medicine and in Behavioral and Biomedical Research. The enabling legislation directed the Commission to study, "the ethical and legal implications of the matter of defining death, including the advisability of developing a uniform definition of death" (42 USC 1802 (1978); Veatch, 1976).

The Commission published its report *Defining Death* in July, 1981. After an extensive review of the theological, philosophical, legal and medical literature and wide consultation with experts and with the public, the Commission recommended that legal jurisdictions enact the following Uniform Determination of Death Act:

> An individual who has sustained either (1) irreversible cessation of circulatory and respiratory functions, or (2) irreversible cessation of all functions of the entire brain, including the brain stem, is dead. A determination of death must be made in accordance with accepted medical standards (President's Commission 1981, 2).

This formulation expresses the Commission's conclusion that death should be considered a unitary phenomenon which can be accurately demonstrated either on the traditional grounds of irreversible cessation of heart and lung function or on the basis of irreversible loss of all functions of the entire brain. At this writing, some 40 state legislatures have enacted the Commission's Recommended Uniform Statute, either as new legislation or by amending earlier statutes, and other states have adopted similar positions through case law. Thus, it can be stated with confidence that the ethical issue that plagued the first decade of organ transplantation has been resolved. Those legal jurisdictions that have not adopted the Uniform Statute can do so in the confidence that this broad consensus exists. In some states political obstacles remain. Even where such obstacles exist, the advantages of this legislation for clarifying a most troubling legal situation and for providing benefits to those in need advise its passage.

Once the distinction between total brain death and persistent coma has been established in conceptual and clinical terms, the question can still be asked whether it is ethical to remove major organs from persons in persistent coma for purposes of transplantation. Presumably, if no ethical objection were raised to such a practice, legal authorization could be obtained by statute. In a widely noted article, "Harvesting the Dead" Gaylin suggested that the proposed benefits would not surpass the costs in intangible effects on our sense of human dignity and respect (Gaylin 1974; Jonas 1974). More recently, Rolston argues against the "vivisection" of an irreversibly comatose person for purposes of transplantation. He proposes that whatever is biologically vital has ethical value and that there is an obligation to respect the body that is still fighting death: "part of the dignity of a living body is revealed in its sustained resistence to death" (Rolston 1982, 332). As we mention below, the legal and ethical preference for the whole brain criteria also eliminates the retrieval of organs from anencephalic infant. At present, this supply of organs is generally considered beyond reach. Thus, the acceptance of the whole brain criterion for determination of death had two effects: it legitimized the salvage of organs from the dead and, at the same time, restricted the supply of organs by rejecting salvage from the irreversibly comatose. This leads to another ethical problem: the distribution of a scarce resource.

THE SUPPLY OF ORGANS

The majority of organs for transplantation do come from cadavers, persons judged dead on the basis of brain-related criteria. In the late 1960s, the Uniform Anatomical Gift Act was passed in every state. This law enables competent adults to indicate their intention to donate the organs of their body at the time of their death by signing a legally valid document. In the absence of such a document, specified family members may authorize the taking of organs, unless the deceased had specifically denied the intent to donate [Uniform Anatomical Gift Act, Uniform Laws Ann 15 (1983)]. In recent years, concern has grown that there is a critical shortage in the supply of organs. Approximately 200,000 persons are declared dead each year on the basis of brain-related criteria; organs are obtained from approximately 2000. Yet, the need for hearts, lungs, kidneys is estimated in the range of 50,000 or more potential beneficiaries (Schwartz 1985).

The Anatomical Gift Act preserves a traditional principle of law and ethics: a person has the right to direct the disposition of her body and its parts; only next-of-kin are permitted to dispose of the cadaver in the absence of the specific directives of the deceased. However, the need for organs for the benefit of others raises doubts about this traditional principle. Can ethical reasoning refute that principle or demonstrate that others than the deceased and immediate family have authority of the disposition of the body?

The Western philosophical tradition contains nothing that would argue against the ethical propriety of a person's willing body parts after death for certain uses, provided those uses were not in themselves reprehensible. At the same time, this same tradition does not appear to demand that removal of organs always be sanctioned by an explicit voluntary donation. Although a long debate surrounded the ethics of autopsy, the question of the decedent's permission to be the subject of autopsy was not a major point of dispute.

Jewish religious law explicitly prohibits mutilation of the dead body. Contemporary developments have refined that position and allowed it to be interpreted as permitting removal of an organ when the life of another can be saved thereby. Even then, care must be taken that contact with the dead not cause religious defilement (Rosner 1979; Tendler 1978). Several other religious traditions are most cautious about transplantation. Islamic beliefs about resurrection require bodily integrity at the time of death. Buddhism also abhors mutilation of the body and transplantation has been viewed skeptically. Nevertheless, in Islamic and Buddhist countries, donation after death has been permitted if the explicit consent of the donor has been obtained before death (Reich 1978, 891, 893, 1171, 137). The only question that deserves fuller consideration is whether organs should be removed and used for transplant, without or even against the explicit wishes of the decedent or the family. Does the cadaver, in some sense, belong to the state or to society? One modern ethical theory, utilitarianism, can provide a plausible argument that any use of the body of a decedent that could benefit society would be mandatory, unless society's revulsion or discomfort at certain uses counterbalanced the advantages.

Still, most ethicists have argued against routine salvaging of organs without personal or familial permission. Ramsey proposed that "the routine taking of organs would deprive individuals of the exercise of the virtue of generosity" (Ramsey 1970, 210). Veatch also states that, in a "society which values personal integrity and freedom, we must be able to control our bodies not only in our lifetime but within reasonable limits after that life is gone" (Veatch 1976, 268).

A philosopher, J. L. Muyskens, argues against both Ramsey and Veatch. Against Ramsey, he maintains that routine salvaging does not deprive persons of the opportunity to exercise the virtue of generosity simply because there are many ways to demonstrate that virtue. Against Veatch, he counters that salvaging does not undermine individual autonomy of the individual and collectivity, since not all powers vested in the state threaten the autonomy of the individual. Thus, "with regard to organs such as kidneys—given the relatively good chances of successful transplantation—we (pragmatically) ought to be (hence, if acting rationally would be) willing to relinquish our right to be buried intact" (Muyskens 1978, 97).

This thesis implies the acceptance of the utilitarian principle, that actions are ethically right if they contribute to the greater good of the greater number. Such a principle would point in the direction of such beneficial use of organs that otherwise would simply corrupt. Even then utilitarianism might recommend respect for individual choice on the basis that salvaging organs without permission might have some social disutility, e.g., undermine in a progressive fashion the inviolability of the human body before death. Also, it might offend the religious or moral feelings of many persons, leading to feelings of outrage and discrimination which are also social disutilities. In addition, it would also be important to acknowledge, if not the absolute authority, at least the privacy and sensitivity of the family.

Caplan suggests another approach to salvaging organs without explicit consent. He proposes that unless a person or a family explicitly objects to removal of organs, it can be presumed that a person is willing to donate for the good of others. Kennedy has made the same suggestion in Great Britain. In France, the law actually approves such an approach: cadaver organs can be taken unless the decedent has objected or the family objects. However, if the right to refuse is taken seriously, it would require record keeping and coordination that would be complex and perhaps impossible. Caplan has recently modified this concept to "required request:" hospital personnel would be required by law to request permission of the family. Several states have already enacted legislation to this effect. However, these proposals to increase the supply of organs do not come to grips with the central ethical issue: does the person, the family, or the state have moral claim on a cadaver when the cadaver can be used for social benefit?

Even if thoughtful philosophical consideration of this issue concludes that social authority over use of organs is ethical and, in general, supercedes the ethical value of individual or familial right to prohibit such use, there might be important policy reasons for not adopting this position. A policy that would afford certain legal protections to the refusal of individuals and families, as well as requiring the permission of next of kin when available might be preferable. It is important that law be devised that will make organs available with ease, while at the same time respecting these limitations. The problems encountered in framing such a statute can be seen in the history of such an effort in Virginia (Caplan 1983, 1984; Hoffmaster 1985; Kennedy 1979; Lombardo 1981; Raymond 1978; Sadler and Sadler 1984).

Would a market for the buying and selling of organs increase the supply? From the earliest years of corneal and renal transplantation, indigent persons have on occasion offered to sell one of their "disposable" organs. A market in blood has flourished alongside the voluntary donation system. Semen has also been sold for artificial insemination. Our society seems to tolerate the buying and selling of bodily parts when the parts can be readily restored. Yet in recent years, the sale of kidneys, particularly by poor persons in underdeveloped nations, has raised serious questions (Freedman 1985; Pittsburgh Press 1985).

Some find no objection to a market in organs. In a recent discussion, a philosopher and a physician approved of the proposal. The philosopher saw no morally relevant difference between selling one's time and selling one's organ and noted that in the transplant situation, the donor is now the only one who does not profit financially. The physician agreed. He remarked that sale would be good for both provider and recipient and doubted that a slippery slope will be started. These views are in the minority, even in the sparse literature on the subject. The contrary position rejects the market in organs, on the grounds that a traffic in organs would be degrading and the profit motive would be likely to reduce care and caution in selection of suitable organs (Frier and Mavrodes 1980; Kennedy 1979). In the most extensive article to analyze the ethics of a market in organs, Perry (1980) reviews the arguments for and against the two options usually discussed, namely, the donation of organs and the harvesting of organs. He suggests that a market be constructed in which there would be reimbursement but not profit.

Weighty objections attend even a policy of reimbursement. Desperate persons might be enticed to offer organs for sale pre- or postmortem. There would be an opportunity for exploitation of the poor. This is an example of the "blocked exchanges" of which Walzer speaks. Certain sorts of human exchange that might be accomplished with efficiency through a market system are not permitted by a society primarily because they are "desperate exchanges or trades of last resort . . . this is a restraint of market liberty for the sake of some communal conception of personal liberty, a reassertion . . . of the ban on slavery" (Walzer 1983, 102). There are other objections. A market system would encourage the development of a class of "middle men" and "entrepreneurs" whose practices might be less than savory. They would be modern counterparts of the 19th century graverobbers. Finally, a market might make it difficult to sustain the sort of quality control over organ accrual that is necessary for the best medical care. In summary, one philosopher writes:

> Allocating life saving organs by the ability of those in need to pay what the market will bear is blatantly unfair to the poor. Nor can medicine morally allow itself to be used by those who would risk their own health out of greed, desperation or ignorance. To argue that the sale of organs is a business motivated by humanitarian concerns for the well being of those in need simply flies in the face of the fact that selling organs can only increase the cost for those who now receive them for free (Caplan 1983).

The supply of organs may be increased by means short of routine harvesting or marketing. Legislation and social arrangements could tip the balance in favor of donation. The law might favor or mandate request to patients or the next of kin of the deceased. Arguments against a market in organs do not rule out certain arrangements that might involve monetary considerations. Tax deductions or reduction in hospital bills might increase the incentive to donate. The idea of organized giving to charity based on similar incentives was frowned upon in the earlier years of this century by those accustomed to giving solely for the sake of charity, unmotivated by anything but generosity.

The critical shortage of organs has prompted unusual proposals, two of which raise interesting ethical questions. The first proposes that animal organs be used, if anatomically and physiologically possible. In 1984 a surgeon transplanted the heart of a baboon into a newborn girl whose heart lacked a left ventricle. The infant died several days later. The operation was much criticized, primarily because the scientific preparation for such a transplant was inadequate, giving dim prospect for success. However, questions about the propriety of exchanging organs between species was raised. Some raised this objection on religious grounds, claiming that God puts an impassable barrier between animals and humans; others objected to the killing of an animal, particularly, one from an endangered species, in order to benefit a human. The religious argument is difficult to defend; a group of distinguished theologians, asked by the President's Commission to study the issue of the impassable barrier in the context of genetic engineering, concluded that Judeo-Christian theology does not contain any specific Divine prohibition against crossing species. In addition, the evolutionary process shows many examples of transfer of genetic material between species. The animal rights arguments have a growing persuasiveness at the present time, but still run counter to strong values that favor benefiting humans even at the cost of animal life. If such benefits could be produced by cross species transplants and if there were not other significant disadvantages, ethical arguments would probably predominate in favor of such activities (Altman 1984).

A second proposal to alleviate the shortage of organs suggests that organs from anencephalics be used for transplantation into newborns and infants in need. Anencephaly is a genetic anomaly in which the higher portions of the brain and the skull remain undeveloped in the fetus; when born, the anencephalic may live for a few hours or even a few days, but will inevitably die. Some 2000 anencephalics are born in the United States each year; it is estimated that approximately the same number of infants are in need of hearts, livers, and kidneys. Such transplants are scientifically and surgically possible. However, the anencephalic, once born, is a living infant, protected by law. Although it lacks higher brain portions, the anencephalic has a functioning brain stem and, so, is not legally brain dead. Salvaging viable organs would, it appears, constitute a direct act of killing the donor infant. Thus, while some ethical arguments suggest that the anencephalic should be treated differently from the all other newborn infants, this proposal, despite its logistical attractiveness, is not likely to win public favor or legal sanction (Harrison and Meilaender 1986).

SELECTION OF PATIENTS FOR A SCARCE RESOURCE

Organs for transplantation are, at present and for the foreseeable future, in short supply. Many persons who might benefit by organ transplantation will not be able to receive an organ. Thus, the ethics of selecting patients to receive a scarce resource arises. On what principle should available organs be distributed so that a fair and equitable allocation is achieved? The question first arose in the late 1960s, when chronic hemodialysis was introduced as a life-sustaining therapy for persons with end-stage renal disease. The few centers in which the skills and machinery existed for this procedure were forced to select a handful of patients from among the thousands throughout the United States that were in need. One center, Northwest Kidney Center in Seattle, devised a method to select patients by submitting the names of all medically suitable candidates to a lay board which was to choose the few fortunate recipients of this life-saving therapy. The Committee became known as the "God Committee," for they had the power to choose those who would live and those who would die. The choice often turned on the "social worth" or "productivity" of candidates.

Renal transplantation, the parallel therapy for end-stage kidney disease, also required allocation of a scarce resource, available organs. Heart transplantation faced the same problem. Thus, the problem of fair and equitable distribution of scarce medical resources came to be widely discussed in the press and by scholars. Scholarly discussion has generally centered on two quite different approaches to the problem of allocation: one favors distribution of the scarce resources based upon the principle of social utility; the other favors egalitarian principles. The egalitarian approach leads its advocates to recommend some system of random selection as the only mechanism consonant with the dignity and equality of all candidates. The utilitarian approach requires explicit assessment of the qualifications of candidates, although it too may allow random selection when faced with two candidates equally in need and equally qualified.

The argument between the utilitarian and egalitarian approaches is carried on at two levels: on the level of the basic principle and on the level of practicality. At the level of basic principles, one confronts the perennial philosophical question of whether the foundation of moral judgment is social utility, viz, the achievement of the greater good for the greater number in a society, or the absolute moral claims or rights of each person to certain radical human goods, such as life and liberty.

In one of the earliest philosophical analyses of this problem, Rescher asserts, "society 'invests' a scarce resource in one person as against another and is thus entitled to look to the probable prospective 'return' on its investment" (Rescher 1969). This statement endorses the principle of social utility. It is one way of viewing the value of individual lives to the society as a whole. However, much as one might respect the life of an individual, the value of that life is, in the last analysis, to be viewed as a factor within the welfare of the society as a whole. Even if the most serious efforts are made to protect and enhance the value of individual lives, the design and limits of those efforts are dictated by the needs of the general good.

On the level of principle, many philosophers offer criticisms of this position. In the debate over patient selection, Childress notes, "the individual's personal and transcendant dignity, which on the utilitarian approach would be submerged in his social role and function, can be protected and witnessed to by a recognition of his equal right to be saved" (Childress 1970). From this viewpoint, society's "investment" is not merely the resources poured into a medical device or procedure; nor is its "return" the measurable usefulness and productivity of certain "social roles and functions." Rather, its investment is the incalculable and multiple contribution that a society makes to the very existence of each individual; its "return" is the very life of individuals, saved and fostered by multiple social interventions.

When applied to the distribution of life-saving resources, the analogy of "investment" is plausible but inadequate. Its plausibility comes from the fact that significant resources of knowledge, time, money and materials are brought to bear on the development of certain medical interventions. Even when these do not come "from the government," they draw, in a collective and cumulative way, from the store of human potential available to any society. Their devotion to one purpose subtracts them from other purposes. This holds true in public and private sectors and in various spheres, such as education, arts, recreation, and commerce. Presumably, the bending of efforts to certain tasks has some purpose, some goal. Some potential value is sought, some good is to be created. Also, those who make these efforts often do so in the hope that their children, their fellow citizens and many others unknown to them will benefit. Thus, the plausibility of the "investment" analogy lies in the recognition that out of significant efforts, significant goods should come.

The analogy, however, is inadequate, for it does not aid much in discovering what good, how much good, and to whom the good should flow. At best, in the debate over life saving medical resources, it suggests that the good should be "health." If the resources are antibiotics, health is freedom from infection; when the resources replace the heart, health is a revitalized cardiovascular system. But, in the utilitarian perspective, the good envisioned by the "investment theory" is not health in the abstract, nor even health as a personal attribute of individuals. It is more likely to be health insofar as health contributes to social productivity. The healthy person is the employed person or the active person contributing to, and not subtracting from, the welfare of society. It is always this overall welfare that the utilitarian principle envisions. This apparently laudable goal is fraught with ethical perils.

These ethical perils appear when authors turn to practical levels. Those favoring the egalitarian approach are highly critical of any effort to assess the qualifications of individuals. Admitting that society does evaluate persons in many ways and for many purposes, they maintain that such evaluation is often inadequate and frequently biased. In the matter at hand, the provision of a life saving resource, evaluation approaches the impossible. In the words of Paul Freund, "the more nearly total is the estimate to be made of an individual, and the more nearly the consequences determine life or death, the more unfit the judgment becomes for human reckoning . . . Randomness as a moral principle deserves serious study" (Freund 1969, xvii).

Authors critical of the utilitarian approach note the impossibility of weighing the multiplicity of valuable human qualities in the same scale—is the shrewd politician who maintains social peace through intricate compromises more valuable than the insightful novelist whose sharp criticism makes society uncomfortable? They call attention to the fallibility of predictions about future contributions by persons whose goals and attributes may change in a society where new needs are always emerging. They cite instances where obviously irrelevant personal characteristics tip the balance—the choice of a church-going Scout leader over a respectable person without strong civic or religious interests. On the bases of these arguments, advocates of the egalitarian approach conclude that any system of selection that requires evaluation of personal qualifications will be flawed by fallibility, bias, ignorance, and capriciousness and, thus, be unfair in its working and results. They are led to recommend various systems of random selection, such as lottery or first come, first served. They see these systems as more consonant with fundamental human equality and as less open to the flaws of an evaluation system. It is possible, however, for an egalitarian to favor certain sorts of criteria, such as age, provided the criteria can be shown to be relevant to the selection and can be fairly applied.

Advocates of social utility do not generally discuss the weakness of assessment of personal characteristics. One author merely comments "the fact that the standard (of social contribution) is difficult to apply is certainly no reason for not attempting to apply it" (Rescher 1969, 619). Another admits that techniques of assessment are "imperfect, but that they succeed better than random chance in maximizing social value of the selected candidates . . . errors are regrettable but . . . more such errors would have occurred had we used any other allocative technique" (Basson 1979, 327). On the contrary, these authors frequently note that the sort of assessment repudiated by egalitarians is intrinsic to evaluating any medical need and medical success. An appropriate diagnosis and prognosis rests not only on physiological information, but on many psychological and social features of a particular patient. The chances for successful treatment often depend upon intellectual and emotional capability for understanding and following a regimen, and upon the "network" of support on which a patient can draw for support. As advocates of the maxim that where society as a whole makes an investment, society has the right to maximum return, they count the return in terms of productive lives saved, persons restored to self support and a life of active contribution to society. Thus, the distribution of a scarce resource in which social investment has been made or by which society may gain or lose in significant ways mandates careful discrimination between persons in order to ascertain those in whom use will be "highest and best." Advocates of egalitarian approach do not deny this but tend to see medical suitability as consisting of more objective data and, if psychological and social evaluations are involved, they recommend that "the attempt to establish fine degrees of prospective response to treatment should be avoided" (Childress 1970, 622).

The concept of a return on social investment does not address another crucial question: who should determine what counts as a suitable return on the investment. If, as these authors assert, society invests in the development of means of health care, presumably, society should determine the level of return. Since society is constituted of individuals who explicitly or implicitly contribute to that investment out of their income and efforts by foregoing other sorts of benefits, it is plausible to suppose that they expect to enjoy that return for themselves or for their children. At least, it is plausible to suppose that persons expect to have a chance equal to others to be beneficiaries of the investment. This line of argument affirms a strong imperative of fair and equal distribution and appears to turn the "social investment" argument on its head: all persons in the present and all future persons should be given an equal chance!

Occasionally, it has been suggested that persons who are responsible for their own illness should not be the beneficiaries of scarce resources. Indeed, insurers and employers are beginning to make decisions about premiums and employment on the basis of judgments about personal responsibility for health, e.g., smokers are considered high risk. However, this claim, which has some ethical plausibility at face value, is countered by the fact that the relationship between voluntary actions and any specific illness is generally statistical. Causes of any illness are complex and interrelated. In most conditions—and certainly for those for which cardiac transplant is contemplated—it is factually impossible to blame any specific individual. Further, even if a casual connection could be established, the behavior in question might not be voluntary in the sense relevant for ascribing responsibility. Thus, the suggestion that persons should be excluded from health care because they have brought about their condition has carried little weight in the ethical literature (President's Commission 1983).

Those favoring egalitarian principles often propose a system of random selection of patients. The lottery is defended as most suitable to human dignity, least open to bias, most palliative of anxiety about "qualifying" and most likely to be chosen, if the society was offered a referendum on various selection systems. In principle, the lottery seems, to many commentators, the only "fair" system. However, the lottery has also been criticized. Far from seeing a human lottery as appropriate to human dignity, some authors have been repelled by the idea. The Jurisprudent Edmund Cahn considers "the stakes too high for gambling and the responsibilities too deep for destiny" (Cahn 1955, 71). Joseph Fletcher calls a lottery "literally irresponsible, a rejection of the burden, refusal to be rational" (Fletcher 1969). Even Katz and Capron, who ultimately favor a lottery, are critical:

> The lottery is more blind than fair, for an evenhanded approach is desirable only insofar as it deals with like classes of individuals (Katz and Capron 1975, 193).

Other authors note the practical problems of a lottery. It requires that a group form before lots can be drawn, a situation that is unrealistic since patients appear serially with a need for help; the patients' condition can also change during the waiting time. One author has stressed the fact that lotteries can be rigged and, in matters of such import, are likely to be (Harris 1975; Willard 1980). Some authors question the contention of those favoring lotteries that random selection would alleviate anxiety and several authors distinguish between the "natural" sorts of random selection, such as first-come, first served and artificial ones, such as lotteries. The queue, some note, is more in accord with the realities of illness and the traditions of health care, but the queue can be "jumped" (Fried 1974; Willard 1980). At the same time, all systems of random selection make it possible for certain socially disreputable and dangerous persons to receive the scarce gift of life, a prospect that critics of the lottery find unpalatable, but proponents consider the price of fairness.

ALLOCATION OF SCARCE RESOURCES

The selection of patients for a scarce resource is not the only problem posed by scarcity. It is also necessary to decide how health resources in general are to be distributed within the population. What sorts of services should be available to what classes of persons at what cost to whom? This is sometimes called the problem of "macroallocation," to distinguish it from "microallocation," the selection of particular persons as recipients of a service. In the United States we have traditionally allowed the market to distribute health care services—people "buy" the services they need through direct payment or insurance—and have supplemented the market with public funding of services for those unable to buy what they need.

The advent of organ transplantation put the issue in a new light. The ability to save specific lives, in a highly visible way, by transplantation raised the question whether any individual should be allowed to die because he or she could not afford the high costs of transplantation.

For some, the attempt to devise a fair system for allocation of scarce resources misses the mark. No principles for such a system exist and, in their absence, the only "fair" approach to distribution is the market. In fact, there is evidence that a market for organ transplantation has come into being. It has been reported that individuals, particularly wealthy foreigners, have been moved to the top of waiting lists for transplants and pay almost four times the amount charged to citizens. Organizations to facilitate market transactions have been formed (Pittsburgh Press 1985).

The market model for health care has been extensively discussed in the economics and policy literature, but, until recently, the ethical implications of a free market have not been explored. Most authors assume, although they seldom demonstrate, that a market in which only individuals who have the resources and the desire to purchase care are able to do so, is obviously unsuitable when the commodity is essential to save and sustain a life otherwise doomed. As Outka writes, ". . . health crises are often of overriding importance when they occur. They appear therefore not satisfactorily accommodated to the context of a free marketplace where consumers may freely choose among alternative goods and services" (Outka 1974, 588).

The market pure and simple does seem to put those without resources at the greatest disadvantage, namely, the loss of their lives. On the other hand, ready resources may be at the command of individuals whose manner of life is hardly beneficial or even harmful to society, but who can draw disproportionately on the pool of scarce life-saving services. Some analysts have suggested that modifications in the market could remedy its defects. However, Katz and Capron, who do examine the feasibility of the market with some care, conclude,

> Modifications in the market—by changing what is bargained for or persons' ability to bargain—do not seem likely to solve the problems inherent in the market system. In particular, we doubt that people's willingness to pay for and undergo a lifesaving treatment corresponds exactly to the value of their lives to society and, even if it did, the market does a poor job of allowing them to express their valuation . . . the premise (that a person's wealth reflects their value to society) would be dismissed out of hand by most people today, both as a factual matter and as a deviation from our collective equality of all persons (Katz & Capron 1975, 188; Menzel 1982).

In 1972, the Congress approved the End Stage Renal Disease Amendments to the Social Security Act, almost without hesitation. These amendments provided broad financial support to all persons in need of kidney transplantation and dialysis. In its first phase, the program appeared modest: 11,000 patients cared for at a cost of 280 million dollars, but it rapidly assumed major proportions. Today, it serves approximately 50,000 patients, at a cost of over one billion dollars. The spontaneous altruism of the Congress has, in the eyes of some, become a social burden, not only because its considerable costs serve relatively few persons, but because it raises the question, "should not this be afforded to all who are in need of any organ transplant?"

In the seventeen years since the enactment of the End Stage Renal Disease Amendments, the costs of medical care and the proportion of the national product devoted to its financing has become a major public concern. In 1978 the Congress asked the President's Commission on the Study of Ethical Problems in Medicine and in Biomedical and Behavioral Research to study the question of access to health care from an ethical viewpoint. Its report, *Securing Access to Health Care*, is the first extended analysis of the problem of justice in health care. Many scholars in philosophy, economics, social policy and sciences and health sciences contributed to its formulation. Considerable data was amassed to provide an empirical basis for discussion. The Report concluded that "Society has an ethical obligation to ensure equitable access to an adequate level of health care without the imposition of excessive burdens" (President's Commission 1983, 4).

"Adequate" is defined as that level of care that will enable individuals to achieve sufficient welfare, opportunity, information, and evidence of interpersonal concern to facilitate a reasonably full and satisfying life. Recognizing that the concept of adequacy is indefinite, the Commission refrained from attempting to specify what adequate care should include. Instead, it suggested characteristics of adequacy that deserve attention in any discussion of an equitable health policy. These characteristics are the relationship between various forms of care and the health needs of an individual, and the relationship between the benefits of care and its costs, including diversion of resources from other socially desirable endeavors. The Commission concluded:

> Consequently, the level of care deemed adequate should reflect a reasoned judgment not only about impact of the condition on the welfare and opportunity of the individual but also about the efficacy and the costs of the care itself in relation to other conditions and the efficacy and cost of the care that is available for them . . . and the cost of each proposed option in terms of foregone opportunities to apply the same resources to social goals other than that of ensuring access [to health care] (pp. 36–37).

The "reasoned judgment" is made by drawing upon such criteria as professional expertise, average current use of health resources, and lists of services deemed necessary. The Commission also recognized the extreme complexity of the problem posed by the principle of ensuring equity of access and recommended a variety of means to resolve them: better data on and analysis of health care needs and the costs and efficacy of forms of care, education of profession and public, and various financial strategies to limit and distribute costs.

Some philosophers are at pains to reject the concept of the "rights" approach to health care. This rejection arises from their awareness that the notion of rights would require dedication of unlimited resources to the health benefits of individuals. Claiming such a right would rule out priority comparison between various sorts of health goods as well as between health goods and those of different sorts. Such a claim is too strong. Thus, these philosophers would repudiate the proposal that any particular health care intervention, such as cardiac transplantation or artificial heart implantation, must be provided as a matter of right to every individual needing such an intervention, even it if is lifesaving (Green 1983; McCullough 1981).

Philosophers do acknowledge that a right to access might be established within a theory of justice. (It is a philosophical commonplace that the term "rights" can stand for the moral claims of individuals prior to social considerations, or, as here, to the conclusions of arguments about justice.) Starting from different definitions of social or distributive justice, many philosophers have concluded that all persons in a society have the right in justice to some level of health care. This conclusion requires some form of state or social intervention in order to assure access. The level to be provided is expressed in various ways: the amount needed to provide a level of health equal to other persons' health, a decent minimum, or an adequate level. Most of these authors affirm that some form of care can be excluded from the level to which all have a right if these forms endanger society's ability to provide all with a "decent" or "adequate" level.

At the same time, only rarely have philosophers made the argument that it is unjust that some, who are able to do so, can purchase care that is not included in the adequate or decent level for all. Several have approved of insurance schemes that would allow persons to expend personal resources on more expensive forms of care, in accord with their own determination of acceptable risk. Philosophers have not, however, examined closely the practical problems of the coexistence of a socially supported level of adequate care and a free market in health care. Still, many of them recognize the desirability of a "one-tiered" system as the best realization of an ethical principle of equal access (President's Commission 1983, Appendix Two).

Thus, on the basis of philosophers' arguments about equity, it can be asserted that an expensive procedure such as cardiac or liver transplantation or artificial heart implantation might or might not be included within the forms of care considered necessary to a decent minimum or adequacy. Acceptability of these procedures depends on the impact they would have on the assured provision of the adequate level of care for all citizens. The fact that it is lifesaving or life-extending is not the most salient or weighty feature in favor of its inclusion in public-supported programs. A Massachusetts Task Force on Organ Transplantation has made a valiant effort to translate these considerations into public policy (Massachusetts Task Force 1985).

The Commission's principle seems to lead to a paradox. On the one hand, organ transplants are potentially life-saving. Persons are threatened with death regardless of race, social class or economic status. It seems radically unfair that, in the face of this great equalizer, only those who can afford this technology should benefit from it. Thus, to rectify this unfairness, we seem obliged to make the life saver available to all. In so doing we add a charge to the publicly supported medical budget that may have the effect of pushing other services—services that deserve to be among those judged adequate—to the fringes, or out of existence entirely. We may find this itself an unfair solution to a problem of unfairness.

The other horn of the paradox then appears. We rightly demand that a technology should not jeopardize access of all to an adequate level of care. We intuitively believe that such things as prenatal care, access to physicians for early diagnosis or reassurance, treatment of the many reversible disorders that would otherwise be lethal or crippling, palliation of ravages of chronic disease—all these must belong in the adequate level. We envision that an expensive new technology made available to all, that is, supported by public funds, may jeopardize or restrict many of these useful and necessary services. But the only place they will do so, with any probability—one might say certainly—is within the segment of health care that is supported by public funds. Medicare is a budget in the real sense (though probably a very complex and messy one). It has a dollar limit, fund balances and a bottom line. Within such a real budget, funds can be reduced, eliminated, or moved from one line to another. On the other hand, the so called "health care budget" of the United States is a fictitious or metaphorical one. Its bottom line is added up from a diversity of sources over which no budget officer has any control. Thus, the addition of a large expense to a real budget implies that, unless new money is added, that budget will be stressed and, in order to balance it, the less visible, less dramatic, less "necessary" items may be threatened (Jonsen 1986).

Thus, in the last analysis, the principle of equitable access is noble. It is probably the best statement of the principle of justice in health care that our present wisdom can generate. But the ability to carry the principle into practice probably eludes us, given our current system. It can go only this far: an expensive technology should not be financed by those tax dollars that now finance presently available health care if it appears that the new technology will derogate from the currently available services. Yet, the new technology will be on the market and can be purchased by those who desire it (at least until we find the will and way to prohibit it, and even then until we succeed in keeping it from being offered in neighboring states and nations). Thus, some will require the embargoed device; others will not, although their need may be the same. Is this unfair or merely unfortunate? (Engelhardt 1984). A Federal Task Force on Organ Transplantation struggled with this question and tended to see it as unfair. It concluded that, for purposes of public policy, major organ transplantation should be financed by government funds. The governmental agencies who would pay the bill may be inclined to see it as unfortunate (DHEW Task Force 1986).

This difficult and profoundly moral question brings this survey to a close. It also brings us back to the profoundly moral question with which the survey opened. We noted that organ transplantation raised the perennial question, "what does one human being owe to another?" The intrinsic morality of transplanting organs has been demonstrated: one human being may accept a risk in order to save the life of another. Similarly, one human being may donate a part of his or her body to save the lives of others. However, beyond those fundamental answers, many questions remain. Does a family have the moral right to countermand a donation—probably not. May organs be taken from those not dead but in permanent coma—possibly, but serious doubts remain. Does the state have the right to take cadaver organs without consent—probably, but with many reservations. Does anyone have a moral claim on the organs of another—probably not. Can a society prohibit or limit life saving transplantations to some in the name of fairness—probably. All of these questions remain open for debate. The merits and demerits of different answers call for reasonable assessment. This is the task of ethics.

REFERENCES

Altman, L. "Learning from Baby Fae." *New York Times,* no. 18, 1984.

Ad Hoc Committee of the Harvard Medical School to Examine the Definition of Brain Death. *JAMA* 205 (1968): 337–340.

Basson, M. "Choosing Among Candidates for a Scarce Medical Resource." *J Med Philos* 4 (1979): 313–334.

Cahn, E. *The Moral Decision: Right and Wrong in the Light of American Law.* Bloomington: Indiana University Press, 1955.

Caplan, A. "Organ Transplants: The Costs of Success." *Hastings Cent Rep* 13, no. 6 (1983): 23–32.

———. "Ethical and Policy Issues in the Procurement of Cadaver Organs for Transplantation." *N Engl J Med* 311 (1984): 981–984.

Childress, J. "Who Shall Live When All Cannot Live? *Soundings* 53 (1970): 339–355.

DHEW Task Force on Organ Transplantation. Washington, D.C.: Department of Health and Human Services, 1986.

Engelhardt, H. T. "Shattuck Lecture—Allocating Scarce Medical Resources and the Availability of Organ Transplantation: Some Moral Presuppositions." *N Engl J Med* 311 (1984): 66–71.

Fletcher, J. The Greater Good. (Unpublished lecture), 1969.

Freund, P. "Introduction to the Ethical Aspects of Experimentation with Human Subjects." *Daedalus* 98 (1969): viii–xiv.

Freeman, B. "The Ethical Continuity of Transplantation." *Transplant Proc* 17 (1985): 17–23.

Fried, C. *Medical Experimentation.* New York: Elsevier, 1974.

Frier, D., and G. Mavrodes. "The Morality of Selling Human Organs." In *Ethics, Humanism, and Medicine,* edited by M. Basson. New York: Liss, 1980.

Gaylin, W. "Harvesting the Dead." *Harpers* 249 (1974): 23–30.

Green, R. "The Priority of Health Care." *J Med Philos* 8 (1983): 373–380.

Harris, J. "The Survival Lottery." *Philosophy* 50 (1975): 81–87.

Harrison, M., and G. Meilaender. "The Anencephalic Newborn as Organ Donor." *Hastings Cent Rep* 16, no. 2. (1986): 21–23.

Hoffmaster, B. "Freedom to Choose and Freedom to Loose." *Transplant Proc* 17 (1985): 24–32.

Jonas, H. *Against the Stream: Comments on the Definition and Redefinition of Death. Philosophical Essays.* Englewood Cliffs, N.J.: Prentice-Hall, 1974.

Jonsen, A. "The Artificial Heart's Threat to Others." *Hastings Cent Rep* 16, no. 1 (1986): 9–11.

Katz, J., and A. Capron. *Catastrophic Diseases. Who Decides What?* New York: Russell Sage Foundation, 1975.

Kelly, G. "The Morality of Mutilation: Toward a Revision of the Treatise." *Theological Studies* 17 (1956): 332–344.

Kennedy, I. "The Donation and Transportation of Kidneys: Should the Law Be Changed? *J Med Ethics* 5 (1979): 13–21.

Lombardo, P. "Consent and Donations from the Dead." *Hastings Cent Rep* 11, no. 6 (1981): 9–11.

Massachusetts Task Force on Organ Transplantation. *Law Medicine and Health Care* 13, no. 1 (1985): 8–27.

McCormick, R. "Proxy Consent in the Experimental Situation." *Perspect Biol Med* 18 (1974): 756–769.

McCullough, L. B. "Justice and Health Care: Historical Perspectives and Precedents. In *Justice and Health,* edited by E. E. Shelp, 51–71. Dordrecht and Boston: Reidel, 1981.

McFall v. Shimp, No. 78–17711. In Equity. C. P. Alleghany County, Penn., 26 July 1978.

Menzel, P. *Medical Costs, Moral Choices.* New Haven, Conn.: Yale University Press, 1982.

Muyskens, J. L. "An Alternative Policy for Obtaining Cadaver Organs." *Phil Pub Affairs* 8 (1978): 88–99.

Outka, G. "Social Justice and Equal Access to Health Care." *J Religious Ethics* 11 (1974): 32.

Perry, C. "Human Organs and the Open Market." *Ethics* 91 (1980): 63–71.

The Pittsburgh Press. "The Challenge of a Miracle: Selling the Gift," 3–8 November 1985.

President's Commission for Study of Ethical Problems in Medicine and Biomedical and Behavioral Research. *Defining Death.* Washington, D.C.: Government Printing Office, 1981.

———. *Securing Access to Health Care.* Washington, D.C.: Government Printing Office, 1983.

Ramsey, P. *Patient as Person.* New Haven, Conn.: Yale University Press, 1970.

———. "The Enforcement of Morals: Non-Therapeutic Research on Children." *Hastings Cent Rep* 6 (1976): 21–30.

Raymond, A. "France, the Automatic Transplant." *Washington Post,* 16 Aug. 1978.

Reich, W. T., ed. *Encyclopedia of Bioethics.* "Organ Transplantation," 1170–1171; "Organ Donation," 1154; "History of Medical Ethics," 891, 893; "Buddhism," 137. New York: Free Press, 1978.

Rescher, N. "Allocation of Exotic Lifesaving Medical Therapy." *Ethics* 79 (1969): 173–186.

Rolston, H. "The Irreversibly Comatose: Respect for the Subhuman in Human Life." *J Med Phil* 7 (1982): 337.

Rosner, F. "Organ Transplantation in Jewish Law." In *Jewish Bioethics,* edited by F. Rosner and J. D. Bleich. New York: Sanhedrin Press, 1979.

Sadler, A. M., and B. Sadler. "Organ Donation: Is Voluntarism Still Valid?" *Hastings Cent Rep* 14, no. 5 (1984): 6–9.

Schwartz, H. S. "Bioethical and Legal Considerations in Increasing the Supply of Transplantable Organs: From UAGA to 'Baby Fae.'" *Am J Law Med* 10 (1985): 397–438.

Strunk v. Strunk, 445 S.W. 2d 145 (Ky 1969).

Tendler, M. D. "Cessation of Brain Function. Ethical Implications in Terminal Care and Organ Transplant." *Ann NY Acad Sci* 315 (1978): 394.

Veatch, R. M. "The Whole Brain Oriented Concept of Death: An Outmoded Philosophical Formulation." *J Thanatology* 3 (1975): 13.

———. *Death, Dying and the Biological Revolution.* New Haven, Conn., and London: Yale University Press, 1976.

———. "What Is a 'Just' Health Care Delivery?" In *Ethics and Health Policy.* Cambridge, Mass.: Ballinger, 1976, 127–153.

Walzer, M. *Spheres of Justice.* New York: Basic Books, 1983.
Willard, D. "Scarce Medical Resources and the Right to Refuse Selection by Artificial Chance." *J Med Phil* 5 (1980): 225–229.
Wolstenholme, G. E. W., and M. O'Connor. *Law and Ethics of Transplantation.* London: Churchill, 1968.

DISCUSSION QUESTIONS

1. What criteria should be used for selecting the recipients for scarce organs? How would such factors as medical need, probability of success, lifestyle, and ability to pay fit into a selection scheme?

2. Should organs be bought and sold on the open market? What would be the economic, social, and medical implications of such a policy?

3. Should organ transplantation be included in the commonly understood notion of "adequate" or "minimal" health care?

4. What are the advantages and disadvantages of the following policies: harvesting organs from cadavers? routine inquiry? presumed consent? Who would be most harmed and who would most benefit? Are fundamental moral rights jeopardized by such policies?

5. Should organs procured from U.S. citizens be used for noncitizens (i.e., nonimmigrant aliens, citizens of other countries who come here to be transplanted, etc.)?

10

Moral Problems in Psychiatry

Loretta M. Kopelman

SUMMARY

This chapter introduces some moral issues that arise in psychiatry, clarifies some of the psychiatric terms and presuppositions used, and distinguishes moral from psychiatric claims. It discusses psychiatric issues about confidentiality, competency, freedom, involuntary commitment, paternalism, consent, research, and uncertainty.

The diagnosis of mental illness in itself raises moral issues since it affects how people are viewed or treated. Psychiatric diagnoses have been understood in many ways: as merely subjective judgments, as subject to value-free confirmation, as requiring proof of an underlying bodily disease, or as only socially determined conventions. All these views are rejected. Diagnosis serves three potentially conflicting purposes: to assure accuracy or integrity of observation and description, to benefit the patient, and to benefit society.

In psychiatric practice, moral problems often arise because of differing opinions about what people ought to be free to do when their mental illnesses impair their capacity to understand, reason, choose, or act. The problems include confidentiality (the duty to maintain it, exceptions for disclosure of information), competence (standards for determining competency, the competency of the suicidal person), freedom (the harm principle, weak paternalism, substituted judgment, and the best interest standard), involuntary commitment (arguments for and against, legal battles), paternalism (how to distinguish when it should be used), gaining consent (its importance, what constitutes proper consent), and research (how to honor and protect the rights and welfare of persons while allowing important research to continue, what is a "minimal risk" study), and uncertainty (how can we acknowledge it properly).

The founders of modern psychiatry, such as Benjamin Rush and Sigmund Freud, changed how society viewed and treated people who were then called "lunatics" and "madmen." In 1812 Rush wrote, "For many centuries they have been treated like criminals, or shunned like beasts of prey; or if visited, it has only been for the purposes of inhumane curiosity and amusement. . . . Happily, these times of cruelty to this class of our fellow creatures and insensibility to their sufferings are now passing away" (1979, 243). As a result of the early work in psychiatry, the behavior of the "lunatics" was reclassified from moral categories such as sinfulness to medical categories of sickness. This meant that insofar as their behavior resulted from mental illness, they need not be held responsible for it, and that compassionate medical treatment and care, not moralizing, was the proper response. The reclassification also meant that these conditions should be carefully described and studied like other illnesses.

Pioneers like Rush and Freud enlarged our notions of illness or disease to include mental illness. Since they both believed major mental illnesses had some physiological base, it was compatible with another important enlargement of the concept of illness or disease that also occurred in the nineteenth century. Rudolf Virchow proposed that the study of disease be extended to the examination of the structure and function of cells.

One criticism of the current notion of mental illness, however, is that it has been enlarged too much. With the growth of psychiatry as a systematic field, Willard Gaylin writes the "definitions of mental illness have expanded to include progressively milder disorders; in that process, inevitably, the number of people that can be termed 'mentally' ill has increased. Confusion was bound to follow" (1982, 270). Episodes of aberrant behavior, the absence of normal behavior, nonfunctioning, and even inhibitions came to be regarded by some as mental illness.

As Gaylin points out, how we understand mental illness (and related notions not distinguished herein such as ailments, abnormalities, maladies, disease, or

EDITOR'S NOTE: I dedicate this to my father Frank M. Criden, M.D., a retired psychiatrist. I wish to thank P. Butchvarov, N. Dahl, T. S. Savitt, J. L. Smith, and R. Lie for helpful comments they made when I was preparing this manuscript.

disorders) has practical consequences. It affects discussions of the moral problems in psychiatry because we usually think it proper to treat people who are seriously sick differently from those who are not. We may decide, for example, someone is not bad but sick, or needs help despite objections. Major mental illnesses diminish the person's capacity to understand, reason, choose, or act, thus affecting the person as a responsible agent.

The purpose of this survey is to introduce moral issues that arise in psychiatry. To clarify some of the terms and presuppositions used, this chapter begins by distinguishing moral and psychiatric claims. After discussing some of the moral issues that arise in the diagnosis of mental illness, moral issues about confidentiality, competency, freedom, involuntary commitment, paternalism, consent, research, and uncertainty are introduced.

MORAL AND PSYCHIATRIC OPINIONS

We begin by distinguishing moral and psychiatric opinions rather than moral and psychiatric activities because psychiatry is a practice with a tradition of moral values, rules, goals, virtues, goods, and principles that are integrated into it. Someone acting within this tradition as a psychiatrist is using skills in a way the practice of psychiatry considers worthy. Like other branches of medicine, these internal virtues, goals, values, and goods concern the relief of suffering; the restoration of health; and the diagnosis, treatment, and prevention of illness. The virtues of a good psychiatrist involve gaining and using skills that are a part of this practice and increasing knowledge to achieve these ends. Like other dynamic traditions, there are differences of opinion about how to fulfill stated goals and virtues (MacIntyre 1981). And like other fast-moving fields in science and medicine, practices considered good even a short time ago may be discredited today.

Consider the following:

Case 1. Peter has applied to medical school. He has a straight A average, excellent letters of recommendation, outstanding test scores, and praise from his interviewers. Dr. R, a physician serving on the admissions committee, knows that Peter has been seen for many years by a psychiatrist for a serious psychotic disorder and has been hospitalized more than once for this. Peter functions poorly when he has to deal with people. He has succeeded academically because his work has been confined to learning material from books and working in the library. Based on what is known about this condition, Dr. R concludes the stress of medical training would be very bad for Peter and that in the unlikely event he finished, he would be an unfit physician. If Dr. R says nothing, Peter will be admitted, and another candidate will be denied admission. What ought Dr. R to do?

Dr. R contemplates four options: (1) Tell the committee what he knows about Peter; (2) tell the Dean of Admissions privately; (3) tell the committee that he knows something about Peter that he cannot share but that makes Peter an entirely unsuitable candidate for admission; and (4) say nothing. Suppose too that given the competitive nature of the admissions process and the esteem with which the committee holds Dr. R, he knows the first three options would result in Peter not being admitted to medical school. Dr. R may not recommend to the committee that they ask Peter about his medical and psychiatric history because institutions receiving federal funds cannot ask otherwise qualified candidates either directly or on the admission form if they have had medical or psychiatric problems (U.S. Rehab Law 1973). Each of the above options has been adopted by admissions committee members; but what has been done does not settle the moral question of what ought to be done. Dr. R wants to select and act on a morally justifiable opinion, not merely state a personal, social, or institutional preference.

To put forth an opinion as moral, one must be willing to defend it in a certain way. Some philosophers have called this practical reasoning, or offering a moral justification. This reasoning is a goal toward which we strive when we claim to be making a moral judgment. None can say with certainty it has been achieved. In a moral justification, one seeks clarity and all relevant information, defends one's choice with reasons, and is willing to apply the reasons universally and impartially. It requires that one is not being egoistic but will apply the reasons to all, even oneself. One also must want to assess one's reasons critically in relation to other relevant (albeit fallible) considerations such as legal, social, and religious traditions or other stable views about how we should act or what we should be. These may hold the preserved wisdom about how to rank values. It also includes a willingness to be sensitive to moral conflicts and problems; to beliefs about what is compassionate; and to the feelings, preferences, and rights of others.

If we assume Dr. R has sufficient information, then Dr. R's problem is more of a moral one than a scientific one. This is because unless the conflict is solved in another way (for example, Peter might volunteer the information), Dr. R has to decide how to rank certain important values. He has to decide whether to honor Peter's privacy and confidences, or to try to select the best candidates for medical training, or to protect people, including Peter, from harm. The way we rank values is sometimes affected by our roles. For example, does Dr. R have a greater duty to be silent if he is Peter's psychiatrist? If Dr. R tells about Peter, then will he help to undermine the important practice of respecting privacy and medical confidentiality? If Dr. R does not tell, is he responsible if Peter becomes sicker in medical school or harms others? Is Dr. R unfair if he denies a more suitable candidate a place in the class?

It is the *method* of reflection, not just the arrived-at opinion, that makes a judgment worthy of being considered a moral judgment. It is also the method used that makes someone's claim worthy of being called scientific. Dr. R presumes knowledge of the diagnosis, nature, and course of Peter's illness well enough to predict that medical school would be an all-around disaster for Peter. Dr. R believes his opinion is psychiatrically correct.

Psychiatry like any other branch of Western medicine is committed to the scientific method. It is a matter of debate how moral judgments differ from factual or scientific claims. Leaving this aside, let us say that *psychiatric opinions* are scientific judgments used in the practice of psychiatry. They are judgments based on data collected or appraised in relation to hypotheses or theories; the purpose of gathering data and building theories in science is to describe, explain, predict, or control events. Such claims serve in medicine as a basis for the activities of diagnosis, prognosis, prevention, or treatment of illness. The practice of psychiatry, however, also includes values, goods, goals, and virtues as an internal part of this tradition. Psychiatric opinions are here understood to be scientific judgments that are necessary but not sufficient for the practice of psychiatry.

Dr. R would not be justified in expressing his opinion about Peter's prognosis as a psychiatric opinion unless he could justify it scientifically. For example, if reliable studies show that 90 percent of those with Peter's condition become acutely ill with the kind of stress found in medical school, then Dr. R could predict problems for Peter with a high degree of certainty.

All scientific claims, including psychiatric opinions, must generally be testable or falsifiable. Certain schools of psychiatry are held to be unscientific because their theories cannot be used to derive testable hypotheses that can be confirmed or refuted. Popper (1962) and Alston (1967), for example, argue that certain psychoanalytic theories are not scientific because they cannot be confirmed or refuted. If this is correct, then, whatever utility such theories may have, insofar as they do not derive testable hypotheses, they are not scientific. Essential to a scientific opinion is that claims are testable or falsifiable and that controversies can in principle be resolved by more data or by better hypotheses, methodologies, or theories. For example, suppose one study found 90 percent of the people with Peter's condition became seriously incapacitated in stressful situations, but another study with similar subjects and methods found that only 5 percent of them did. Investigators would not be satisfied with these different findings and would try to give some account of the different results. For in science, it is usually assumed that similar situations result in similar findings and consequences. That similar conditions generally result in similar results is one of the framework assumptions of the sciences usually called the assumption of the uniformity of nature. Diversity of views and opinions in science generally set a problem to be solved by investigators. Some debates on the level of quantum theory or cosmology may be difficult to resolve factually. In science great emphasis is also placed on systematic power, elegance, and simplicity in resolving disagreements when two accounts square with what is known.

While there are many controversies in the sciences, it is generally assumed that they can in principle be resolved by more data; by better methodologies, hypotheses, or theories; or by further studies. In contrast there may be diversity of opinion in the moral life that cannot be resolved by these means. This does not mean rational discourse is any less important in morality than it is in science or that science is value-free or theory-neutral. It means that reasoned differences of opinion in the moral life can occur and that they may result from differences in the balance given to conflicting goods, rights, duties, goals, principles, virtues, or values. Insofar as more than one ranking of them can be justified at a given time, different reasoned views of what we ought to be or do may be appropriate. Thus, even when we do not agree in our moral opinions, we can sometimes recognize that alternative views have merit and that tolerance of diversity of opinions may be appropriate. This does not mean, however, any opinion is as good as any other.

Morality or ethics is a field of philosophy especially concerned with conflicts of important values, rights, principles, duties, goals, or ends where reasonable and informed people of goodwill can reasonably disagree. Sometimes these differences of opinion can be resolved by gaining more relevant information, by clarifying the language we use, by examining the worthiness of our reasoning, by looking at the consequences or implications of our reasoning, or by identifying the nature and ranking of the importance of principles proposed as justifiable and worthy.

This philosophic interest in moral conflicts and forced rankings can lead to a certain bias in the problems studied by philosophers. For while the vast majority of moral problems that arise in psychiatry are resolvable in a fairly straightforward manner, philosophers tend to be especially interested in conflicts of important values, rights, duties, principles, ends, or goals that are hard to resolve whether or not they are rare. For example, studies show that persons with mental illness are as a group probably no more or little more dangerous than the general public (Zembaty 1982). Yet theoretical discussions often focus on the rare cases where a person may be a danger to self or others in order to test the fair limits of liberty or the power of the state to intervene, constrain, or coerce citizens. Furthermore, many reasonable people are interested in resolving or avoiding the head-to-head conflicts that force such rankings.

Let us consider some of the differences and similarities between calling something a "moral opinion" or a "psychiatric opinion." Attaching the honorific title "moral" or "psychiatric" to one's opinion means one believes a certain method of reasoning has been used and used well. It means the view is not just a matter of preference, mores, traditions, aesthetics, or social approval. If one calls one's view moral, it means a method of moral justification is used; if one's view is called a psychiatric opinion, it means that the scientific method has been used. Moral and psychiatric judgments are alike in seeking consistency and the use of the best available data. A dissimilarity is that different reasoned views in science are generally seen as a problem to be solved. Moral problems are often but not always solved by better data, studies, methods, or theories. Sometimes reasonable and informed people of goodwill may rank important values differently. Insofar as they do, it may be proper to be tolerant of different views. It is possible, therefore, to disagree while acknowledging that alternative choices are rational, and as far as we know, and moral. In the next section, we discuss a misconception about how they are different that has had consequences for moral issues that arise in psychiatric diagnosis. This is the mistaken view that science and scientific opinions are value-free and that morality and moral opinions are not.

PSYCHIATRIC DIAGNOSIS

Illnesses or diseases are bad because they cause or increase the risk of suffering; they are unpleasant, not useful, restrict freedom, or diminish the nature and quality of people's lives. Although some diseases are symptomless especially in their early stages, they are involuntary conditions associated with pain, loss of well-being, increased morbidity or mortality, and decreased function. They have some sustaining cause (Culver and Gert 1982). Our notions of illness and disease are complex, and this by no means offers a sufficient characterization for all their uses.

Like physicians in other branches of medicine, psychiatrists treat a broad range of illnesses and problems. These problems range from mild disturbances that would likely correct themselves in time, to chronic debilitating conditions (such as schizophrenia), and to life-threatening disorders (such as anorexia nervosa and severe depression). Some psychiatric patients are competent people seeking counseling for the problems of living that thwart them, such as how to cope when they feel trapped by a job, marriage, or school; how to respond to an abusive person in their life; or what to do when they feel very sad. Psychiatrists also see patients who are extremely impaired. They may be suicidal or violent. Some are unable to act as they wish and cannot, for example, leave their homes without experiencing great anxiety. Others are not responsible for their actions or may have a picture of reality distorted by hallucinations, delusions, or irrational misconceptions. Psychiatrists seek to diagnose, study, prevent, and treat these conditions, and, as in other branches of medicine, they do so with varying degrees of success.

Given the range of disorders from mild to severe, when is the label "mentally ill" justifiable? A diagnosis of mental illness can help people or harm them. It can help them if it results in treatment that reduces suffering, restores their well-being, or excuses them from blame. It can also harm them. For example in Case 1, it would be a terrible injustice to Peter if he were capable of medical training, but Dr. R told the committee Peter is unfit based solely upon a haphazard diagnosis.

Since diagnoses of mental illness can affect how people are viewed or treated, an important moral issue is to clarify when the diagnoses are done well or badly. In this section, we consider views about how psychiatric diagnoses should be understood. It seems incorrect to say that they are reducible to factual, psychiatric opinions because describing people as mentally ill also seems to be a value-judgment. It means they fail (not morally but through sickness) to meet certain norms or ideals considered good, desirable, or worthwhile. Such descriptions together with medical practice seem value-laden in a different way because they create obligations for those given the authority to make them. In the first section, we examine views on whether diagnoses convey normative judgments that are nonetheless subject to rational confirmation or rejection. In the second, we discuss the special obligations of those given the authority to diagnose others.

Views About Psychiatric Diagnoses

One view is that judgments about mental illness are merely subjective and cannot be given a rational defense. A consequence of this view, for example, would be that we have no way to evaluate, confirm, or reject the judgment of a minister who in 1860 decided his wife was mentally ill and committed her to an institution for no other reason than that she disagreed with him (Szasz 1970). If diagnoses are just a matter of opinion, then diagnosing cannot be done well or badly or for good or bad purposes. But if this is so, then there is no scientific basis or moral justification for saying people have mental illness or for psychiatry as a profession. This view is obviously unacceptable.

A *second* view is that judgments about psychiatric diagnoses are subject to rational confirmation or rejection only when they are purged of value judgments. Some claim that the statistical-frequency model can result in value-free testing and judgments (Mercer 1973). According to this view, distribution of a trait (e.g., fearfulness) is determined on the basis of a standardized test, and those judged two or more deviations from the mean are considered abnormally low or abnormally high.

But this method is not value-neutral at all. Researchers must make certain choices and they may do so well or badly, or for good or bad purposes. Values are introduced in the selection of norms judged appropriate for the purpose of the test, in the selection of the test instrument itself, in the uses to which the test is put, in the selection of a significance level, and in the interpretation of the results. For example, a teacher selects what to test and what grade is failing somewhat like a researcher decides what to test and what cutoff is abnormal. This may be done well or badly, fairly or not. Hence, this view is also rejected.

A *third* view is that psychiatric diagnoses are defensible only if there is a known bodily disease. Otherwise, "mental" illness is a metaphor to describe or control behavior we do not like (Szasz 1970). Physical illnesses are real, and mental illnesses without a demonstrated physiochemical pathology are social fictions. If this view is correct, it is wrong to diagnosis people like Peter in Case 1 as having an illness unless we know this condition to be a physical disease. This view has important moral consequences because if people are not sick then they cannot be excused for what they do on the grounds of mental illness.

There are serious problems with this view. First, we do not use notions of diagnosis of diseases in this way, even if we limit ourselves to physical illnesses. (Thus, it seems a misnomer to call this the "medical" model as some do.) When people have unexplained but similar symptoms such as in asthma, multiple sclerosis, and schizophrenia, physicians diagnose them as diseases before knowing their physical causes. The pattern of illness is sufficient to say something is an illness or disease even before satisfactory physical explanations of them are found. Thinking of illness or disease as a pathophysiological process began with Virchow. Virchow, like Rush and Freud, however, expanded but did not invent the concept of disease. The older notion was understood in terms of the patterns in people's complaints, suffering, and dysfunction. Virchow's insight, while of great importance to the ushering-in of the age of research and scientific medicine, cannot be the single basic notion of disease. In order to seek and define a process or function *as* pathological, we need to identify a pattern of illness. Moreover, even if we did adopt this recommendation, it would be impractical. It may take many decades to learn what the underlying pathology of diseases may be and how they are affected by environmental, social, and genetic factors. It also shifts attention away from people's suffering as the pivotal notion to their physiology.

Second, if we look at the practice of medicine, it seems inappropriate to sharply distinguish mental and physical illnesses. Mental and physical illnesses seem inter-related. For example, depression can bring on physical illness, and physical illness can cause depression. Psychiatric practice has traditionally focused on ailments where suffering involves impairment of a person's ability to understand, reason, choose, or act. Sometimes physical lesions or processes are found to explain these. Psychiatrists would be unwilling to say they are interested in mental as opposed to physical illness. First, they have always been interested in diseases of the brain such as Alzheimer's disease where it has been clear that there are underlying physical pathologies. Second, some ailments once regarded as mental conditions are now regarded as having physical causes, but they are treated in psychiatric practice. This seems to be the case with certain forms of manic-depressive illness and schizo-phrenia.

The third objection to the view that a rational defense of psychiatric diagnoses requires proof that they are physical disorders is that there are inherent problems within the reductionist or materialistic view it presupposes. One assumption made by these reductionist or materialistic accounts is that the human point of view can be eliminated from scientific inquiry. Yet this is problematic because one needs a perspective in order to conduct studies or evaluate claims. These accounts also presuppose that universal covering laws can explain human behavior and illness and do so without exception. Yet no successful example of this has ever been produced. Some suggest there are good reasons for supposing these assumptions cannot succeed (Chisholm 1956; MacIntyre 1981; Margolis 1966).

A *fourth* view is that diagnoses about mental illness are only socially deter-mined conventions. But if diagnoses are just socially determined, then it does not permit us to say that those in another culture diagnose well or badly, or do so for good or bad purposes. Yet, this seems possible and even appropriate. For example, there has been harsh worldwide professional criticism of some psychiatrists in the Soviet Union because they label mild character disorders as "schizophrenia" and treat those who exhibit no signs of serious illness as mentally ill (Block 1981; Reich 1981). Psychiatric diagnosis has been employed, critics charge, as a weapon by the Soviets since the 1950s to repress dissidents. It has been used, non-Soviet psychia-trists claim, to involuntarily detain and "treat" Soviets advocating human rights or nationalism for republics within the Soviet Union as well as persons seeking to emigrate, having religious convictions, or embarrassing the Soviet government (Block 1981). The Soviets argue that the criticisms are unfounded. They say these people are sick because they are maladjusted, nonconformist, and abnormal within their society, and this is demonstrated by their deviant and inappropriate social behavior. Soviet psychiatrists are taught to view such behavior as mental illness. If all diagnoses and practices are social acts framed by society's own norms and values, then arguably these are sick people in Soviet society, even if they might not be in other societies. This view presupposes great uniformity within and significant differences between cultures. However, the first criticisms of these practices came from Soviets, and a growing reform movement there now openly challenges the political misuse of psychiatry, the view that social deviance is mental illness and the national control of professions. Thus contrary to the assumptions of cultural relativists, vibrant societies cannot be represented by simple uniform views, and cultures may be similar enough so that rational comparisons can be made.

This defense given by some Soviet psychiatrists employs the argument that psychiatric diagnoses and practices are socially determined and that it is not meaningful to talk of their accuracy or utility independently of a specific culture. If true, it means there can be no cross-cultural psychiatric organizations with independent or scientific means of controlling their language and practices. Yet if it seems correct to say that some purposes for diagnosing others in other cultures is wrong or that accuracy is an independent professional duty, then these judgments are not merely a socially framed act.

A *fifth* view and the one that seems correct is that psychiatric diagnoses can be used in a variety of ways, and we have to look at how they are used to say what they mean. We can use "he is a psychopath" to express many things including a psychiatric judgment, fear, humor, hate, prejudice, or cultural views. When used as a psychiatric opinion, however, then the authority for accuracy belongs to the psychiatric profession; but they can be criticized. Diagnoses can be used as psychiatric opinions to describe, explain, or predict events. For example, if someone is described as anorexic, we would expect to see a thin person who has an eating disorder. But diagnosing something as an illness also conveys an evaluation about that condition. It is bad to have anorexia nervosa. On the one hand, diagnosing in psychiatric practice has a factual, scientific base that needs to be justified; on the other, it conveys normative judgments that also must be clarified and justified. But these estimates may be controversial or change. For example, Benjamin Rush held the established medical view that sexual promiscuity was a deplorable and pathetic disease of the mind causing such physical illnesses as "pulmonary consumption, dyspepsia, dimness of sight, vertigo, epilepsy, hypochondriasis, loss of memory, monologue, fatuity and death" [1812 (1979), 347]. The fact that estimates change or vary does not lead to hopeless relativism if there are methods for evaluating our opinions. The scientific method and moral reasoning offer two means for rational evaluation. Admitting one's point-of-view is a first step toward being critical about it. Religious counselors and psychiatrists such as James Knight (1982) sometimes use the concept of the wounded healer to divest people of the notion that patients alone have limitations.

In the last section, it was argued that psychiatric practice is both a moral and scientific enterprise. The psychiatric profession is committed to standardize the vocabulary of technical terms and to restrict the diagnosis of mental illness to conditions that seriously affect behavior (APA 1980). This professional choice has a scientific purpose because unless we use the same names for conditions, we cannot study them. It also has a moral purpose because it minimizes the inappropriate labeling of others due to mistakes, inconsistency, or politics. This affords an objective basis for saying a diagnosis is correct or incorrect. It was on these grounds that world psychiatric organizations condemned the Soviet psychiatrists for using labels such as "schizophrenia" for persons who do not show signs of serious illness.

As a practical matter, clearly personal and cultural values can influence our assessments of health and illness. Consider the following:

Case 2. Mr. and Mrs. Q seek counseling from Dr. B. Mr. Q is a graduate student from a country Dr. B believes to favor the subjugation of women's interests to men's. Mrs. Q, as a result of living in this country while her husband goes to graduate school, wants to attend school and achieve more personal independence. Her husband forbids this, regarding these recent views to be either evil or symptoms of mental illness. Dr. B believes Mrs. Q is depressed because she is angry about the way her husband says she must live her life, and she seeks more freedom. Mrs. Q expresses anger, guilt, and doubt about what she should do or be.

In general, professionals should assess diagnoses critically in many ways. For example, some have criticized the characterization of women presented by Sigmund Freud as infused with uncritical views about a woman's role in society. Joseph Margolis argues that psychotherapy employs a mixed model that has "clear affinities with the models that obtain in physical medicine and at the same time with the models of happiness and well-being that obtain in the ethical domain" (1966, 81–82). Margolis argues that some attempts to expand the notion of mental illness, especially in psychoanalytic schools, do construe social or moral ideals in medical terms. He agrees the concept of illness has been enlarged in many useful ways as a result of the growth of the field of psychiatry. He recommends, however, that attempts to enlarge the concept should be evaluated individually.

Cultures may to some degree justifiably draw the line between health and illness differently. For example, because one society is richer than another, it may be more willing to excuse mildly sick people from work. The problems of where to draw the line between health and disease and when to use or avoid diagnoses that are potentially stigmatizing arise in other areas of medicine. For example, at some point hunger becomes malnutrition, and at some point neurological discharges become excessive enough to be called epilepsy. To help address the problems of bias, unrealiability, and cultural differences, professional organizations try to reserve "mental disorder" for very serious, well-defined conditions and press for standard worldwide acceptance of psychiatric nosology (APA 1980) and for more research support. Consider the statement in the *Diagnostic and Statistical Manual of Mental Disorders,* Third Edition (*DSM–III*):

> . . . a mental disorder is conceptualized as a clinically significant behavioral or psychological syndrome or pattern that occurs in an individual

and that is typically associated with either a painful symptom (distress) or impairment in one or more important areas of functioning (disability). In addition, there is an inference that there is a behavioral, psychological, or biological dysfunction, and that the disturbance is not only in the relationship between the individual and society. (When the disturbance is *limited* to a conflict between an individual and society, this may represent social deviance, which may or may not be commendable, but is not by itself a mental disorder) (1980, 6).

By stressing severity, pain, impairment and dysfunctions that are not merely social deviance, *DSM–III* tries to avoid some of the problems we have mentioned. Yet Culver and Gert criticize it for failing to distinguish disabilities and inabilities and for allowing us to include some things that do not seem to be diseases (normal grief) (1982). As in other areas of medicine, controversies persist about how to understand when something should be regarded as a disease.

To understand how diagnoses are used, we also must consider the professional obligations engendered by those with authority to diagnose others. Psychiatrists, psychologists, and others are granted such authority by society and with it come special duties. These duties include consideration of accuracy, commitment to the patient's welfare, and in some cases public safety.

Moral Purposes of Diagnoses

If psychiatric diagnoses can be used well or badly and for good or bad purposes, then it is important to understand when they are used in these ways. Three important purposes of diagnoses follow (Kopelman 1984) with references to how each of them can sometimes be abused.

One reason for labeling or diagnosis is for *accuracy* or *integrity of observation and description*. If a man believes his thoughts are being controlled by satellites, then he should be described as delusional. This should help in diagnosing and planning his therapy. Investigators also need accurate individual descriptions in order to understand patterns of illness and then explain and treat it. As scientists, psychiatrists are committed to accurate observation and description. Soviet physicians were condemned by psychiatric organizations for deliberately using diagnoses inaccurately for political purposes.

Accuracy is important to many including the diagnosed individual, the payer (often an insurance company), the researcher, and the courts. Accuracy and integrity require good data and criteria. But when are standards good and data sufficient? And for what purpose? Investigators and journal editors typically require a probability of at least 0.95 as a ground for holding that "sufficient reason" exists to regard information collected in a well-designed study as reliable. The 0.95 standard, although a reasonable and well-established convention is, nonetheless, evaluative in itself. It is a trade-off between ending a study too soon and getting unreliable results and continuing it too long and denying good care or data to others

(Wikler 1981). Thus, deeply embedded in scientific medicine are evaluative as well as epistemological views about when we should say we know something.

Some have charged that psychiatrists are more willing to recognize abuses due to inaccuracy of diagnoses in the Soviet Union than in their own countries (Reich 1981; Szasz 1970). Reich charges that what the Soviets do is different in degree but not in kind from what we see in this country. Psychiatrists have used diagnosis of mental illness to help people "circumvent the law, . . . get abortions or to help them evade the military draft. Psychiatrists often saw little danger from such human-itarian deeds, and responded to the requests willingly. But the danger was there, and we only need look to Russia to appreciate its extreme potential" (Reich 1981, 84). Even if Reich is correct in saying both are abuses, it is not obvious that they merely differ in degree but not in kind. For there seems to be one relevant difference in his own description of the two. Namely, the "patients" in Russia get the diagnosis against their will so that others may restrict their freedom, but the western "pa-tients" Reich describes seek the diagnosis to gain certain freedoms or evade certain constraints.

A more widespread abuse is the unwitting *redescription* of people in psychi-atric terms to disvalue them or their reasoning. People are sometimes called "de-pressed," "paranoid," or "psychotic" because others do not like their views.

Case 3. Mrs. J is 57-years-old and has just learned she has a cancerous, rapidly growing brain tumor. She is already blind and knows that people with her condition usually die within six months; none have survived a year. She knows she will become increasingly disabled both mentally and physically. She refuses to agree to any procedure that would prolong her life and says she wants to take her own life. Her physician seeks a psychi-atric consultation. The psychiatrist said her choice was neither impaired nor the product of mental illness but the nurses and her physician persisted in thinking her decision showed she was depressed.

A second important reason for diagnosing a person as mentally ill is to *benefit the person* by signaling he or she has important and unique needs. The diagnosis can be very useful to access special care programs or financial aid. It can also be helpful as a means of displacing inappropriate reactions such as anger or blame. Moreover, descriptions of the number of people who are mentally ill can help them collectively by showing that we need more funds for facilities, treatment, or re-search. If benefit to the person is given as a reason for diagnosing others by those with special authority to do so in our society, then people have a right to expect that the diagnosis will produce more good than harm for them. Considerations of bene-fits include that tested care or therapies are available. It might also include consid-eration of a variety of risks including psychosocial dangers (e.g., the loss of status or freedom), misconceptions (e.g., that mentally ill people are dangerous), irrational attitudes (e.g., the thinking of mental illness as punishment for sin), and the "spread" effect or the tendency to view disabled persons as more handicapped than they are. Abuses of diagnosis using alleged benefit to the person may take many forms. It may focus on too narrow a set of benefits or harms and ignore other relevant values. For example, consider this research intended, in part, to benefit subjects by a diagnosis: At one time the XYY genotype was thought to be associated with aggressive behavior. A study was done where one reason given for screening and identifying infant boys with the XYY genotype was that it would allow caretakers to help them by watching for and correcting any indication of aggressive behavior. A hot debate arose over investigators' assurances that this study would benefit the XYY boys. First, there was no proof that the psychiatric follow-up would be beneficial to the boys. Second, it seemed very likely the study was potentially far more harmful than beneficial to the boys. Aggressiveness might be a self-fulfilling prophesy because people would be predisposed to "see" the boys as aggressive. Third, risky research that does not hold out direct benefit to the subjects should not be done on children. Fourth, a retrospective study could have been done with consenting adults. In fact, it was done and showed that the XYY genotype was not associated with aggressiveness (Kopelman 1978). Research may hold out benefit for the subjects, and/or it may be a means to benefit society by gaining new knowledge.

Third, accurate diagnosis may be done *to benefit society*. First, it may serve as a research goal to help us learn about illnesses. Second, epidemiological information can aid resource allocation. Third, people who pose a serious danger to themselves or others should not be permitted to roam free in society. Restricting the freedom of others for the sake of social utility should require a heavy burden of proof. The exact nature of the harmful effects to be avoided or the beneficial consequences to be achieved and the probability of their occurrence must be demonstrated as a reasonable basis for the restriction.

In general terms, these three interrelated and sometimes conflicting reasons for diagnosing—integrity of observation and description, benefit to the person, and social utility (including research)—all use values and create obligations that must be justified. Abuses could result if people ignored the moral responsibility of justifying these values or purposes in the ascription of mental illness or handicap.

In this section, it is argued that diagnoses of mental illness can be rationally confirmed or rejected but that they convey evaluative judgments. Justification of diagnoses in general or of that given to a particular individual requires a moral and scientific defense. This is also true of the justification of a procedure as a treatment.

PSYCHIATRIC TREATMENT

Therapy is an activity primarily intended to benefit persons by providing care for them during an illness. Good intentions, however, are not always sufficient. For example, Benjamin Rush had the most compassionate goals, yet his intentions were more humane than his methods. He popularized "therapies" of copious bleeding and purging, strapping people to "tranquilizing" chairs, and spinning them in gyrating chairs to "treat" them for the congestion of blood in the brain which he believed to be the cause of mental illness (Alexander 1966). He did not test these treatments in a systematic way. The testing of therapies in a controlled way is a recent mid-twentieth century medical practice.

Therapeutic practices, in addition to being intentional, are also part of a scientific tradition. The intention must be to benefit the patient, but they ought to have some likelihood of working. In this section, some of the moral problems arising in psychiatric practice are introduced. These problems often arise because there are different opinions about what people ought to be free to do when they are so mentally ill that they may be impaired in their capacity to understand, reason, choose, or act. The problems may be complex because of uncertainties or conflicting values or because people impaired for some purposes may not be for others. Even very sick people might have reasonably objected to some of Rush's "treatments" despite assurances they were being treated by an esteemed and compassionate physician. Sometimes, of course, there is good evidence that treatment over someone's objections will restore health and freedom or alleviate suffering. It is sad and frustrating to be unable to help people who from our point-of-view are really in need but who refuse treatment. Sometimes actions over people's objections save them or others from pain. In Case 1 Dr. R considers breaking confidentiality to save Peter as well as others from harm.

Confidentiality

Freud saw psychiatric patients in his office, but he scheduled them so they would never meet in order to ensure privacy. Thus almost from the beginning of modern psychiatry, extraordinary precautions were taken to ensure privacy and confidentiality. Part of the reason for this is that the old stigmas associated with psychiatric illness have not yet died. But part of the reason is because the information is sensitive owing to the nature of the illness. It would make for interesting gossip and nervous clients to learn that a stockbroker suffers from a manic-depressive illness or that a college president has a psychosexual disorder.

The duty to maintain confidentiality is honored in special ways in psychiatric practice because diagnostic information can be very sensitive. Hospitals often separate psychiatric charts in order to restrict access to them. Some psychiatrists hold two files, keeping one with the more sensitive information safely locked away from those who have general access to records. Medical confidentiality is not only threatened by the type of indiscretion and gossip properly condemned by the Hippocratic oath, but also by access to patient information in computerized databanks and by chart reviewers, third-party payers, physicians, nurses, administrators, social workers, nutritionists, students, and other health-care specialists who may have access to a patient's records. Privacy can be more easily maintained in private offices than in hospitals, but the old days when a patient told a physician information that went absolutely no further are largely gone (Grossman 1977; Siegler 1982). In many jurisdictions, patients have a right to review their charts. Special restrictions are sometimes added for psychiatric patients presumably because this information might harm some of those who are mentally impaired.

According to the ancient tradition in medical practice, a patient's confidences must be held in secret, and reasons for making exceptions must be compelling. The burden of proof is on the person who wishes to break medical confidentiality. This tradition honors a person's right to privacy and self-direction. Moreover, patients have come to expect that information learned from or about them will be kept secret. The practice of keeping confidences is useful and generally beneficial because it encourages patients to disclose sensitive information that may be crucial for making good health-care decisions. Maintaining confidentiality also benefits physicians. Patients would be reluctant to seek out or keep any physician who had the reputation of violating patient confidentiality.

There are well-established exceptions to the duty to maintain confidences. These include reporting knife and gunshot wounds; serious infectious diseases such as AIDS, tuberculosis, or venereal diseases; and suspected child abuse. The least controversial exception to the duty to honor confidentiality is where there is a clear, immediate, and grave threat of harm to other persons. For example, consider the following:

Case 4. Dr. T is a psychiatrist counseling Mr. and Mrs. N. They tell her that they keep their three-year-old child locked in the attic for long periods of time as punishment.

Dr. T is obligated to report suspected child abuse to the authorities for investigation whether or not it makes her clients angry or relieved. This is considered justifiable because protecting the child is more important than maintaining patient confidentiality. This exception to confidentiality has been well-established in our laws and our society since pediatricians began to work for such laws in the 1960s. Before that, child abuse was rarely recognized or reported. If you agree it was good to change laws and social attitudes that permitted child abuse to be ignored, then you should also agree that moral opinions cannot be reached simply by appealing to social laws or mores.

The more uncertainty that exists about the probability and magnitude of the harm predicted or benefit to be gained, the more controversy there exists over whether to break confidentiality. Reasonable and informed people of goodwill may disagree about whether the probability and magnitude of the harm to be avoided or the benefit to be gained justifies exceptions. Different views may represent different weights given to the duty to protect people and the duty to respect the rights of privacy and confidentiality.

Great controversy was generated by the decision in the precedent-setting case *Tarasoff v. Regents of the University of California* (1976):

Case 5. A patient, Prosenjit Poddar, confided to Dr. Moore, a psychologist, that he intended to kill his former girlfriend, Tatiana Tarasoff. Dr. Moore believed him and notified his superior and the police. No action was taken to warn the woman, whom Poddar eventually killed. The California Supreme Court ruled in favor of the family who later sued claiming that the psychiatrist and psychologist had a duty to warn her. "When a therapist determines, or pursuant to the standards of his profession should determine, that his patient presents a serious danger of violence to another, he incurs an obligation to use reasonable care to protect the intended victim against such danger" such as warning the intended victim, notifying the police or "Whatever other steps are reasonably necessary under the circumstances" (1976, 204).

This is a controversial precedent because therapists argue that the standard used is difficult to apply. In therapy many patients express great hostility to others, even saying they will kill them. Therapists claim they cannot predict which of the very few among the many who say such things really mean it. Psychiatrists have argued that they are being required to deliver psychiatric opinions about who is a genuine threat when there is insufficient data to make such predictions. This offends them as scientists who do not have a reliable means of making such predictions and puts them in the untenable position of being forced to pose as experts in matters where they cannot claim expertise. They charge that forcing them to report too widely (for example, due to fear of litigation) would undermine the important practice of confidentiality as well as the patient-therapist relation. The debate in law and medicine over the Tarasoff ruling continues. And it is possible this ruling may be applied to other problems such as the duty to warn third parties that they are at risk of getting diseases such as AIDS.

Another important class of exceptions to the duty to honor medical confidences concerns the person who poses a risk of harm to self.

Case 6. Mr. D is taken to his internist, Dr. S, who learns Mr. D has become thin and withdrawn since the death of his son two months earlier. Mr. D in despair blames himself for his son's death. Assurances that he was in no way to blame cannot touch his unshakable belief. He thinks he is worthless, talks openly about how he could go about killing himself, but forbids his physician to say or do anything to stop him. He believes himself unworthy of treatment or hospitalization. Mr. D's physician does not regard his desire to die to be rational. He views Mr. D as depressed and suicidal. Dr. S believes Mr. D's condition is treatable and that he needs to be protected from harming himself. Dr. S seeks psychiatric treatment for Mr. D over Mr. D's objections.

The greater the risk and the less the evidence for the psychiatric opinion that the probability or magnitude of harm is great, that the condition is reversible, or that the person is impaired, then the less the justification for regarding the situation as an exemption to medical confidentiality. If Mr. D's condition is reversible and if there is evidence that great harm can come to Mr. D because of his impaired reasoning, then Dr. S's decision is more likely to be viewed as justified.

Suicide is a means some people use to escape pain and improve their lot (Heyd and Block 1981). Both Mr. D in Case 6 and Mrs. J in Case 3 sincerely want to commit suicide. But there is no evidence that Mrs. J's decision, unlike Mr. D's, is the product of mental illness or that her condition is reversible. How can we determine when people are competent enough to make certain decisions?

Competency

Some of the most difficult moral problems that arise in psychiatry are generated by disagreements over or uncertainty about someone's competency.

Case 7. Mr. V is 52 and has lived on the streets of Boston for four months. He was released from a mental hospital six months ago to a "half-way house," but he disliked it and stayed only two months. He carries his belongings and sleeps in the park when it is warm and over hot air grates when it is cold. He begs for money and food and lives on what others discard. It is a bitterly cold January, and people explain that he must enter a shelter to keep from freezing to death. He curses at them telling them to leave him alone. They are convinced he does not understand his danger and that he might improve if he were hospitalized and treated. Others say he should live as he wishes.

Case 8. Miss M is 21 and has been seeing Dr. Z as a psychiatric outpatient. Miss M has anorexia nervosa and weighs 70 pounds. Dr. Z believes if Miss M does not enter the hospital she will soon be dead. Dr. Z explains to Miss M that her prognosis is poor even if she enters the hospital, but that there is a 20 percent chance she can recover if she is hospitalized and cooperates.

> Miss M is cheerful, intelligent, and accurately discusses the risks and bene-
> fits of hospitalization, but she refuses to enter the hospital.

Mr. V and Miss M each are capable of expressing intentions or desires. Someone's capacity to *express an intention or desire,* however, is an inadequate general
standard of competency. Seriously impaired and incompetent people (like the depressed and suicidal man in Case 5) may express preferences that are the product of
mental illness. Another inadequate standard is that we decide if people are competent based on whether we happen to like *the nature of the person's choice.* Competent people may make choices many people do not like, and incompetent people
make "choices" people do like. Thus, this cannot be the standard for determining
competency or capacity.

In contrast to these two clearly inadequate standards, competency and incom-
petency may be judged *functionally.* That is, the judgment focuses on a person's
capacity to comprehend, reason, or act in relation to a specific task. Persons who
are seriously mentally impaired may still be competent to make many decisions for
themselves. The President's Commission recommends that determination of incapacity be based on a functional approach. In the Commission's view, incapacity to
make certain decisions means the person "lacks the ability to understand a situation
and to make a choice in light of that understanding" (1982, 172). It specifies three
requirements to judge capacity, "Decision making capacity requires, to greater or
lesser degree: (1) possession of a set of values and goals; (2) the ability to communicate and to understand information; and (3) the ability to reason and to deliberate
about one's choices" (1982, 57).

The functional approach, however, has problems. Who decides what tests
and thresholds to use to determine if someone is competent to do certain tasks?
Sometimes our decisions about another's competence will be affected by our purposes and how we rank certain values. For example, civil rights lawyers with the
goal of protecting individual rights might argue that either or both Mr. V in Case 7
and Miss M in Case 8 should be allowed to live as they wish because they have
sufficient capacity to be regarded as legally competent. Physicians with the goal of
trying to help those in need, might argue that either or both are incapacitated by
illness and could benefit from treatment; they might argue both fail to appreciate the
high probability and magnitude of their danger and this failure to appreciate the
risk is related to the nature of their respective illnesses. Physicians sometimes argue
the criteria for judging capacity or competency when someone refuses extremely
important care should vary directly with the risk and likely benefit of treatment
(Appelbaum and Roth 1982; Roth, Meisel, and Lidz 1977).

When physicians are uncertain if patients are competent, they usually seek a
psychiatric consultation. There are standard tests for assessing this. They test persons' orientation to person, place, and time; their remote and short-term memory;
their intellectual capacity including abilities to reason, to learn relevant facts, and to

understand consequences of ordinary acts; and their mood and affect. They also examine them for suicidal ideation, delusions, hallucinations, and illusions and determine if their behavior is anxious, agitated, or disoriented. They determine if there are changes in their behavior such as disruption of established eating, sleeping, or living patterns. These tests, however, do not always give clear answers. Consider the following:

Case 9. Mr. W, age 44, has been incapacitated by schizophrenia for many years and has had repeated hospitalizations. He is somewhat less incapacitated than usual, but he and others expect this is temporary. He has repeatedly said such things as "My suffering is greater than anything you can imagine, far worse than the pain of my heart attack last year." He plans to kill himself now because he now has the capacity to do it and wants to save himself from his horrible existence. He sees his life as a terrible burden to himself, his family, and his community. Most of the psychiatric staff who have known him over the years believe they would feel exactly as Mr. W does if they were in Mr. W's place. Should he be hospitalized for suicide prevention?

Is Mr. W, who in many ways is severely impaired, able to make this decision? Are others able to understand his anguish? The decision about whether a person is competent to make a certain decision or do certain things is important in determining whether it is morally permissible to interfere. The more momentous and irreversible the choice, the more we should want to examine the competency of someone's choice.

Some argue that the desire to commit suicide is always wrong or always should be prevented. These arguments may take various forms. First, religious arguments may hold suicide is a violation of divine law because only God may take a life. Second, some hold that suicide is an unnatural act because it is an act of self-destruction. Third, some have held it is always an irrational act since it seeks to improve a life by destroying it. Fourth, some have held that suicide is immoral and ought to be prevented because it harms the community that permits it by diminishing the value of all human life. Fifth, some hold the desire to commit suicide in itself shows mental illness.

Each of these reasons has been challenged. First, appeals to God's will or to divine laws are unconvincing because we disagree on what positions these appeals support. They have been used for and against slavery, universal suffrage, abortion, and many other controversial issues. Moreover, beliefs that one's opinion is shared by God hardens people's hearts to the need to subject their opinions to critical and rational examination. Moreover, David Hume argued that suicide does not violate divine law because God permits it. Assuming God is all powerful in governance of all things, suicide must conform to God's will and laws. Second, Hume also argued that it does not violate natural laws because it is possible. Furthermore, if it violates natural laws then we might be led to the absurd conclusion that saving a life also violates natural laws. Third, Hume argued that the act of suicide may be rational when a person, "hunted by pain and misery, bravely overcomes all the natural terrors of death and makes his escape from this cruel scene" [Hume (1784) 1965, 300]. The fourth argument is also attacked by Hume. He argues it does not harm society when the person can no longer contribute to society. Hume argues, then, that suicide is not a crime against our duty "to God, our neighbors or ourselves" [Hume (1784) 1965, 298]. Fifth, this argument simply assumes, but does not show, that the desire to commit suicide is a sufficient sign of incapacitating mental illness. Mrs. J's decision in Case 3 does not seem the product of impairment or mental illness, however.

Of course, these objections are not entirely convincing to some. For one thing, Hume makes the bold assumption, "I believe no man ever threw away life, while it was worth keeping" [Hume (1784) 1965, 305]. This glosses over the fact that some conditions, which seem hopeless to the person because he is sick, are reversible. Mr. D in Case 6 (unlike Mrs. J in Case 3) has a condition that is probably reversible and makes a decision that seems impaired due to his mental illness. Moreover, if Mr. D has family members who love and depend on him, some would doubt Hume's claim that the interests of others are not affected by his choice to end his life.

The position favored by many psychiatrists is to vary the standard of competency with the risk-to-benefit ratio (Appelbaum and Roth 1982; Roth, Meisel, and Lidz 1977). If the treatment or intervention has a low or uncertain likelihood of helping the person, then a lower test of competency is acceptable. Forcing treatment on Mrs. J in Case 3 who has a terminal and horrible illness has a low or uncertain benefit. Furthermore, she is competent by a high standard. Thus, it is wrong to interfere. If treatment is likely to help then a higher standard of competency for refusal is used. Treatment is likely to help Mr. D in Case 6, and he seems very sick. Thus, it is wrong not to interfere. Accordingly, when we ask if someone is competent, we need to ask for what? The danger exists, however, that we may paternalistically adjust the level of competency by whether we like the choice. Thus, while a functional approach seems reasonable in calling for flexibility, it fails to indicate who decides and how or what tests, thresholds, values, or purposes to adopt. It does not solve the problems but clarifies them.

To summarize, various *de jure* and *de facto* standards are used to judge competency or capacity. Inadequate standards include simply using a person's ability to express a preference or simply deciding whether others like the choice made. In contrast, many prefer a functional approach to judge decisionmaking capacity. We can disagree, however, about how to apply this functional standard because we disagree over the potential harms, benefits, or capacities of the person relative to specific tasks and circumstances. Disagreements about when people are competent or capable are important because they affect the decision about whether their liberty should be restricted.

Freedom

When people become mentally ill the illness in itself may cause a loss of freedom. They may have the same freedom of action as they did when they were well in that no one interferes with them. Yet on balance they are less free because they are less able than before to understand, choose, or act (Feinberg 1978). These illnesses may rob people of freedom not unlike external constraints and compulsions. If someone is sick and agrees to treatment that leads him to become better, then no violation of self-determination occurs, and the result is that the person is freer. The difficulties arise when we have to choose between respecting someone's refusal of treatment and trying to enlarge someone's liberty by forcing them to undergo certain treatment (Feinberg 1978).

One important standard for deciding when it is justifiable to interfere with the liberty of others was urged by John Stuart Mill. He held that competent adults should not be restrained or compelled against their will unless to prevent harm to others (Mill 1859). Mill made exceptions to this rule. He held that those who were not competent to exercise control over their lives were exempt. Mill's "exceptions" included children and persons incapacitated by mental illness or retardation.

The issue of when to restrict freedom is extremely important in psychiatry. Forcing treatment or hospitalization may help people when they badly need it, or may violate their freedom to control their lives. In this section, some liberty-limiting principles are explicitly reviewed (some of them were appealed to earlier), and then suggestions are made regarding how decisions should be made for incompetent or incapacitated persons.

Many principles have been proposed to justify interference with the liberty of others. They include preventing harm to others, *the harm principle,* and preventing "self-regarding harmful conduct only when it is substantially nonvoluntary or when temporary intervention is necessary to establish whether it is voluntary or not" (Feinberg 1971, 113), *weak paternalism.* That these or other principles have been used does not settle whether they are all equally justifiable or when they are justifiable.

The harm principle is probably the most widely accepted and least controversial principle for limiting the liberty of others. Yet it can be controversial in at least two ways. First, we may disagree about whether the harm is sufficient in magnitude and probability to justify the restriction of another's freedom; second, we can disagree about what to do with the genuinely borderline cases. The following is a clear application of the harm principle.

Case 10. A two-year old boy, John, has been admitted to the hospital with multiple fractures, cuts, and bruises. His father, Mr. U, claims he has been sent from the future to destroy John, who will be the next Hitler if he is allowed to live. Mr. U says he must also destroy all John's friends because they will be the next Gestapo leaders.

Those who pose a serious threat of physical harm to others, like Mr. U, clearly need to be restrained.

A second principle used to justify limiting the liberty of others is *weak paternalism*. The physician in Case 6 used weak paternalism to have the incompetent, depressed, and suicidal Mr. D committed against his will. Genuine disagreement might arise about whether such reasoning could properly be used to hospitalize Mr. V who lives in the street in Case 7 or Miss M who has anorexia nervosa in Case 8. A weak paternalist would permit interference with the liberty of others to determine if they are competent or capable of making a rational choice. The weak paternalist might recommend hospitalizing Mr. D and Miss M to evaluate their competency. If found competent and capable, the weak paternalist favors noninterference with the person's liberty as long as they do not harm others.

Interference with someone's liberty is sometimes a duty. We ought to protect or to promote the good of those who cannot take care of themselves, such as children and those incapacitated by major mental illness, dementia, or retardation. Paternalism when applied to competent people, however, gives what most take to be insufficient importance to the value or right of self-determination. Mill argued that competent people should be regarded as the best judge of what is in their own interest.

If a person is incompetent or incapacitated, then how ought decisions be made for him or her? Two important standards that have been discussed are the *substitute judgment standard* and the *best interest standard*. The substitute judgment standard holds that the person deciding for an incompetent person (such as Mr. D in Case 6), should make the kind of judgment the person would have been likely to make if that person were capable of reflecting on his or her present state. An advantage of the substitute judgment standard is that it honors the person's right of self-determination as well as can be done. It requires, however, having known the person well enough when competent to extrapolate what he or she would now choose. For example, the family of a patient with advanced Alzheimer's disease and pneumonia may know that were he competent he would prefer to die by pneumonia and be released from his life of dementia.

There are difficulties with this standard. First, people often claim to know and to be using the person's preferences and values when they are really using their own. Even with good intentions, it is hard to separate our interests, preferences, and values from those we imagine the person might express. Second, some of us have physicians or family members whom we would not want to make any choices for us. It might be best if we designate proxies to make decisions for us if we become incompetent, but this is rarely done. A third problem is that this standard cannot be used if the person was never competent. Fourth, the standard requires extrapolating a decision. And that judgment becomes increasingly suspect the more we move from the person's expressed views. Fifth, in the case of a person who changes significantly because of brain disease or dementia, we can ask in what sense we are following the wishes of the same person.

Another standard that has been offered as a way of reaching decisions for incompetent persons is the *best interest standard*. According to this standard, one bases one's decision, all other things being equal, on the action that is likely to produce the greatest balance of benefit over harm for the individual. We say "all other things being equal" because what is really best might not be possible; it might really be best to hire a full-time psychiatrist to provide care for someone, but it might not be possible. There are advantages to the best interest standard. First, it has us consider as central the individual's needs and situation. Second, it directs us to focus on the duty of beneficence (doing good and preventing harm). But there are also criticisms of this standard. It tends to be a very conservative standard with conventional social mores usually selected as "best."

It may be that the substitute judgment and best interest standards each have a place in different circumstances. Where people have expressed views or left advance directives about their care, then the substitute judgment standard may be appropriate. The best interest standard might be proper and useful for someone who never expressed relevant views or was never competent. While placing the patient's wishes or interests first seems appropriate, an ongoing problem is how to rank these in relation to other considerations such as the burden to the family, other patients, or society; the allocation of resources; or the health or safety of others.

To summarize, when we ask if someone is competent or capable of living as they wish, we need to ask, competent or capable for what? Someone may be competent or capable in one area, but not in another. Mr. W, the man with schizophrenia in Case 9, is capable of handling almost nothing in his life, but perhaps he is the only person who can say whether it is worth living. In contrast, Miss M in Case 8 seems competent to handle almost everything in her life, except perhaps the intake of food. Should our decision about whether to interfere with others be affected by the momentous nature of their choice such as the finality of suicide? Should it be affected by beliefs about the reversibility of their condition? The kinds of standards we adopt reflects how much we value liberty or fear abuses of liberty-limiting standards.

Interference with the liberty of adults requires a heavy burden of proof to show they are incapacitated, incompetent, or a threat to others. It requires proving first that the probability and magnitude of the harm merits this interference; second, that the means to do so are effective and the least restrictive available; third, if the reason given is to prevent harm to or benefit the person, then there must be adequate evidence that on balance it will prevent harm to or benefit the person; fourth, if the reason given is to prevent harm to or benefit the society, then there must be adequate evidence that on balance it will prevent harm to or benefit the society.

Involuntary Commitment

Committing persons involuntarily to a psychiatric unit or giving them treatment against their will is a severe restriction of their liberties. Laws exist that permit courts to do this if people are regarded as dangerous or neglectful to themselves or others. Jurisdictional statutes differ, but they are very specific and have many safeguards. They generally permit involuntary commitment when there is good reason to believe that people are a danger to themselves or others, or that they are gravely disturbed; this means they are too sick to provide themselves with the basic necessities of life (Holder 1985).

The debates about when involuntary civil commitment to a mental hospital may be justified to keep an individual from harm raise very difficult problems. On one hand, making rules flexible might allow the complexities of individual situations to be considered but also might allow abuses. On the other hand, making the rules inflexible might minimize certain kinds of abuses but leave us with policies that make no sense in certain situations. Thus, unless we can trust people to use policies with equity, there may be a dilemma from which we cannot recover. That is, either the policies are so restrictive that they do not apply in certain specific cases or they allow flexibility and thus allow indiscretions. Part of the difficulty over current policy is that in the past there have been well-documented abuses of the involuntary commitment procedures. Some seek to cure the abuses by abolishing or severely restricting the practice of involuntary civil commitment. This has left many psychiatrists troubled that the cure is worse than the disease and that patients will be harmed by making it difficult to protect them or making it very easy for them to get discharges when they need longer hospital stays (McGarry and Chodoff 1981).

A very important case was *O'Connor v. Donaldson* decided by the United States Supreme Court in 1975. In this divided decision, the court ruled that "a nondangerous individual who is capable of surviving safely in freedom by himself or with the help of willing or responsible family or friends can not constitutionally be confined" (1975, 287). The court ruled, "A finding of 'mental illness' alone cannot justify a state's locking up a person against his will and keeping him indefinitely in simple custodial confinement" (1975, 287). The court ruled that J. G. O'Connor, the superintendent of the institution, acted malevolently to violate Kenneth Donaldson's constitutional right to freedom.

Case 11. Kenneth Donaldson, after making a political comment, was knocked unconscious by fellow workers in 1943. A judge, on the request of his parents, committed him to a mental institution for treatment. He was given an eleven-week treatment of electroconvulsive therapy (ECT) and released. In 1956, at the request of his father, Donaldson was arrested, jailed, and diagnosed as "paranoid schizophrenic." Two physicians interviewed him very briefly and a judge informed him he would be sent to the Florida State Hospital. He stayed there fifteen years, during which time Donaldson petitioned various courts asking for a hearing. When it was finally reviewed in 1971, Donaldson was regarded as no longer incompetent and was released. He sued for having been committed without treatment. The jury found that two physicians acted in bad faith by being guided by what Donaldson's parents wanted rather than what would have been in Donaldson's interest.

Courts have ruled that people in mental institutions must get appropriate treatment and be housed in proper facilities. Psychiatrists who may get sued when this is not provided worry that they are "becoming scapegoats for the inadequacies of public mental health facilities" (McGarry and Chodoff 1981). In some cases, psychiatrists and mental health facilities are caught in a squeeze between the courts that order proper treatment and housing and legislatures that allocate insufficient funds for this purpose.

Some have charged that those seeking to save money and those fostering legal activism to protect civil liberties have joined forces to seek release of large numbers of mental patients. They claim that the result is not always in the best interest of mental patients. Many patients were discharged from institutions in the 1970s because the institutions were crowded or did not provide treatment or because it was argued that the patients, like Donaldson, were capable of making it on their own especially with the help of friends. But many of these patients, like Mr. V in Case 7, became "street people." Some psychiatrists charge that activists, in their enthusiasm for either saving money or defending civil liberties, have forgotten that there also exists a duty to protect people who need help or who cannot take care of themselves (McGarry and Chodoff 1981). Even Mill, with his strong statement of the importance of individual liberties, exempts people who cannot take care of themselves.

Some have argued, however, that involuntary civil commitment in any circumstance is wrong. One reason given for this view is that such laws have been abused. People who were no threat to self or others were committed for long periods of time. A second reason offered is that the interests of justice would be better served if the criminal justice system were used to deal with dangerous people, like Mr. U who beat up his son in Case 10. Often these critics object to the insanity defense. If people are dangerous and violent, they should be tried and put in prison. Or, according to Thomas Szasz, with whom these views are closely associated, they should be put in a prison-hospital where medical and psychiatric treatment could be provided along with incarceration. A third reason why Szasz and others argue that those considered mentally ill ought not receive special treatment is because they say mental illness is a fiction (Szasz 1963).

Each of these reasons given for doing away with involuntary civil commitment is problematic. A difficulty with the first reason is that all laws can be abused, but this does not mean we should abolish laws. It is not (alas) a reason for doing away with taxes. Therefore, citing outrageous violations does not settle the issue of whether there should be such laws. What proponents for this view would have to show is that such laws are always inappropriate, like laws fostering racial segregation or sexual discrimination are always inappropriate. They must show laws allowing persons to be hospitalized or treated over their objections are always wrong. But it does not seem obvious that the interests of justice would be better served by disallowing such laws. Should Mr. D in Case 5 who is depressed over his son's death be left to live as he wishes—and likely commit suicide—or should there be a legal means (with many safeguards) to treat him for what is probably a reversible condition?

The second reason also has problems. If people are put in prison for doing bad things, then why should they have to get psychiatric treatment? If Mr. U, who beats up his child in Case 10, is bad, it is appropriate to punish him for what he has done but not subject him to psychiatric treatment without his consent. But if he is sick and for that reason could not help what he did, then why is it appropriate to punish him by putting him in prison? Most psychiatrists believe Szasz' proposal to use the criminal justice system in place of civil commitment procedures would be far more detrimental to mental patients than the possible abuses that could result from the misuse of the involuntary civil commitment procedures (McGarry and Chodoff 1981).

A third reason Szasz and others oppose involuntary civil commitment is because they deny the reality of mental illness. Szasz argues that if we know of an underlying physical cause to explain someone's bizarre behavior, such as a brain tumor, we can treat him as sick; but we cannot treat him as sick if no underlying physical cause can be found by us. We have reviewed difficulties with this view earlier.

Those who oppose the involuntary civil commitment laws often do so on civil libertarian grounds. They argue that involuntary commitment for treatment is neither fair nor compassionate. But psychiatrists typically argue that the alternative frequently proposed, using the criminal justice system, would be far less fair or compassionate. Another area of controversy is whether children should have the same legal protection as adults. Parents may commit children without judicial review. Some argue that this allows too little protection for children (Holder 1985).

Paternalism

Most people want help when they are sick and miserable. Health professionals are committed to helping them if they can, sometimes as a good parent helps a child. Paternalism (parentalism) may be a duty when either people cannot make decisions for themselves, suffer incapacitating mental illness, show involuntary, self-destructive behavior, or make choices so inappropriate to their own established life-long goals that we doubt their autonomy. In the presence of nonautonomous, self-destructive behavior or when means are used that are irrational, unreasonable, and uncharacteristic, interference seems warranted.

Paternalism that properly protects individuals from harm or helps them under the above conditions is good; paternalism that improperly treats people as children is bad. The problem is how to distinguish them. Views about how to do this have direct practical consequences for psychiatric practice.

What should be done if the intended intervention is really in the patient's best interest, but the person does not want it? For example, Mrs. Yetter, a mentally incapacitated woman, consistently refused needed surgery for suspected cancer (*In re Yetter* 1973). The court agreed with her physicians and family that the surgery was in her best interest and that her reasons for refusal were delusional. Yet the court ruled that her being steadfast in her fear of death during surgery, not the delusions, was her primary reason for refusing surgery, and it honored her right to refuse surgery even though judging it was in her best interest to have it. Thus, determining that something is in someone's best interest is not sufficient to impose it even on someone who is unquestionably mentally ill. Probably her family and physicians were frustrated by her steadfast refusal. But they (correctly) let the courts decide what to do rather than either forcing surgery on her or abandoning her to her decision. It can be a terrible burden not to be able to help those who need it.

Physicians recognize a duty to act in the best interest of patients. This duty of beneficence (to do good or avoid harm) is an ancient medical tradition and is sometimes said to promote unwarranted paternalism. It would be unjustly paternalistic, if it said that all one has to do is to decide sincerely what one believes is in the patient's best interest and then to do it (Veatch 1981). Then, it would not matter what the standard of care was, what patients thought, or what the laws required. Believing that one is acting in the best interest of another shows sincerity of purpose. This is important because it may never be correct to go against one's conscience. One's conscience, however, may be informed or not, prejudiced or not, empathetic or not, or partial or not. Thus doing what is best or what one thinks is best is not sufficient to justify actions. If the injunction to act in the patient's best interest is understood as a test of conscience of the virtuous practitioner, as a rule of action having a *ceteris paribus* clause, or as a *prima facie* duty, then it does not entail paternalism.

Disrespect to others can take many forms. This includes not only unwarranted paternalism but indifference or abandonment of people who make irrational or impaired choices. I do not think Mrs. Yetter's physicians would have shown her more respect if they had left unchallenged her impaired refusal. Thus, while the best interest standard can be abused, there seems no clear reason to suppose it entails or systematically promotes abuses in the form of unwarranted paternalism. The best interest standard may even be necessary to promote an empathetic system of health care (Kopelman 1985a). It can be abused, however, by making avoidable scientific or factual errors or by uncritically using one's own value system to decide what is best.

Psychiatrists as a group have a great deal of power. Because of their area of expertise as well as to their professional commitment to act in patients' best interest, their views have weight. With considerable influence they can, for example, recommend or oppose people being hospitalized or treated against their will, being found innocent of criminal charges by virtue of insanity, or being judged incompetent to make certain decisions. Still, they only make recommendations to the courts. Actual decisions are shaped by policies, laws, and professional standards including regulations about due process, gaining consent appropriately, when to seek court orders, and how invasive therapies must be tested or may be used. Judge David Bazelon writes that it is the courts' job to test publicly these decisions. "Today every profession is being challenged by those who believe that trust should rest not on mystique but rather on what the public knows about its exercise of its expertise. . . ." [(1974) 1979, 193]. The laws, policies, or court decisions are no final appeal in determining what scientific or moral views are correct. But they are sometimes the "least worst" alternative because they offer a means of public review and criticism. Bazelon writes, "The law must also reconcile competing values that seem irreconcilable. In this task it does not seek final solutions; it recognizes the ongoing nature of deep-rooted conflicts. A judge reviews and develops criteria for resolving each case as it comes before him. The criteria are made known to the public in written opinions in which the competing values are ventilated. The court's decisions are never fixed and frozen; they are altered in response to new information, new understanding and public demands. The law itself does not provide wisdom. It offers a method for seeking wisdom" [(1974) 1979, 186].

In the past, courts and physicians have acted in ways we today would find unjustly paternalistic. Only recently has there been legal and medical recognition of the duty to consult patients about their care and to honor a competent patient's right to refuse treatment (Miller 1980). It would be paternalistic to use a high standard of competency for no other reason than that we do not like someone's choice and a low one simply because we do. Of course, it may be appropriate to explore refusals of treatment that have momentous consequences more carefully than those that do not. One of the cases most frequently discussed in this regard is that of Dax Cowart:

Case 12. In the film *Please Let Me Die* (1974), a patient, Dax Cowart, is interviewed ten months after being burned over 65 percent of his body. Blind, disfigured, and without fingers, he has consistently insisted on his right to refuse medical treatments. These include extensive surgery and extremely painful procedures that will result in a quality of life he finds unacceptable. He would die quickly without treatment but also talks of committing suicide. Two psychiatrists find him competent and hold that his decision is not the product of mental illness. He cannot get a court hearing he wants and is treated over his objections. His refusals have been unwavering for ten months but are discounted as incompetent, childish, manipulative, or insincere. Ten years later in *Dax's Case*, (1985) he uses similar reasoning to defend the right to refuse treatment. Cowart is now a lawyer working to help patients gain their rights.

With the best intentions people may be entirely wrong about what harms or benefits a patient. They may be wrong for factual or evaluative considerations. Patients have some protection from the paternalistic enthusiasms of others because of policies about competency, consent, involuntary commitment and how invasive therapies and drugs may be used. Some of these policies exist because of past abuses. For example, early methods of psychosurgery in the 1940s were crude, done without consent or testing, and irreversibly harmed many people without any compensatory benefit (Macklin 1982). Until recently in every area of medicine, invasive and powerful procedures were used without consent and without what we today would consider adequate criteria or testing. The psychoactive drugs that caused near miraculous changes in psychiatry in the 1950s were widely used before much was known about their side effects. These drugs alter mood, behavior, and thought, but some unknown percentage of users get side effects such as tardive dyskinsea (a loss of motor control) that may be irreversible.

The development and use of these invasive technologies have raised additional serious questions about the limits of paternalism. First, should competent adults have to get permission from psychiatrists to use mind-altering drugs they believe will enhance their lives; if they do not harm others, why should these drugs be controlled substances? Second, the worse the mental illness, the more reasonable it may be to consider using risky, invasive, uncertain, or irreversible therapies; but the worse the mental illness, the less patients are probably able to assess competently for themselves the risks and benefits of treatments. And, as therapies become more risky, invasive, uncertain, or irreversible, it becomes harder for others to claim clear moral authority for making these decisions for them.

Consent

Gaining consent is important because it honors the person's right to personal integrity and self-determination and because it is useful to have the person's cooperation in a therapeutic program. Meaningful consent has three necessary features. The person must be sufficiently informed, acting voluntarily, and competent. Physicians have a duty to gain proper consent unless there is an emergency or unless disclosure itself would be likely to cause great harm. Major mental illness affects one's ability to understand, reason, choose, or act. Consequently, each of the three necessary features of consent may present unique problems in psychiatric practice. For example, a suicidal patient may welcome hazardous or painful procedures yet his "choice" may be nonvoluntary and due to illness. In discussing psychosurgery, Gaylin described the problem as one in which "the damaged organ is the consenting organ" (Macklin 1982, 17).

When dealing with persons with major psychiatric illness, consent can be a problem because the very skills needed for proper consent are impaired (understanding, reasoning, choosing, or acting). Still some recommend that all patients including psychiatric patients be encouraged to make their own treatment choices. For example, Charles Culver and Bernard Gert concede that patients with a major depression have difficulty making decisions, yet urge them to choose between the different therapies available. Physicians should give their expert advice and discuss the treatments' risks and benefits but promote patient choice (1982).

How one regards the right to consent to or refuse treatment is often shaped by how one thinks about rights generally. Are rights morally indispensable, redundant, confrontational, minimalistic, or unnecessary in a caring relationship? (Gewirth 1986). For example, should consent and refusal be seen as a patient's just claim on someone that creates a correlative duty on others, as a process of mutual decisionmaking, or as both? Cowart's problems in Case 12 may illustrate the weakness of a notion of consent that does not incorporate a right to refuse treatment. Yet these hopelessly unresolvable situations seem rare. Where nature did not solve the problem, people of goodwill often seem able to find a plan all can accept. Tolerance and a willingness to appreciate the views of others can often lead the principals to find acceptable strategies. Such negotiating occurs frequently in all medical practice as patients, physicians, and sometimes nurses, social workers, family, and friends try to influence each other about treatments or hospitalization. Perhaps all the problems presented herein could have been solved if people used the methods of moral reasoning to seek a plan with which they could live. Peter in Case 1 might be persuaded that studying philosophy would suit him better than medicine; Mr. and Mrs. Q in Case 2 might agree to a plan whereby they act one way in this country and another at home.

But at what point is "successful negotiation" a compromise of principle and when is "influence" undue pressure, manipulation, or coercion? Influence may take the form of encouragement, education, indoctrination, persuasion, bargaining, pressure, manipulation, or even coercion. Mill (1859) and Feinberg (1978) have argued that efforts to influence people that fall short of manipulation or coercion may be appropriate.

Since the 1970s great emphasis has been put on gaining documentation of consent from patients. Whether for medicolegal or moral reasons, psychiatrists routinely seek consent for risky or invasive therapies. The physician has a duty to make a reasonable attempt at seeing that the patient or guardian comprehends appropriately. These requirements have been elaborated on in detail because we need to have clear guidance about such things as what information is material for a choice or when pressure defeats meaningful consent. But some procedures are so irreversible and invasive that they create special doubts about consent. For example, surgeons will no longer agree to do psychosurgery without consent, and some are unwilling to do it even with consent. What constitutes proper consent for very risky or permanently altering behavior modification?

Case 13. A judge has contacted a surgical group at the request of two prison inmates. The surgeons discuss if they should do as the judge and inmates propose. One inmate with pedophilia, convicted of sexual abuse of children, seeks castration. The other inmate is extremely violent and seeks psychosurgery. Both hope to shorten their incarceration. The surgeons refuse because they hold "no one can give meaningful consent. Anyone mentally disturbed enough to need it, doesn't have the capacity to give it. And no third party should be allowed to give consent in these circumstances."

There is a good deal of controversy about what constitutes proper consent as the risk of therapy or investigation increases. Appelbaum and Roth (1982) offer four important standards of competency to consent. These are expressing a choice, understanding the issues, manipulating the information rationally, and appreciating the nature of the situation. Mr. V who lives on the streets of Boston in Case 7 may not understand what is at stake; Miss M in Case 8 who does may fail to appreciate the nature of the situation.

RESEARCH

Increasingly, therapists have had to justify that treatments would benefit persons by providing care or a cure for their illness, for diagnosis or for prevention of illness. Therapy has both beneficial and intentional goals. Its goal is beneficial because it seeks to benefit or remove harms, and its goal is intentional because it focuses on the beliefs or intentions of people who try to do this. Herbalists, folk-doctors, suggestologists, and rolfists may sincerely intend to provide therapy but fail to have any scientific basis for their claims. Controlled testing is necessary to evaluate proposed therapies. Because of research, each decade of this century has transformed many medical and psychiatric practices. In short, with a rate most would find surprising, new medical therapies become available, old therapies become discredited, and alternative therapies with different risks or benefits are acceptable in medical practice. Earlier forms of electroconvulsive treatment (ECT), psychosurgery, and drugs with permanent debilitating side effects were once widely used without explicit criteria, without adequate testing, and without informed consent (Macklin 1982). People sincerely believed in them. But great harm is often the result of using invasive procedures without adequate testing in any area of medicine. This is why there are now so many regulations about testing therapies.

In scientific medicine, there is a moral requirement to test therapies. Such information is needed to justify its beneficent and therapeutic intent and to gain consent that is adequately informed. A moral problem is how to honor and protect the rights and welfare of persons while allowing important research to continue. Recent guidelines reflect moral and legal views that patients' rights and welfare are higher values than medical progress. In the United States, "Guidelines for Research on those Institutionalized as Mentally Infirm" were proposed for those who have impairments such as, or similar to, mental illness, senility, psychosis, mental retardation or emotional disturbances (HEW 1978). To try to balance the social utility of research with respect and protection of the person, the guidelines stipulate that the greater the risk, the more rigorous and elaborate the protections and consent requirements. In general, no research that presents more than a minimal risk is permitted on subjects who cannot give meaningful consent unless there is evidence that the intervention holds out the prospect of direct benefit to the subjects. A "minimal risk" is understood as the kind of risk encountered in daily life or in a routine physical examination and includes consideration of physical and psychosocial risks. [This definition is problematic as some daily risks are not minimal and highly sensitive information can come to light in routine office visits (Kopelman 1981).]

According to these guidelines the consent or assent of the mentally infirm person must be sought. None who refuse may be enrolled in any study that does not hold out direct benefit without authorization from the courts. Otherwise, a guardian may consent for nontherapeutic studies only if the person cannot give consent, the risk is minimal, and the person does not object.

Some believe it would be just and compassionate to prohibit nontherapeutic testing on those who cannot give meaningful consent. The problem with prohibiting all nontherapeutic studies is that it would rule out some very important, nonrisky studies. Examples of important low-risk, nontherapeutic studies might include epidemiological surveys of the infectious diseases in an institution; questionnaires about how patients might prefer to be treated; whether people tend to lose or gain physical strength while patients in mental institutions, whether certain illnesses tend to occur at a certain time or circumstance, how long they last, what is their course, whether there is a familial pattern, what complications tend to occur, and so on. Some claim nontherapeutic studies without consent are always an abuse, but others have argued they have not made their case if the reasonable person would not object and if the research is not risky (Kopelman 1985b).

A very controversial study sought to compare the effects of drug therapy and psychosurgery on criminal sexual psychopaths. The court ruled in *Kaimowitz v. Department of Mental Health for the State of Michigan* (1973) that "psychosurgery should never be undertaken upon involuntarily committed populations, when there is a high-risk, low-benefit ratio as demonstrated in this case. This is because of the impossibility of obtaining truly informed consent from such populations." The court refused to permit a willing subject to participate. The court's ruling in *Kaimowitz* has been praised for limiting psychosurgery. It has also been criticized for making it appear that a person is incompetent simply because the environment is potentially coercive (Appelbaum and Roth, 1982; Murphy 1979).

Research studies have great utility and are rarely risky or burdensome; participation can even provide an interest for people who must spend long, dreary days in an institution. Even before the days of regulations and Institutional Review Boards (IRBs), few investigators failed to put the welfare of subjects anything but first (Beecher 1966). Without controlled testing of therapies, there is often no way to determine which interventions are useful, useless, or harmful, and we would return to the days of prescientific medicine. Investigators have made great progress in developing therapies in just a few decades because they are trained to acknowledge uncertainty and try to defeat their own hypotheses and theories in testing.

UNCERTAINTY

Many of the moral problems in psychiatry we have discussed have features that cannot be settled with certainty but have important consequences for people. Judge Bazelon indicates some of the fundamental questions frequently raised in the courts:

"Who can be morally convicted of a crime? Who can be ordered into a hospital for compulsory treatment, and for how long? What kinds of treatment can be imposed without the consent of patients? These questions engage the overriding question of the balance between the state and the individual. The effort by the courts to strike a balance requires the knowledge and expertise of the experts in the behavioral sciences, particularly psychiatry" [(1974) 1979, 185]. Unfortunately, he writes, we need more knowledge and expertise.

Jay Katz has argued that we do not do a good enough job in acknowledging and disclosing uncertainty: "It is a fact of life that human beings find it difficult to maintain a consistent, self-conscious appreciation of the extent to which uncertainty accompanies them on their daily rounds and to integrate that uncertainty with whatever informs their conduct" (Katz 1984, 84). We deny uncertainty when we are uncritical about our own views or claim greater justification for our hypotheses, theories, or treatments than the data allow. Moreover, scientific claims are, by their nature, general. Medical like moral and judicial decisions require fitting general knowledge to individual settings. Such interpretations necessarily introduce more uncertainty.

Another way uncertainty arises concerns how to use reasons or principles. Stephen Toulmin has argued that debates about moral issues often suffer from excesses of generality: "These days, public debates about ethical issues vacillate between, on the one hand, a narrow dogmatism that confines itself to general assertion dressed up as 'matters of principle' and, on the other hand, a shallow relativism that evades all firm stands by suggesting that we choose our 'value systems' as freely as we choose our clothes" (Toulmin 1981, 31). Scientific, moral, and legal rules and theories, practices or principles, as important as they are, cannot by themselves generate moral judgments about individual situations. They too have to be interpreted in being used. Moreover if, on the one hand, they are highly specific, they are not likely to allow the discretion needed to make equitable decisions in all sorts of particular situations. On the other hand, if it is sufficiently general to cover every kind of case, they are unlikely to offer clear direction about what to do (Margolis 1984). Toulmin argues that our response to inadequate rules, theories, and practices should not be inflexible rules, but rules that direct us to make equitable and discriminating judgments, that is, that allow for discretion. To create rules and policies that leave little discretion is in itself a denial of uncertainty. For it presupposes that in forming rules and principles, we can think of every kind of situation that may come before us.

This review of the moral problems that arise in psychiatry suggests how moral problems should not be solved. They should not be solved simply by appealing uncritically to one's mere opinion, conscience, traditions, beliefs about God's will, social mores, or laws. Rather, we should identify and acknowledge the reasons for which we act, evaluating them critically in terms of formal criteria of consistency and universalizability and in terms of the available data, consequences, and other considerations that are part of the methods of moral justification. This should also include acknowledging the uncertainty surrounding these matters that so deeply affect people's lives.

REFERENCES

Alexander, F. G., and S. T. Selesnick. *The History of Psychiatry*. New York: Harper & Row, 1966.

Alston, W. P. "Psychoanalytic Theories, Logical Status Of." In *The Encyclopedia of Philosophy*, Vol. 6, edited by Paul Edwards, 512–516. New York: Macmillan/Free Press, 1967.

American Psychiatric Association. *Diagnostic and Statistical Manual of Mental Disorders*, 3d ed. (*DSM–III*). Washington, D.C.: APA, 1980.

Appelbaum, P. S. and L. H. Roth. "Competency to Consent to Research." *Arch Gen Psychiatry* 39 (1982): 951–958.

Bazelon, D. 1974. "Psychiatry and the Adversary Process." In *Biomedical Ethics and the Law*, 2d ed., edited by J. M. Humber and R. F. Almeder, 185–193. New York: Plenum Press, 1979.

Beecher, H. K. "Ethics and Clinical Research." *N Eng J Med* 274 (1966): 1354–1360.

Block, S. "The Political Misuse of Psychiatry in the Soviet Union." In *Psychiatric Ethics*, edited by S. Block and P. Chodoff, 321–341. Oxford, England: Oxford University Press, 1981.

Chisholm, R. "Sentences About Believing." *Proc Aristotelian Soc* 56 (1956): 125–148.

Culver, C. M., and B. Gert. *Philosophy in Medicine*. New York: Oxford University Press, 1982.

Dax's Case. Concern for Dying, New York, 1985. Videotape.

Duff, A. "Psychopathy and Moral Understanding." *Am Philos Q* 14, no. 3 (1977): 189–200.

Dworkin, G. "Can Convicts Consent to Castration?" *Hastings Cent Rep* 5 (Oct. 1975): 17–18.

―――. "Autonomy and Behavior Control." *Hastings Cent Rep* 6 (Feb. 1976): 23–28.

Faden, R. R., and T. L. Beauchamp. *A History and Theory of Informed Consent*. New York: Oxford University Press, 1986.

Feinberg, J. "Legal Paternalism." *Can J Philos* 1 (1971): 105–124.

―――. "Freedom and Behavior Control." In *Encyclopedia of Bioethics*, Vol. 1, edited by W. T. Reich, 93–101. New York: Free Press, 1978.

Frankena, W. K. "Value Judgments." In *The Encyclopedia of Philosophy*, 2d ed., vol. 8. New York: Macmillan, 1967, 229–232.

―――. *Ethics*, 2d ed. Engelwood Cliffs, N.J.: Prentice-Hall, 1973.

Freud, S. *Collected Papers*, Vol. 1–5. New York: Basic Books, 1959.

Gallie, W. B. "Essentially Contested Concepts." In *Philosophy and the Historical Understanding*. New York: Schocken, 1964.

Gaylin, W. "In Matters Mental or Emotional, What's Normal?" In *Social Ethics*, 2d ed., edited by T. A. Mappes and J. S. Zembaty, 269–271. New York: McGraw Hill, 1982.

Gewirth, A. "Why Rights Are Indispensible." *Mind* 95 (July 1986): 329–344.

Grossman, M. "Confidentiality in Medical Practice." *Annu Rev Med* 28 (1977): 43–55.

Hare, R. N. "Principles." *Proc Aristotelian Soc* 73 (1972–1973): 1–18.

Heyd, D., and S. Block. "The Ethics of Suicide." In *Psychiatric Ethics*, edited by S. Block and P. Chodoff, 185–202. Oxford, England: Oxford University Press, 1981.

Hume, D. 1784. "Of Suicide." In *Hume's Ethical Writings*, edited by A. MacIntyre, 297–306. New York: Macmillan, 1965.

Holder, A. R. *Legal Issues in Pediatrics and Adolescent Medicine*, 2d ed. New Haven, Conn.: Yale University Press, 1985.

Jonsen, A. R., M. Siegler, and W. J. Winslade. *Clinical Ethics*. New York: Macmillan, 1982.

Kaimowitz v. Department of Mental Health for the State of Michigan. Circuit Court Wayne County, Civil Action No. 73–19434–AW, 10 July 1973.

Katz, J. "Why Doctors Don't Disclose Uncertainty." *Hastings Cent Rep* 14 (Feb. 1984): 35–44.

Knight, J. "The Minister as Healer, the Healer as Minister." *J Religion and Health* 21, no. 2. (Summer 1982): 100–114.

Kopelman, L. "Ethical Controversies in Medical Research: The Case of XYY Screening." *Perspect Biol Med* (Winter 1978): 196–204.

————. "Estimating Risk in Human Research." *Clin Research* 29 (1981): 1–8.

————. "Respect in Retardation: Issues of Valuing and Labeling." In *Ethics and Retardation*, edited by L. Kopelman and J. C. Moskop, 65–86. Dordrecht, Holland: D. Reidel, 1984.

————. "Justice and the Hippocratic Tradition of Acting for the Good of the Sick." In *Ethics and Critical Care Medicine*, edited by J. Moskop and L. Kopelman, 79–103. Dordrecht, Holland: D. Reidel, 1985a.

————. "Paternalism and Autonomy in the Care of Chronically Ill Children." In *Issues in the Care of Children with Chronic Illness: A Sourcebook on Problems, Services and Policies*, edited by N. Hobbs and J. M. Perrin, 61–86. San Francisco: Jossey-Bass, 1985b.

MacIntyre, A. *After Virtue.* Indiana: University of Notre Dame Press, 1981.

Macklin, R. "Mental Health and Mental Illness." *Philos Sci* 39 (Sept. 1972): 341–365.

————. "The Medical Model in Psychoanalysis and Psychotherapy." *Compr Psychiatry* 14 (Jan./Feb. 1973): 49–69.

————. *Man, Mind and Morality: The Ethics of Behavior Control.* Englewood Cliffs, N.J.: Prentice-Hall, 1982.

Margolis, J. *Psychotherapy and Morality: A Study of Two Concepts.* New York: Random House, 1966.

————. "Applying Moral Theory to the Retarded." In *Ethics and Mental Retardation*, edited by L. Kopelman and J. Moskop, 19–36. Dordrecht, Holland: D. Reidel, 1984.

McGarry, L., and P. Chodoff. "The Ethics of Involuntary Hospitalization." In *Psychiatric Ethics*, edited by S. Block and P. Chodoff, 203–219. Oxford/New York/Melbourne: Oxford University Press, 1981.

Mercer, J. *Labeling the Mentally Retarded.* Berkeley: University of California Press, 1973.

Mill, J. S. *On Liberty.* 1859.

Miller, L. J. "Informed Consent: I." *JAMA* 244 (7 Nov. 1980): 2100–2103.

Murphy, J. G. "Therapy and the Problem of Autonomous Consent." *Inter J Law Psychiatry* 2 (1979): 415–430.

O'Connor v. Donaldson. Supreme Court of the U.S., 422 U.S. 563, 95 S. Ct. 2486, L.Ed. 2d 396, 1975.

Please Let Me Die. Galveston: Department of Psychiatry, University of Texas, 1974. Videotape.

Popper, K. R. "Science, Conjectures and Refutations." In *Conjectures and Refutations: The Growth of Scientific Knowledge.* New York: Harper & Row, 1962.

Rawls, J. *A Theory of Justice.* Cambridge, Mass.: Harvard University Press, 1971.

Reich, W. T., "Psychiatric Diagnosis as an Ethical Problem." In *Psychiatric Ethics*, edited by S. Block and P. Chodoff, 61–88. Oxford, England: Oxford University Press, 1981.

Roth, L. H., A. Meisel, and C. Lidz. "Tests of Competency to Consent to Treatment." *Am J Psychiatry* 134, no. 3 (1977): 279–284.

Rush, B. 1812. *Medical Inquiries and Observations upon Disease of the Mind.* Birmingham, Ala.: The Classics of Medicine Library, 1979.

Siegler, M. "Confidentiality in Medicine—A Decrepit Concept." *N Engl J Med* 307, no. 24 (1982): 1518–1521.

Szasz, T. *The Myth of Mental Illness.* New York: Hoeber–Harper, 1961.

————. *Law Liberty and Psychiatry: An Inquiry into The Social Uses of Mental Health Practices.* New York: Macmillan, 1963.

————. *Ideology and Insanity.* New York: Doubleday, 1970.

Tarasoff v. Regents of the University of California. 131 California Reporter 14, 1 July 1976.

Toulmin, S. "The Tyranny of Principles." *Hastings Cent Rep* 11, no. 6 (Dec. 1981): 31–39.

U.S. Department of Health, Education and Welfare, National Commission for the Protection of Human Subjects of Biomedical and Behavioral Research. "Research Involving Those Institutionalized as Mentally Infirm: Report and Recommendations." Publication (05) 78–0006 and Appendix (05)78–0007. Washington, D.C.: HEW, 1978.

United States President's Commission for the Study of Ethical Problems in Medicine and

Biomedical Behavioral Research. *Making Health Care Decisions,* Vol. 1 Report. Washington, D.C.: Government Printing Office, 1982.

United States Rehabilitation Act. P.L. 93–112.29, U.S.C. 74, 1973.

Veatch, R. *A Theory of Medical Ethics.* New York: Basic Books, 1981.

Wikler, D. "The Ethics of Clinical Trials." *Semin Oncol* 8 no. 4, (1981): 437–441.

In re Yetter. Court of Common Pleas of Northampton County, Pennsylvania, Orphans' Court Division, 1983, 62 Pa. D. & D., 2nd 619, 1973.

Zembaty, J. S. "Introduction: Mental Illness and Individual Liberty." In *Social Ethics,* 2d ed., edited by T. A. Mappes and J. S. Zembaty, 263–268. New York: McGraw-Hill, 1982.

DISCUSSION QUESTIONS

1. To what extent and in what ways do psychiatric diagnoses involve moral and other evaluative judgments? Would you view the following to be diseases or simply unusual behaviors: grief, premenstrual syndrome, homosexuality, drug addiction, alcoholism, borderline personality disorder, antisocial personality disorder, sadistic personality disorder, dependent personality disorder?

2. Of what importance is it to determine whether a psychological problem has an underlying physical basis? Are psychological problems with no identifiable underlying physical basis part of medicine? What difference does it make? Are they less real because there is no known physical basis?

3. Under what limitations, if any, is a psychiatrist justified in using his or her professional skills for the benefit of societal goals? Would it be justifiable to treat a soldier suffering severe psychological problems from being in a battle for the purpose of returning him to the battlefield even if it is not in his interest to return?

4. Under what circumstances, if any, is a psychiatrist justified in breaking confidentiality in order to benefit other persons? Would he or she be justified in warning a potential homicide victim? In reporting a confessed murderer to the police? In reporting a pathologically angry AIDS victim who confesses his intention to infect as many people as possible before he dies? In telling a fiancee of a person's strong homosexual tendencies?

5. Under what circumstances is it morally legitimate to commit someone to a mental institution against his or her will? Is it a violation of confidentiality for a psychiatrist to disclose in court his or her belief that a patient has mental problems making that person a danger to himself?

11

Health-Care
Delivery and
Resource Allocation

Allen Buchanan

SUMMARY

Increasingly medical ethics involves decisions concerning the allocation of health-care resources and the institutional arrangements for making those decisions. Such key concepts as health-care resources, allocation, and cost need to be defined because they shape the moral and policy discussion. This chapter considers different criteria for evaluating allocations of health-care resources. To do this, two types of models of allocation are examined—efficiency models and the ethical models.

In efficiency models of allocation, utility-maximization, cost-benefit, or cost-effectiveness are the standards for judgment. Efficiency criteria are not by themselves sufficient for evaluating allocations; ethical criteria are also necessary. Two case studies, rationing chemotherapy and the allocation of human heart for transplantation, illustrate the differences in the two approaches.

Broader issues relating to the ethics of resource allocation also are presented. Among these are the problem of access to health care and controversies over rival specifications of the right to health care, including utilitarian, egalitarian, equality of opportunity, and "decent minimum" views.

Recently attention has shifted to include beneficence as well as justice. Issues central to approaches that emphasize beneficence include the nature of societal obligation, the free-rider problem, the assurance problem, and the enforcement of obligations. Although many strategies have been offered for making ethical evaluations of health-care resource allocation, none so far is fully adequate or uniquely attractive.

INTRODUCTION

The Central Role of Allocational Issues in Medical Ethics

Virtually every significant problem in medical ethics either includes ethical issues concerning the allocation of scarce resources or is shaped by allocation decisions that are subject to ethical evaluation. For example, to decide whether to prolong the life of a severely disabled newborn when doing so will involve great financial burdens (for her parents, the hospital, and the public coffers), the decisionmaker—whether it be a parent, a court-appointed legal guardian, the physician, or a hospital administrator—is in effect choosing to allocate scarce resources to this particular baby rather than to someone else or something else. Unless prior allocation decisions had been made to channel resources into neonatal research and into the construction of the neonatal intensive care units in which the results of research were applied, then the need for the allocation decision that will determine this particular baby's fate would never have arisen.

This chapter is a critical survey of several major views on the ethical evaluation of decisions concerning the allocation of health-care resources, and the institutional arrangements established for making those decisions.

Preliminary Analysis of Key Concepts: Health-Care Resources, Allocation, Cost

HEALTH-CARE RESOURCES

In the most inclusive sense, health-care resources are any goods or services that can reasonably be expected to have a positive effect on health. Thus health-care resources include, but are not restricted to, medical resources. Furthermore, health-care goods and services are not limited to those that are produced by persons ordinarily recognized as health-care professionals, such as physicians and nurses. Resources used for pollution control, shelter, food required for normal growth and functioning, and not just medical drugs, procedures, and treatments, are also health-care resources.

ALLOCATION

To allocate is to distribute resources among alternative uses. Allocation in this broad sense does not presuppose an allocator (an individual or a group) who deliberately distributes the available resources. Thus a competitive market allocates social resources, through the interactions of individual exchangers, each of whom only makes allocation decisions concerning his or her own resources in the pursuit of his or her own particular ends. Allowing a market for the buying and selling of organs, for example, is just as much an allocation decision as the adoption of an explicit rationing policy that allocates organs according to a criterion of social contribution or personal desert.

Even when an allocation of resources results directly from a social (rather than an individual) decision, the allocation is often a by-product of the pursuit of other goals (rather than an intended result). For example, a law stating that nurse-midwives must be supervised by physicians if their services are to be reimbursed by third-party payers has an allocational effect: It transfers income from nurse-midwives to physicians because the latter charge the former for the service of supervision and it restricts the available number of practicing nurse-midwives to however many are able to secure such supervision. Similarly, a decision to pump millions of dollars of public funds into cancer centers affects the allocation of physicians among specialty training programs. If more money is available for residencies in oncology than for primary-care residencies, then more medical students may become oncologists and fewer may become primary-care specialists. In neither of these examples is it necessary that any decision be aimed at the allocational effect in question. Allocations are subject to ethical assessment, however, whether they are the objects of explicit allocation decisions or not.

COST

In the sense most pertinent to reasoning about allocation, the cost of something may be defined as the value of the most preferred alternative foregone. Suppose that one has to decide how to spend one's weekly entertainment budget. In the order one prefers them, alternatives are (1) seeing the ballet; (2) attending a football game; and (3) going out to dinner. Because one's budget is limited, if the ballet is chosen one loses the opportunity to attend the game and dine out. Since the game is the next most preferred alternative after the option one actually takes, its value is the cost of one's decision to see the ballet. In the sense just specified, all costs are "opportunity costs." Given that resources—including time—are limited, deciding to use a resource for one purpose forecloses opportunities for alternative uses.

Types of Allocations

Discussions of allocation often utilize a distinction between macro and micro allocation. This distinction is, however, of limited use, and can be misleading unless its relative nature is clearly recognized. A decision by the U.S. Congress to allocate N

billion dollars for Medicare and $N + m$ billion for national defense is perhaps the paradigm of a macro allocation decision. A micro allocation is a decision made by a particular physician when she decides to utilize the one available bed in her burn unit to Mr. Jones rather than to Ms. Smith. But there are, of course, many types of allocation decisions that are smaller-scale than the former but larger-scale than the latter. In response to this complexity, it is tempting to say that whether an allocation is micro or macro is determined by the *level* of decisionmaking authority or the level of available resources to be distributed. Talk of levels, however, is misleading to the extent that it encourages the fiction that there is an overall system, of a hierarchical character, within which micro and macro decisions are interconnected in some principle way. Whether or not any existing society is in fact this highly structured in its mechanism for allocation may be a matter of controversy, but it is fair to say that the United States, perhaps more so than many industrialized countries, currently lacks anything that could realistically be called an allocation system with regard to health-care resources.

It is perhaps more useful to begin instead with a classification of fundamental types of allocation problems that leaves open the question of what sort of allocational system, hierarchical or otherwise, will be needed to solve them. James F. Childress offers the following list:

1. What resources (time, energy, money, etc.) should be put into health care and into other social goods such as education, defense, eliminating poverty, and improving the environment?
2. Within the area of health (once we have determined its budget), how much time, energy, money, etc., should we allocate for prevention and how much for rescue and crisis medicine?
3. Within either preventive care or rescue medicine, who [if anyone] should receive resources such as vaccines or artificial hearts when we cannot meet everyone's needs? (Childress 1982)

CRITERIA FOR EVALUATING ALLOCATIONS

Existing, predicted, or proposed allocations may be evaluated on grounds of either efficiency or ethics, or both. It is unfortunate that discussions of the ethics of health-care resource allocation typically ignore the efficiency evaluations that dominate the work of real-world policy makers and policy analysts, who in turn often convey the impression that by exclusively employing efficiency criteria they are approaching allocation issues in a nonethical or value-neutral way. Both approaches, as we shall see, are mistaken.

Allocation decision processes may also be evaluated ethically and for efficiency. A decision process may be inefficient due to excessive expenditures of material resources (e.g., equipment for information gathering and processing), time, or human resources, or because the costs of the social conflict the process engenders is excessive. Even if an allocation decision is itself ethically unassailable, the process by which it was reached may be challenged from an ethical standpoint for procedural unfairness or on the ground that the decisionmaker lacked appropriate authority. For example, an adequate ethical evaluation of an allocation decision may require an assessment of the procedural fairness of the decisionmaking process (from which that allocation issued) because there is no consensus among reasonable persons as to whether the allocation, considered by itself, is ethically acceptable.

Efficiency Criteria

The dominant conception of efficiency among economists is that of Pareto Optimality. A state of a system is Pareto Optimal if and only if there is no feasible alternative state in which at least one person would be better off and no one would be worse off (Buchanan 1985, 4–13). A move from a state which is not Pareto optimal to one which is is a Pareto improvement and the latter state is Pareto superior to the former.

Many economists and policy analysts find the Paretian conception of efficiency attractive. One important reason for its appeal is that it avoids what many consider insurmountable obstacles to making the interpersonal utility comparisons that would be required if the Principle of Utility, a criterion of utility maximization, were employed instead. According to the Principle of Utility, allocational states are to be ranked according to how much net, overall utility they produce. The net, overall utility of a particular allocation is calculated by summing up the net utility for each individual affected. The net utility for each individual is the sum of the benefits that allocation produces for him or her, minus the costs (or "disbenefits") to him or her. An allocation maximizes utility if and only if the net, overall utility it produces is at least as great as, if not greater than, the net, overall utility produced by each of the feasible alternative allocations. In order to determine whether an allocation maximizes utility, it is necessary to sum up utilities and disutilities (or costs and benefits) across different individuals, and these, interpersonal utility comparisons require that we be able to locate everyone's state of well-being along a single numerical scale. The obstacle to achieving this is that there appears to be no nonarbitrary method for selecting a common zero point or baseline from which different individuals' utilities could all be measured, nor for determining a common unit of measurement. Even if a utility scale could be constructed for each individual by recording the choices he or she makes among various options, this seems to provide no basis for relating their respective utility scales to one another in a way that allows the needed aggregation (Brock 1973, 245–49; Sartorius 1975). In order to ascertain whether an allocation is Pareto Optimal (or to determine whether a change from one allocation to another would be a Pareto improvement), however, it is not necessary to make interpersonal utility comparisons. All that is required is that each person's well-being under a particular allocation be comparable to his or her own well-being under alternative feasible allocations.

Although an allocation may be Pareto optimal and still not maximize utility, a move from one allocation to another that constitutes a Pareto improvement at least entails an increase in utility, since at least one person's utility increases and no one's decreases. Consequently, use of the Paretian conception of efficiency can be seen as a kind of second-best alternative to the utility-maximization criterion.

If the Paretian conception of efficiency is seen in this way, relying on it as the exclusive or primary standard for evaluating allocations is no more plausible than a similar reliance on utility maximization would be, if the problem of interpersonal utility comparisons were solved. But there are strong objections to the Principle of Utility, quite apart from the difficulty of interpersonal comparisons.

First of all, it would be a mistake to view the Principle of Utility simply as a principle of collective rationality that is an uncontroversial extension of the principle of individual rationality prevalent in economic theory. The latter simply defines efficiency as taking the least-costly, effective means to one's end, that is, as individual utility maximization. Some who assume that utility maximization would be the appropriate criterion for evaluating allocation (were it not for the problem of interpersonal comparisons) and view Pareto optimality as a second-best approximation to it, may be under the impression that the Principle of Utility is an uncontroversial extension of the Principle of Individual Utility Maximization. This, however, is an error. First, if it is assumed that what is rational for an individual is to maximize his own utility, then whether or not it is rational for anyone to seek the maximization of overall utility will depend upon whether, as a matter of contingent fact, that is the best way for him or her to maximize his or her own utility. Clearly there are many instances in the real world in which maximizing one's own utility and maximizing overall utility diverge. Whenever they do, the economic definition of rationality as individual utility maximization undermines, rather than supports, the claim that overall utility maximization is the rational standard for evaluating allocations.

Second, the Principle of Utility fares no better if it is understood not as the principle of individual rationality extended to society, but as an ethical principle. To assume that the Principle of Utility is the appropriate standard for evaluating allocations is to make the ethically controversial assumption that society is to be viewed as an apparatus for maximizing overall utility. Such a view of society may be incompatible with according proper respect to individual persons, who ought not to be regarded merely as contributors to ends that are not their own (Buchanan 1985). A particular allocation, or a complete social system, might maximize overall utility and yet be grossly unfair or unjust, violating the most fundamental rights of some individuals. Rawls and others have observed that a system in which some persons were slaves would in fact maximize overall utility, as long as the gains to the masters exceeded the losses to the slaves (Rawls 1971). That the criterion of utility maximization would not only allow but indeed require such a system if it did in fact produce the most utility is taken by many to be a telling objection to Utilitarianism.

This extreme example illustrates the more general objection that opponents of Utilitarianism often raise: evaluating social arrangements, including allocations, simply according to their tendency to maximize overall utility neglects fairness as a fundamental ethical value. Similarly, Utilitarianism has frequently been criticized for ignoring another key ethical value: personal desert. That one individual deserves some good, while another does not, is never itself a reason for the utilitarian to allocate the good to the former person; all that matters is how much utility can be gained.

These ethical objections also apply to attempts to evaluate allocations using the Paretian criteria for efficiency. An allocation may be Pareto Optimal, yet grossly unjust or unfair (for example, it may be impossible to improve the condition of some of the slaves without worsening the condition of some of the slave holders). Similarly, the pursuit of Pareto improvements recognizes no role for personal desert as such—all that matters is whether a change can be made that improves the condition of some without worsening the condition of any, regardless of who deserves the benefits conferred.

It follows that those policy analysts who evaluate allocations solely by the standard economic (i.e., Paretian) criterion of efficiency are either mistakenly assuming that they have avoided controversial ethical issues or are offering a fundamentally incomplete evaluation that must be supplemented by ethical criteria. If the Paretian standard of efficiency is employed as the sole criterion for evaluating allocations, then what is required is nothing short of a full-scale defense of Utilitarianism, which, as we have just seen, is a very controversial ethical theory.

If, on the other hand, the Paretian standard is offered not as the sole criterion for evaluation, but as one standard among others, including those that embody ethical values such as justice, fairness, and personal desert, then what is needed is a theory, a systematic account, of how much weight should be given to efficiency relative to these other standards of assessment.

Cost-Benefit and Cost-Effectiveness Analyses

In part because the direct and unrestricted use of the utility-maximization criterion requires staggering amounts of information about the consequences of all feasible alternatives and in part because in the more vexing policy decisions none of the feasible alternatives is likely to be Pareto Optimal (typically there will be losers as well as winners no matter what is done), policy analysts have developed other efficiency criteria. The most widely discussed of these are cost-benefit analysis (CBA) and cost-effectiveness analysis (CEA), which M. C. Weinstein and W. B. Stason concisely define and contrast as follows.

> The key distinction is that a benefit-cost [or cost-benefit] analysis must value all outcomes in economic (e.g., dollar) terms, including lives or years of life and morbidity, whereas a cost-effectiveness analysis serves to place priorities on alternative expenditures without requiring that the dollar value of life and health be assessed (Weinstein and Stason 1977).

The preceding definition restricts CBA to a comparison of the health benefits of a particular allocational decision with the costs of implementing that decision. If this restriction were lifted, so that all costs and benefits of a particular decision were compared with all costs and benefits of each feasible alternative, then CBA would be identical with the use of the utility-maximization criterion. Although CBA in the sense defined by Weinstein and Stason is narrower than utility-maximization because it only compares health benefits with costs, it nonetheless in principle allows quite diverse programs to be ranked. For example, CBA purports to tell us whether a program to educate teenage females about prenatal care would produce a greater ratio of health benefits (for pregnant teenagers and the children they bear) to financial costs of the program than the ratio of health benefits (for persons with hypertension) to the costs of a hypertension screening program. According to CBA, resources are to be allocated to those uses that have the highest health benefit/cost ratios.

As should be apparent, the chief objections to utility-maximization apply with equal force to CBA. Even in the narrow sense, CBA requires interpersonal utility comparisons since the cost-benefit ratio for a given allocation is determined by substracting the total financial cost from the sum of all the health benefits to all persons affected. Similarly, the most obvious ethical objections to utility-maximization apply to CBA, even when restricted to health benefits: neither criterion for allocation takes into account fairness or personal desert.

There are, in addition, special difficulties with the methods that cost-benefit analysts have proposed for assigning a dollar value to lives saved or to life-years gained as a result of the alternative allocations whose cost-benefit ratios are to be compared. The two most common methods are (1) future earnings (or human capital) and (2) willingness to pay.

According to the former, the monetary value of each individual's life, for purposes of calculating a cost-benefit ratio, is his or her total expected life-time income. Critics of the future earnings approach point out that it places a higher value (on average) on the lives of men than on the lives of women. The difficulty is not simply that women who work in the home typically receive no reported wages for their labor—this could be remedied by calculating the market value of their domestic services and counting it as income. The real problem is that even when women receive income for their services, they often receive lower pay than men performing comparable work. Hence to value women's lives for purposes of determining allocations of health-care resources according to their expected future earnings is simply to compound the unfairness of an already unfair social system.

As we have already seen, to allocate resources strictly according to which allocation has the highest overall benefit/cost ratio is to assume that Utilitarianism is the correct ethical theory. Even if this controversial assumption is left unchallenged, however, future earnings are an inadequate measure of the value of human life for purposes of calculating overall utility simply because the effect an individual's life (or the loss of it) has on overall utility is not equivalent to his or her future earnings. For one thing, an individual's earnings represent (at best) the utility his or her services produce for those who pay for them, not the total utility—or disutility—produced by his or her rendering of those services. In other words, the future earnings approach does not take into account the effects of "externalities", whether positive or negative, on overall costs or overall benefits. An externality is a "spill-over," or "neighborhood effect," or "third-party effect" of an exchange. For exam-ple, air pollution from a chemical plant is an externality (a negative one in that it results in harm to people, wildlife, and plants), a cost that is not reflected in the exchange between the chemical plant and its customers. Finally, even if an indi-vidual's future earnings were an adequate approximation of his or her contribution to social utility, it can still be objected that it is unethical to view society as a kind of grand machine for producing ever more utility and human beings as cogs in the machine (or "factors of production" in a productive enterprise).

Quite apart from its ethical defects, the future earnings approach is flawed as an account of how people do in fact value not only their own lives but the lives of others as well. The value a parent places on her child—and the loss she feels at the child's death—typically has little to do with what the child's life-time income would have been had he or she survived. Similarly, the value an individual places on his own life typically reflects the value he places on the future experiences and activities he will be deprived of, not the loss of future earnings (Brock 1986). The future earnings approach, then, is not only ethically deficient, but descriptively inaccurate as well.

The second method assigns value to a life or to prolongation of a life according to the amount of money the person whose life it is would pay in order to avoid the loss of his life (or to reduce the risk of losing it) or to prolong it for some specified period. The chief attraction of the willingness to pay approach is that it is subject-centered: the value assigned to a life is determined by the preferences of the indi-vidual him- or herself, not by others. Unfortunately, however, willingness to pay does not avoid the ethical objection raised earlier against future earnings. It, too, systematically reproduces whatever injustices in the distribution of wealth already exist, because how much a person is willing to pay to avoid death or reduce the risk of death will depend upon how great his or her resources are. If the current distribution of wealth is unjust or unfair, then relying on the willingness to pay approach to make allocation decisions will be unfair and unjust as well.

Although the foregoing problems are extremely serious, it would be a mistake to conclude that CBA has nothing of value to bring to decisionmaking concerning the allocation of health-care resources. Understood in the most general way, CBA is an indispensable procedure for practical reasoning in general, not just for matters of resource allocation. In its broadest outlines, it is simply the attempt to make the gains and losses of alternative courses of action explicit and, to the extent that this is possible, to make them sufficiently commensurate with one another so that at least an approximation of a maximizing strategy can be formulated. Any theory of prac-tical reasoning which recognizes that there is a plurality of goods, that at least some gains are not costless, and that values are at least sometimes roughly commensu-rate, will utilize CBA in this generic sense, and this includes nonutilitarian ethical theories.

In the latter, moral values that represent constraints on overall utility-max-imization can be reflected in the weights that are assigned to different gains and losses. For example, an ethical theory that rejects Utilitarianism and takes certain individual rights as fundamental, but which recognizes that rights may conflict, might nevertheless find it illuminating to use a cost-benefit procedure, in the broadest sense, to arrive at reasonable trade-offs between basic rights when they conflict.

The preceding objections to CBA are not to be understood, then, as a rejection of all practical reasoning that attempts to weigh losses against gains and in some sense maximize gains. Instead, they are criticisms of attempts to use specific maximizing techniques that either ignore or beg important ethical questions about the proper scope of maximizing reasoning and the appropriate weight which different values (for instance, fairness versus efficiency) ought to be given when a maximizing procedure is appropriate.

There are two quite different ways to construe the ethical objections to both the future earnings and willingness to pay approaches. One is to argue that even if one or both adequately captures the economic value of life, attending only to the economic value of life is an insufficient basis for calculating overall benefit, even if we accept the principle that we are to maximize overall benefit in making allocation decisions. In this first view, future earnings and willingness to pay are incomplete measures of the value of lives, where value is objective and commensurate in the way required for a maximizing calculation. On the second reading, a critic of these two approaches can admit that one or both of them adequately captures the economic value of lives and that the only objective and commensurate sense of value is economic, yet also maintain that there are ethical considerations (for example, of fairness) that place limits on the extent to which the value of a person's life (in this objective and commensurate sense) ought to determine his or her share of resources. On the first view the charge is that willingness to pay and future earnings are inadequate measures of the value of lives; on the second it is that maximizing value is not the sole consideration in allocating resources.

Unlike (cost-benefit analysis), CEA does not require that health benefits, including lives saved or prolonged, be measured by the same units (dollars) as the costs of the allocation of resources that provides those benefits. All that is necessary is that all the health benefits expected from a particular allocation be measured by a common unit, usually, "quality-adjusted life years," and that all costs be measured by a common unit (dollars). CEA allows a ranking of alternative programs for producing a given level of health benefits according to the dollar costs of each for producing the desired effect.

There are three major limitations on the usefulness of CEA. The first, needless to say, is the difficulty of formulating a reasonable, objective conception of quality of life for determining the unit of benefit-measurement, the quality-adjusted life-year. Perhaps the chief issue is the extent to which the quality of an individual's life (or of a life-year) is to be understood in a subjective fashion, that is, according to his or her own estimate, or objectively.

The second is simply a variant of the major ethical objection to CBA and to utilitarian approaches more generally: CEA itself recognizes no ethical concerns about how benefits are distributed, except so far as the distribution affects the total benefit produced. In other words, to determine allocations exclusively according to CEA is to beg fundamental allocation questions. CEA might tell us, for example, that a program that establishes mobile coronary care units will produce more health benefits for the money than a liver transplant program, but it cannot tell us what proportion of total social resources should be allocated to health care and what proportion to education or defense. This is a serious limitation since at the present time there are many who believe that the health-care sector has been draining a disproportionate share of social resources away from other areas.

ETHICAL CRITERIA

The Need for Ethical Criteria: Two Case Studies

We have seen that efficiency criteria are not by themselves sufficient for evaluating allocations; ethical criteria are also necessary. Often allocation decisions, especially those toward the "micro" end of the continuum, are made in a much less systemic way than advocates of CBA or CEA would prefer. But here, too, the need for ethical, as well as efficiency criteria, is apparent. Two examples will be discussed briefly here: the allocation of human hearts for transplantation and the selective use of cancer chemotherapy. In the former case the ethically controversial nature of the process is apparent: there are not enough transplantable human hearts for everyone who needs one, problematic choices are being made, and the effects of these decisions, if not the decisionmaking processes themselves, are often exposed to public scrutiny by the harsh glare of the media. In the latter, the usual situation is *not* one in which a limited quantity of a cancer drug is available to a physician and he or she must decide which patients will get it. Nevertheless, ethically controversial decisions are made daily as to which patients will receive certain cancer drugs and in some cases it is clear that the high cost of these drugs plays a role in decisionmaking (though often in indirect and complex ways). Rationing occurs, both with human hearts and cancer drugs.

RATIONING CHEMOTHERAPY

In their controversial book *The Painful Prescription* (subtitled *Rationing Hospital Care*), Aaron and Schwarz contrast the use of cancer drugs for various classes of cancer patients in the United States and England. They note that England spends about 70 percent less per capita on cancer-fighting drugs then the United States (Aaron and Schwarz 1984, 47) and that the most dramatic difference lies in the tendency of American physicians to treat, and British physicians not to treat, patients with metastatic solid tumors who have few symptoms that might be relieved by chemotherapy and for whom chemotherapy rarely produces an extension of life and even less frequently a cure. Aaron and Schwarz report that the rate at which American physicians treat such patients is five to six times greater than that for British physicians (Aaron and Schwarz 1984, 48).

British physicians interviewed in the study justified their practice on the grounds that for this group of patients the disability and discomfort that are often side effects of chemotherapy are not worth the small chance or benefit. American physicians, in contrast, seemed more frequently to be committed to treating such cancer aggressively even though they admitted that the prospects for success were very small.

The responses of some British physicians support the hypothesis that financial considerations are playing a role in this pronounced difference in patterns of practice (Aaron and Schwarz 1984, 50). British physicians know that they are in a sense custodians of a scarce public resource—that the British National Health Service must operate within a limited budget. American physicians operate under no such overall budget constraint and, as Aaron and Schwarz point out, American cancer specialists under the third-party, fee-for-service system have a strong financial incentive to treat patients aggressively.

However, Aaron and Schwarz neglect to mention that American physicians in some cases are already beginning to find themselves subject to budget constraints that give them incentives to take a harder look at *how much* benefit can reasonably be expected from chemotherapy. The director of an oncology department at a hospital owned by a large HMO (Health Maintenance Organization) in the United States reported that he only ordered extremely expensive new cancer drugs if their expected benefit exceeded a certain threshold—say a 0.2 probability of "significant" improvement in terms of life extension with "reasonable" quality of life.[1] Unless some such rationing device were employed, he stated, his oncology unit, by using every new cancer drug which promised some net benefit, would bankrupt the entire HMO in a month's time. Although this case comes from an HMO, it could have occurred in any hospital in which close attention is paid to how resources are allocated among different services.

These differences in prescribing patterns for chemotherapy illustrate two important points. First, the question of what level expected benefits to the patient is high enough in relation to costs to the patient (in terms of side-effects) to justify the treatment is *not* a medical question. For those who value the extension of their life very highly, gaining a rather small chance of longer survival may be worth considerable disability and discomfort, while others may have a more demanding standard for what counts as an acceptable quality of life. Even when all the medical facts are in, a decision as to whether, strictly from the patient's standpoint, chemotherapy is appropriate, will depend upon personal values. Second, the greater the extent to which physicians come to regard themselves as operating under budget constraints—imposed by society or by their own hospital administration—the more likely it is that the cost-benefit threshold they will use to determine whether to prescribe expensive drugs will be influenced by broader cost considerations, not simply by what is best for this particular patient.

As cost-containment pressures mount, one of the most vexed questions con-

---

[1] This was reported to the author in a personal communication with the director of the oncology unit.

cerning the allocation of health-care resources is then becoming this: how can the physician play an effective role in efforts to ration scarce resources responsibly without undermining his or her traditional and valued role as advocate for the individual patient? Once the fact that rationing decisions are not only morally permissible but morally required for the fair and efficient use of scarce social resources, it will become harder to sustain the illusion that different practices concerning the use of cancer drugs or other expensive therapies simply reflect differences in medical judgment.

ALLOCATING HEARTS

The system—or rather the inconsistent patchwork of processes—by which human hearts for transplantation are allocated in the US is neither efficient nor fair according to any reasonable standard (Mathieu 1988). There are several sources of inefficiency. A recent study by the national Task Force on Organ Transplantation (a committee appointed by the U.S. Department of Health and Human Services) found that regionalization of heart transplant centers, rather than the current proliferation of centers as individual physicians and medical centers compete for dollars and prestige, would save resources and increase the quality of care (Report of the Task Force on Organ Transplantation 1986). Perhaps just as importantly, a coordinated, regionalized system of transplant centers would provide better prospects for developing and monitoring more ethical and more efficient procedures for allocating hearts. At present hearts are sometimes allocated to patients who will almost certainly die even though they receive a heart, despite the fact that there are other potential recipients who have a much better chance of living if they were to receive the heart.

This inefficient—and morally irresponsible—use of the public resources used in the development and deployment of transplant technology can occur because of the defective way in which the human heart allocation "hotline" works. A registered transplant surgeon who wants a heart for his patient may call the "hotline" and request a heart. The most abusable feature of this system is that the physician who makes the request unilaterally classifies his patient according to a priority classification. In one recent case, a transplant surgeon designated his patient a "priority 1" on the grounds that he would die almost immediately if he did not receive a heart. Although this was true, it was in fact not a sufficient reason for bestowing the heart on this patient instead of another. The patient's condition had already so deteriorated that competent medical opinion agreed it was virtually certain that he would die even if he received the heart (Mathieu, 1988). An allocation system that allows "urgency"—without consideration of relative expected benefit—to determine priority, and that relies upon interested parties to make priority classifications can only be expected to waste precious social resources.

Quite aside from the problems of inefficiency, the current processes by which human hearts are allocated also can be criticized as unfair. The chief criticism is that morally arbitrary factors often play a decisive role in determining who lives and who dies. The most obvious of these is ability to pay: most transplant centers require as much as $60,000 "cash up front." Further, some centers give first priority to in-state residents, so that where one happens to live may mean that one will not get a heart, even if one's medical need and potential benefit are greater than that of one fortunate enough to be living in the right state. This geographical discrimination is especially suspect since millions of federal tax dollars (not state funds) were spent to develop the technology. Finally, some transplant centers are in effect selling hearts to the highest bidders—in many cases foreign nationals (chiefly Saudis and Greeks, according to one study) (Mathieu 1988).

Ethicists who recognize the need for a more satisfactory method of dealing with the problem of allocating scarce organs for transplantation have recognized two polar approaches (Rescher 1974). On the one hand, an exclusive concern with efficiency, or with producing the most benefit possible, requires that allocations be made simply according to what would maximize quality-adjusted life-years. Such an approach, as we have seen, simply assumes the correctness of Utilitarianism as a moral theory and is subject to the charge that it disregards all issues of fairness. Perhaps most important, it can be argued that a strictly utilitarian system for allocating scarce organs would fail to show proper regard for the equal worth of persons, a worth which cannot be equated with their contribution to social utility.

Some who reject Utilitarian allocation systems on the latter ground suggest that the only way to show proper regard for the equal moral status or worth of persons is to give them equal chances to receive the scarce good, either by using a fair lottery method in which each has an equal probability of winning, or by using a first-come, first-serve system to approximate the randomness of a lottery. The latter proposal is clearly flawed: The poor would be disadvantaged by a first-come, first-serve system not only because they tend to be less educated and informed about medical matters but also because they are less likely to see a physician and be advised of the need to get in line for a transplant.

The lottery method (assuming the lottery is fair) would avoid this problem and could be seen as showing equal respect for persons, but it surely goes too far in eschewing entirely all considerations of how much benefit an allocation will pro-duce. Unless some initial threshhold of expected benefit to the patient is used as an eligibility requirement for participation in the lottery, use of this randomizing meth-od will mean that lives of extremely poor quality will be prolonged, perhaps only briefly, at the expense of much longer lives of higher quality.

One ethicist has suggested that a three-tiered system for allocating hearts would better express the conviction that both efficiency (or maximizing benefit) and equal respect for persons are important values (Mathieu 1988). First, potential recipients would be selected according to a standard of "medical suitability": only if their expected benefit (in terms of quality-adjusted life-years) exceeds a specified threshhold would they be placed on the list of potential recipients. Second, those among this first group whose need was most urgent—those who will die soon if they do not recieve a heart—would be given top priority. Third, if the number of available hearts is greater than the number of people in the top priority group, then the remainder of those who passed the "medical suitability" test (that is, the minimal expected benefit threshhold) would receive hearts on a first-come, first-serve basis.

This sketch of a system is not intended to solve all the problems of allocation for hearts—it does not address the issue of whether a person whose immune system rejects a first heart should receive another, for example, nor does it address the objection that a first-come, first-serve method may discriminate against the poor. But it does illustrate how one system might incorporate both efficiency and fairness (or equity) considerations in a coherent way. An alternative would be to rate each potential recipient according to expected benefit (number of quality-adjusted life-years), but allow expected benefit to be decisive only if there is a difference in expected benefit that exceeds some rather high threshhold. In effect, such a system would show strong—not unlimited—regard for the equal worth of persons by allocating hearts randomly unless some nonrandom allocation would produce a very marked increase in benefit (Brock 1988). Although both of these allocation models would be an improvement over the current arrangements inasmuch as each recognizes that both efficiency and fairness are relevant values, neither by itself avoids the perplexing issue of exactly what the trade-off should be when the two values are in conflict.

The "Access Problem" and the Ethical Evaluation of Large-Scale Allocation Patterns

Ethical theorizing about large-scale allocation patterns has arisen in part from the recognition that macro decisions shape micro problems and that the more piecemeal approaches (such as those sketched in the discussion of the preceding two case studies) are inadequate. In addition, two powerful social factors motivate the search for coherent ethical criteria for evaluating large-scale allocation patterns. On the one hand, there is the growing perception that the rapid rise in health-care expenditures constitutes a "crisis"—and that serious cost containment measures are a necessity. On the other hand, there is the sobering recognition that between 30 and 37 million Americans lack any health-care coverage, either through private insurance or public programs such as Medicare and Medicaid, and that as many as 22 million more have coverage that is inadequate by virtually any reasonable standard (President's Commission 1983). Systematic theorizing is needed, first, to determine when differences in access to health care for various individuals or groups constitute ethically objectionable inequalities, and second, to determine which cost containment measures are ethically acceptable.

RIGHTS TO HEALTH CARE

Until very recently, the prevailing view has been that in order to resolve the important large-scale allocation issues in health care, it is necessary to determine whether there is a moral right to health care, and if so, what is its content. However, this assumption is now being challenged by those who maintain that it is unduly restrictive to limit the discussion to matters of justice and, more specifically, of individual rights. Their point is that allocations may be criticized for being uncharitable or ungenerous even if they are not unjust and violate no one's right. Just as respecting others' rights is not the whole of moral virtue for an individual, so justice, even if it is the first virtue of social institutions, is not their sole virtue. We shall first critically survey the main views on the right to health care before examining "nonjustice" approaches.

Positions on the right to health care range from the denial that there is a moral right to health care to the claim that there is a strong egalitarian right, a right of each to an equal share of health resources. Another view holds that the right to health care is derivative, based exclusively on considerations of utility-maximization. The opposing thesis is that the right to health care is independent of and "trumps" (that is, overrides) all appeals to utility-maximization. To appreciate these disagreements over the existence or scope of a right to health care it is first necessary to clarify the general import of the assertion that someone has a right to something. The distinctive features of such "right" are typically said to be as follows (Buchanan 1984b, 63; Feinberg 1979, 87):

1. If Jones has a right to X, then he has a valid claim or entitlement to it. This is not captured by saying that Jones would benefit from X or that Jones's having it is desirable (to him or others). Since to have a right is to have a basis for making a claim to the thing in question, the appropriate posture for the right-holder is not that of the supplicant pleading for a favor, but rather that of someone demanding what is due to him or her.
2. Consequently, if Jones' right is violated it is not merely that an unfortunate or less than morally optimal situation has occurred; in addition, Jones has been wronged by those who failed to fulfill their obligations and is therefore the appropriate recipient of compensation or restitution.
3. If Jones has a right to X, then someone or some collectivity (society, the government as the agent of society) has an obligation to make X available to Jones.
4. The existence of Jones's right provides a strong prima facie justification for enforcing these obligations if necessary.

Many discussions of rights assume a fifth feature (alluded to earlier):

5. A valid right-claim overrides appeals to utility maximization; in other words, the mere fact that failing to respect the right would maximize utility is not itself a sufficient reason for doing so (Dworkin 1977, 184–205).

Although writers who focus on the fifth feature sometimes fail to point out—it is quite compatible with viewing rights as being derivative upon and ultimately justified by appeals to utility-maximization.

A Utilitarian (Derivative) Right to Health Care

Utilitarianism purports to be a comprehensive moral theory, of which a utilitarian theory of justice, including an account of justice in health care, would be only one part (Buchanan 1981, 4–5). There are two main types of comprehensive utilitarian theory: Act and Rule Utilitarianism. Act Utilitarianism defines rightness with respect to particular acts: an act is right if and only if it maximizes net utility. Rule Utilitarianism defines rightness with respect to rules of action and makes the rightness of particular acts depend upon the rules under which those acts fall. A rule is right if and only if general compliance with that rule (or with a set of rules of which it is an element) maximizes net utility, and a particular action is right if and only if it falls under such a rule.

The most prevalent form of the theory, sometimes called Classic Utilitarianism, (Buchanan 1981)[2] defines the rightness of acts or rules as maximization of aggregate utility. The aggregate utility produced by an act or by general compliance with a rule is the sum of the utility produced for each individual affected. "Utility" is defined as pleasure, satisfaction, happiness, or as the realization of preferences, as the latter are revealed through individuals' choices.

The distinction between Act and Rule Utilitarianism is important for a utilitarian theory of justice, since the latter must include an account of when institutions are just. Thus, institutional rules may maximize utility even though those rules do not direct individuals as individuals or as occupants of institutional positions to maximize utility in a case by case fashion. For example, it may be that a judicial system which maximizes utility will do so by including rules which prohibit judges from deciding a case according to their estimates of what would maximize utility in that particular case. Thus the utilitarian justification of a particular action or decision may not be that it maximizes utility, but rather that it falls under some rule of an institution or set of institutions which maximizes utility.

Some utilitarians hold that principles of justice are the most basic moral principles because the utility of adherence to them is especially great. According to this view, utilitarian principles of justice are those utilitarian moral principles which are of such importance that they may be enforced, if necessary. Some utilitarians also hold that among the utilitarian principles of justice are principles specifying individual rights, where the latter are thought of as enforceable claims that take precedence over appeals to what would maximize utility in the particular case.

A utilitarian moral theory, then, can include rights principles that themselves prohibit or "trump" appeals to utility maximization, as long as the justification of those principles is that they are part of an institutional system that maximizes utility. In cases where two or more rights principles conflict, considerations of utility may be invoked to determine which rights principles are to be given priority. Utilitarianism is incompatible with rights only if rights exclude appeals to utility maximization

---

[2]This discussion of Utilitarianism that follows, as well as some of the material on Libertarianism and Rawls, is drawn from this author's essay "Justice: A Philosophical Review" with permission from D. Reidel Publishing Co.

at all levels of justification, including the most basic institutional level. Rights founded ultimately on considerations of utility may be called derivative, to distinguish them from rights in the strict or fundamental sense.

Whether or not an overarching total institutional system that maximizes net utility will include a right to health care will depend upon a wealth of empirical facts not deducible from the Principle of Utility itself. A utilitarian system of (derivative) rights will pick out certain goods as those which make an especially large contribution to the maximization of net utility. It is reasonable to assume, on the basis of scientific empirical data as well as common sense experience, that health care, or at least certain forms of health care, is among them. Consider, for example perinatal care, broadly conceived as including genetic screening and counseling (at least for special risk groups), prenatal nutritional care and medical examinations for expectant mothers, medical care during delivery, and basic pediatric services in the crucial months after birth. If empirical research indicates (1) that a system of institutional arrangements that maximizes net utility would include such services and (2) that such services can best be assured if they are accorded the status of a right, with all that this implies, including the use of coercive sanctions where necessary, then according to Utilitarianism there is such a (derivative) right. The strength and content of this right relative to other (derivative) rights will be determined by the utility of various forms of health care relative to one another as compared with other kinds of goods.

It has been argued that Utilitarianism is not capable of providing a secure foundation for a universal right to health care—a right to at least some minimal core of health-care services for everyone (Buchanan 1984a, 60). Certain classes of individuals might be excluded from virtually all health-care services. The class of newborns with Down Syndrome (formerly called Mongolism), for example, might well be excluded from the "decent minimum" of health care (and other goods and services) which others should receive as a matter of (derivative) right on utilitarian grounds. These retarded individuals, who often suffer from serious physical disabilities as well, tend to require a rather large outlay of social resources over the course of their lives. Relative to the costs of caring for them, the contribution these individuals make to social utility may not be large, at least so far as we are limited to a conception of contribution that permits quantification. If this is the case, then Utilitarianism will permit—indeed will require—that these individuals be excluded from the right to health care.

To understand why this is taken to be a serious criticism of Utilitarianism, two points require emphasis. The first is that these infants are generally capable of enjoyment, purposeful activity, and meaningful interpersonal relationships, and can often attain something approximating a normal life span. In these respects they are unlike more severely disabled individuals, such as those who become permanently comatose due to disease or trauma, anencephalics (babies born with no brain above the brain stem or with no cerebral cortex), or even profoundly demented patients with Alzheimer's Disease. If Utilitarianism only rendered problematic the claim that these latter sorts of individuals have a right to health care it would be significantly less ethically problematic, since the moral status of such individuals, our obligations to them, and even their capacity to benefit from our aid, are more dubious.

Second, utilitarian calculations may require the Down Syndrome babies (or other groups of moderately disabled people) be excluded, not just from extremely expensive, "exotic" medical technology, but also from the most basic care. In sum, Utilitarianism may mandate that even for basic and relatively inexpensive goods and services, what is guaranteed for most should not be provided for some, even though their needs are as great and they would benefit very much from them.

This criticism of the utilitarian account of the right to health care is simply an application of the more general objection that Utilitarianism fails to provide a secure foundation for any of the most important moral rights as rights of all, not just some, persons. Rawls has argued that the case for equal, basic civil and political rights for all should not depend, as it does according to Utilitarianism, upon contingent assumptions about what will in fact maximize overall utility. He also contends that this deficiency, as well as Utilitarianism's inability to accord proper recognition to the values of fairness and desert, stems, ultimately, from its failure to take seriously the "separateness of persons" (Rawls 1971). According to Utilitarianism, the ultimate objects of moral concern in the universe are desires or preferences, not the persons (or even sentiment organisms) whose desires or preferences they are. For the utilitarian, persons are mere receptacles or loci for utility.

These fundamental ethical objections to Utilitarianism as a general theory count heavily not only against the attempt to base a right to health care on strictly utilitarian grounds, but also against exclusive reliance on the Principle of Utility as a guide to more limited allocation decisions both within and outside health care. None of this, however, supports the more extreme conclusion that utilitarian considerations should have no weight whatsoever in allocating health-care resources. In virtually every ethical theory other than Libertarianism (in its more extreme forms), and in common sense moral thinking as well, maximizing overall utility is often a weighty consideration, even when it is not the sole or even the preponderant factor. This is hardly surprising, assuming that ethics is concerned in some fundamental way with human welfare.

Libertarianism: The Challenge to All Welfare Rights, Including the Right to Health Care

There are a number of different types of theories that are sometimes called libertarian, but Robert Nozick's is often taken to be paradigmatic.[3] Nozick begins by assuming, not arguing for, a very strong right to private property, a right to exclusive control over whatever one can attain through voluntary exchanges in the market (assuming that both parties in fact own what they exchange), through gifts

---

[3]In some respects this may be misleading, since Nozick's view is more extreme than that of some who are frequently labeled libertarians, such as F. A. Hayek, who admit that enforced contributions to provide a minimal welfare safety net are sometimes justifiable.

voluntarily bestowed by others, and by appropriating previously unowned things by "mixing one's labor" with them, so long as (a) one's appropriation does not worsen the condition of others by creating a situation in which they are "no longer . . . able to use freely [without exclusively appropriating] what [they] . . . previously could" or (b) one properly compensates those whose conditions is worsened in the way specified in (a) (Nozick 1974).

Apart from the special case of rectifying past injustices, Nozick's view strictly prohibits any coercive efforts to redistribute wealth, even for the purpose of providing the most minimal welfare rights, including all forms of a right to health care. The legitimate role of the state, on this view, is restricted to the protection of so-called negative rights. The state may wield its coercive power only to protect citizens from assault, theft, and fraud, and for national defense.

According to Nozick, the competitive market with private property is the only social structure compatible with respect for these individual rights. Consequently, for Nozick there is no need for a theory of the just allocation of resources in general, including health-care resources. Resources will be allocated by market processes and so far as people exchange or give what they have rightfully acquired, whatever allocation of resources results is just.

While Nozick's libertarianism has been effectively criticized on a number of grounds, there are two major objections that are especially potent. First, it has been noted that Nozick fails in his attempt to show that every principle of justice that requires redistribution either (a) is either intuitively unjust or (b) would require unacceptable disruptions of people's expectations by frequently appropriating their holdings for the sake of preserving the overacting pattern of distribution specified by the principle.

To support the first prong of his attack on redistributive principles of justice Nozick tries to persuade us that it is counter-intuitive to think that injustice could arise merely from voluntary exchanges among people each of whom owns what he exchanges and that consequently any principle of justice that requires allocations arising from such exchanges to be overturned must be unjust.

As several critics have pointed out, however, Nozick's intuitions here will not be shared by anyone who takes seriously the problem of cumulative harms. Once the cumulative negative effects on both welfare and liberty are appreciated, the need to avoid or minimize these negative externalities can provide strong ethical grounds for limiting the individual's right to acquire and exchange goods—and thus for challenging the virtually unlimited private property right Nozick merely assumes without argument. For example, strictly voluntary exchanges of property may lead to such extreme concentrations of wealth that the rich are able, even through largely legal means, to undermine the civil and political liberties of the poor (Cohen 1978).

The second prong of Nozick's attack is weak as well. It is true that a very demanding principle of justice that required, for example, strict equality in resources, might necessitate frequent redistributions that would be intolerably coercive and disruptive. It is much less plausible to argue, however, that all redistributive principles suffer from this defect. Implementing a principle requiring only that everyone is to have a "decent minimum" of certain basic goods, including food, shelter, and a core set of important health-care services need not result in frequent or severe disruptions. Long-standing, publicized laws specifying predictable tax obligations can be and are used to fund such a core of welfare goods.

Another major objection to Nozick's libertarianism turns against him his own provocative suggestion that the ultimate foundation for his strong right to private property (and hence for the denial of welfare rights it entails) is an appreciation of the central role of autonomy in the leading of a meaningful life. So far as this vague suggestion has any substance at all, it seems to backfire on Nozick. An autonomous person who wishes to lead a meaningful life—which for most of us would not be a life in which poverty limits our aspirations to securing the next meal, finding shelter for the night, and coping with suffering and disability due to health problems that could have been avoided—will require at least a modicum of material resources, including access to health care. An autonomous person values opportunity, and our opportunities can be limited not only by deliberate interferences by others but also by lack of resources, by illness, and by disability.

Libertarians such as Nozick have a reply to the charge that justice as they see it shows too little concern with the human welfare and with the material resources for meaningful, autonomous living. They emphasize that justice is not the whole of morality and that the harsh effects of the libertarian ban on enforced redistribution can be moderated by voluntary adherence to principles of beneficence. However, as we shall see later, when we examine approaches to health care allocation that rely chiefly on principles of beneficence (or "humanity," or "charity"), rather than on principles of justice, there are serious obstacles to efficient, coordinated voluntary redistribution that libertarians tend to overlook.

Rawls's Theory and the Right to Health Care

In his widely acclaimed book *A Theory of Justice,* John Rawls offers a new and highly sophisticated version of the traditional theory of the social contract, as developed by Hobbes, Locke, Rousseau, and Kant. Although Rawls supplies several distinct lines of justification for the principles of justice he advances, it is this hypothetical contract argument for them that is most distinctive.

> The principles of justice for the basic structure of society are the principles that free and rational persons concerned to further their own interests would accept in an initial position of equality as defining the fundamental terms of their association. These principles are to regulate all further agreements; they specify the kinds of social cooperation that can be entered into and the forms of government that can be established. This way of regarding the principles of justice I shall call justice as fairness (Rawls 1971, 11).

One of the chief functions of this hypothetical choice situation, which Rawls calls the original position, is to capture a particular conception of impartiality or fairness. Thus the parties in the original position must choose principles of justice from behind a "veil of ignorance" that deprives them of information about their own socio-economic class, race, or gender—facts which might bias their choice by enabling them to tailor the principles to their own particular advantage. The basic idea is that fair principles of social cooperation are those that would emerge from a choice situation that is fair to all individuals as autonomous persons who have a highest-order interest in being free to choose and revise their ends and to pursue them effectively.

Rawls produces a number of arguments to show that the parties would agree upon the following principles of justice.

First Principle:
Each person is to have an equal right to the most extensive total system of equal basic liberties compatible with a similar system of liberty for all.
Second Principle:
Social and economic inequalities are to be arranged so that they are both:
  a. to the greatest benefit of the least advantaged, and
  b. attached to offices and positions open to all under conditions of fair
     equality of opportunity.

Rawls calls the First Principle "The Principle of Greatest Equal Liberty." The Second Principle includes two parts. Part a is the Difference Principle. It states that social and economic inequalities are to be arranged so that they are to the greatest benefit of those who are least advantaged. Part b is the Principle of Fair Equality of Opportunity. It states that social and economic inequalities are to be attached to offices and positions that are open to all under conditions of fair equality of opportunity.

There is now a vast literature on Rawls's theory and a number of serious criticisms of his view have emerged. It has often been noted, for example, that the Difference Principle would be chosen in the original position only if, as Rawls assumes, the choosers have such an extreme aversion to risk that all they care about is avoiding a situation in which, should they turn out to be among the worst off, they have a lesser share of primary goods than they would have if they were the worst off in some other arrangement. In other words, they care only about minimizing losses should they turn out to be among the worse off, not a bit about reaping the higher gains they might make if they were among the better off under a less egalitarian principle than the Difference Principle. Once this implausibly strong assumption about the attitude toward risk is dropped, it can be argued that a principle requiring only that everyone be guaranteed a "safety net" or "decent minimum" of welfare goods, rather than the Difference Principle, would be chosen.

Even if this and other major objections to Rawls's general theory can be met, however, it is far from clear that Rawls's theory as he himself presents it, contains the conceptual resources for justifying a right to health care that is specific enough to provide a useful goal for policy. To understand this limitation on Rawls's theory, let us suppose that health care is either itself a primary good covered by the Difference Principle or that health care may be purchased with income or some other form of wealth which is included under the Difference Principle. In the former case, depending upon various empirical conditions, it might turn out that the best way to satisfy the Difference Principle is to establish a state-enforced right to health care. But whether maximizing the prospects of the worst off will require such a right and what the content of the right will be depends upon what weight is to be assigned to health care relative to other primary goods included under the Difference Principle. Similarly, a weighting must also be assigned if we are to determine whether the share of wealth one receives under the Difference Principle would be sufficient both for health-care needs and for other ends. Until we have some solution to the weighting problem, Rawls's theory can shed only limited light upon the question of priority-relations between health care and other goods and among various forms of health care.

It is important to see that the informational constraints imposed by Rawls's "veil of ignorance" preclude a solution to the problem of weighting health care against other primary goods because the solution will depend upon facts about the particular conditions of the society in which the notions in question are to be applied. At best Rawls's hypothetical contractors would choose a kind of "placeholder" for a principle establishing a right to health care, on the assumption that the content of the right can only be filled out at later stages of agreement in the light of specific information about their particular society.

However, nothing in Rawls's conception of rational decision suggests that once the relevant, concrete information is available, rational persons will agree on a single assignment of weights to the primary goods. It follows that Rawls's theory does not itself supply any content for the notion of a right to health care. Instead, at best, it lays down a very abstract structure within which this content will be worked out through the democratic political processes specified by the list of equal basic liberties. Given this, Rawls's theory advances us very little beyond the idea that there is a universal right to health care (Buchanan 1984a, 61–62).

Equality of Opportunity as the Basis for a Right to Health Care: Norman Daniels's Rawlsian Theory

In his book *Just Health Care* Norman Daniels develops a substantive account of the right to health care by relying upon Rawls's Principle of Fair Equality of Opportunity. Although Daniels offers no justification for that principle, he indicates that he believes that Rawls's contractarian derivation of it is plausible and also contends that there is a considerable consensus, at least within liberal democratic political philosophy, that equality of opportunity is a central element of justice (Daniels 1985).

According to Daniels the right to health care is derived from the following principle of fair equality of opportunity:

> E. Basic institutions that affect the allocation of health care resources are to be arranged so that, as far as is possible, each person is to enjoy his or

her fair share of the normal opportunity range for individuals in his or her society.

The normal opportunity range for a society is the full set of individual life-plans that it would be reasonable for individuals in that society to pursue, assuming that they enjoy normal species functioning. Although Daniels makes it clear that normal species functioning as he understands it is a strictly objective, biological, nonnormative concept, he does little to say just what it encompasses. However, he does state that disease and disability are to be understood as departures from normal species functioning (Daniels 1985, 28).

For Daniels, an individual's fair share of the normal opportunity range is that set of life-plans that it would be reasonable for that individual to pursue, given his or her particular "talents and skills," were the development of those talents and skills not impeded by departures from normal species functioning; that is, by disease or disability (Daniels 1985, 34), or by features of the social system (such as discriminatory hiring practices and inequalities in the social class into which one is born) that are arbitrary from a moral point of view. The allocation of health care resources, then, is one important tool for ensuring that everyone has fair equality of opportunity, because health-care resources serve to prevent, minimize, or compensate for departures from normal species functioning and because departures from normal species functioning (i.e., disease and disability) constitute one important barrier to fair equality of opportunity understood as having one's fair share of the normal opportunity range.

Daniels's account is designed to help answer two important questions central to an ethical theory of health care–resource allocations: (1) What makes health care morally special? and (2) How should various kinds of health care be ranked relative to one another in terms of priority? The answer to the first question is that health care affects the attainment of normal species functioning and that lack of the latter is one important barrier to fair equality of opportunity. The answer to the second is that those kinds of health care that have the greatest impact on preventing, minimizing, or compensating for departures from normal species functioning should have the highest priority, at least at the level of designing basic health-care institutions, including mechanisms for allocation.

There are, however, several serious problems with Daniels's approach quite apart from objections to the more general Rawlsian account of justice on which it builds. First, and perhaps most importantly, Daniels's fair equality of opportunity principle, (E above), especially if it is given lexical priority over all principles of distributive justice (other than a principle distributing basic liberties, like Rawls's First Principle), seems to place too great a demand on overall social resources in the name of implementing a right to health care. What it requires is that we continue to pump social resources into health care as long as doing so continues to bring individuals closer to the ideal of normal species functioning—which is nothing less than a life free of disease and disability, since the latter are defined as departures from normal species functioning. The only constraint on this imperative to channel all available resources into health care is that doing so must not undermine other efforts needed to achieve fair equality of opportunity by eliminating impediments to one's fair share of the normal opportunity range other than disease and disability (and with satisfying a lexically prior principle of greatest equal liberty).

The objection is that the demand for fair equality of opportunity, understood according to Daniels's principle E, makes the health-care sector a kind of "black hole" capable of sucking in almost unlimited quantities of social resources because, especially for some of those with grave disabilities and diseases, there is virtually no limit to how much could be done, granted continuing technological advances, to bring them closer to the goal of normal species functioning. For example, being born blind, mentally retarded, and deaf is surely one of the most severe impediments to being able to pursue effectively that set of life plans that it would be reasonable for one to pursue in this society, given the talents and skills one would have, were the development of one's talents and skills not impeded by disease or disability. If this is so, then efforts to remedy or compensate for these severe departures from normal species functioning should have high priority in overall efforts (inside and outside the health-care sector) to ensure that every individual enjoys equality of opportunity. The commitment to providing such resources might be so demanding that honoring it would amount to a virtually unlimited right to health care.

Second, Daniels's principle not only seems to create an excessive drain on resources, it also does not appear to provide guidance as to how we are to make priority decisions within efforts to achieve fair equality of opportunity through allocation of health-care resources. It is silent on the question of whether we should first try to improve the condition of the worst-off—those whose disease or disability is so severe that they are the furthest from the ideal of normal species functioning— even if doing this means that the better off will get access to virtually no health-care resources, or whether everyone is to receive at least some of the basic health-care resources.

It is important to understand that Daniels's view that the normal opportunity range is society-relative does little to blunt the force of the "black-holes" objection. The normal opportunity range is society-relative, for Daniels, in the sense that whatever life-plans are reasonable for various people in a society to pursue will be influenced by the resources, cultural attitudes, etc., of the society in question. But in response to a critic who pointed out that the distribution of health-care resources that exist in a particular society will also determine which life-plans it is reasonable to pursue (Buchanan 1984a, 64), Daniels explicitly states that the normal opportunity range is that array of life-plans it would be reasonable for people to pursue in that society if they enjoyed normal species functioning, that is, if they were free of disease and disability. And normal species functioning, Daniels emphasizes, is not society-relative (Daniels 1985, 28–29). Thus even if everyone in a particular society suffered from a certain disease, say a kind of anemia, having that disease would still be a departure from normal species functioning and would be an impediment to everyone's attaining his or her fair share of the normal opportunity range, since the normal opportunity range is that set of life-plans it would be reasonable to pursue in that society in the absence of departures from normal species functioning. As Daniels puts it:

> The anemia in this case is a disease which keeps each individual from adequately carrying out *any* life plan that otherwise would be reasonable in his society. Remember, our reference point is normal species—functioning functional organization, not functioning in a certain society (Daniels 1985, 55).

A third problem with Daniels's fair equality of opportunity principle is that it, like Rawls's narrower principle concerning access to offices and positions, is based on the fundamental belief that opportunity should not be limited by "morally arbitrary" factors. Yet it, again like Rawls's Principle, arbitrarily takes an individual's "talents and skills" as a fixed baseline. In Daniels's case, the baseline is hypothetical: the talents and skills one would have were their development not impeded by disease or disability. The problem is that, as Rawls and Daniels both admit, there are factors other than disease (and social position) that influence the development of talents and skills, but that are equally arbitrary from a moral point of view. The most obvious of these is one's normal genetic endowment. Neither Rawls nor Daniels gives any reason why efforts to achieve fair equality opportunity should not deal directly with this important, "morally arbitrary" determinant of opportunity. Moreover, new advances in genetic engineering may soon make such an extension of their notions of fair equality of opportunity technically feasible. Daniels believes it to be an advantage of his theory that it takes skills and talents (as they would be absent the effects of disease and disability) as the baseline for determining fair share of the normal opportunity range and ". . . does not require us to 'level' all differences among persons" (Daniels 1985, 52). However, the same fundamental concern to eliminate the influences of morally arbitrary factors on opportunity that leads Daniels to require that resources be used to minimize departures from normal species functioning and the effects of socioeconomic class position also seem to require the use of resources for increasing the opportunity of those who are not genetically disabled or diseased but who are nonetheless at a genetic disadvantage relative to the more fortunate.

Less Systematic Accounts of the Right to Health Care

Some ethicists have attempted to approach the right to health-care issue in a somewhat less systematic fashion. Instead of undertaking the ambitious task of first developing a comprehensive theory of justice and then drawing its implications for the right to health care, they have operated mainly at the middle-level of ethical theorizing, offering one or more general principles concerning the distribution of health care and providing less formal arguments for them that do not rely upon complex theoretical backdrops.

An Egalitarian Right to Health Care

Those writers who advocate an egalitarian right to health care have generally taken this less formal approach (Gutman, 1983). They contend that the right to health care is not to be understood simply as a guarantee of a certain "safety net," "decent minimum," or core set of basic health-care services. Instead they advance a much stronger right claim: everyone having equal need for a health-care service or resource is to have equal access to it. In some cases this alleged egalitarian right to health care is advanced as a corollary of a more general egalitarian welfare right: all resources are to be distributed so as to approximate, as nearly as possible, a condition in which everyone's net welfare over a life-time is equal (Menzel 1983, 21; Veatch 1981, 264–268).

Such a view can be criticized in either of two ways. On the one hand, those who provide a more systematic account of a less egalitarian right to health care can appeal to the strengths of the background theory from which that is derived and point to the lack of a well-articulated supporting theory for the egalitarian right. On the other hand, the egalitarian position on the right to health care can be criticized using two less formal sorts of arguments. The first attacks the more general egalitarian welfare rights principle simply by noting that it would be irrational for anyone—including the worst-off—to insist on equality if allowing certain inequalities would improve everyone's situation. Suppose, for example, that it is true that a system that gave higher salaries to physicians than to most other workers would stimulate more intelligent and able people to become physicians with the result that a higher quality of medical care were available to all. Absent a convincing systematic theory to support egalitarianism, it is hard to see why anyone would find such an arrangement objectionable, as long as the greater income of physicians did not have negative effects that outweighed the gain in quality of care to those who have lesser salaries.

Of course, the egalitarian might object by saying that as a matter of fact there will be a preponderance of negative effects in most real-world cases in which income-differentials (or other inequalities) are allowed for the sake of increasing benefits for the worse off: those with higher incomes will wield undue political influence, the self-esteem of the lower-paid will suffer, etc. This defense of the general egalitarian principle is in a sense, however, a retreat from it. For what it amounts to is the claim that even though inequality is acceptable and perhaps even preferable to equality in principle, striving for the goal of equality is a more appropriate practical goal in an imperfect world.

The second objection is directed against those who do not hold that there is an egalitarian right to welfare goods in general but only an egalitarian right to health care. The egalitarian right to health care requires that no one is to have access to any health care that is not also available to everyone else in similar need. The objection takes the form of a dilemma (President's Commission, Vol. One 1983, 18–19). Either the level of health care to which everyone is entitled—and more than which no one is allowed to have—is set as high as is technically possible or it is set lower than that. If the former, then the commitment to providing everyone with the very best care technically possible for every condition will place an unacceptable strain on overall social resources and the loss of opportunities to secure important non-health care needs would be too great.

If, on the other hand, the equal level of health care is set sufficiently below the technically possible optimum to avoid an irrational allocation of overall resources, then, so long as there are inequalities in income and differences in preferences for health care, some people will be prohibited from purchasing higher levels of (or better quality) health care even though they wish to do so with their own resources. Such a situation would be inefficient, since lifting the stricture that levels of health care must be equal would allow a Pareto improvement: those who are better off and have a preference for more or better care would gain by being allowed to satisfy it, and the worse off would not lose so long as they received an adequate share of the nonhealth benefits that could be reaped by keeping the level of health care guaranteed to all lower than the technically possible optimum. But quite apart from this objection on grounds of inefficiency, an egalitarian right to health care that sets the level lower than the technically possible optimum would require unacceptable interferences with individuals' liberty to use their after-taxes income to purchase the health care they desire while permitting them to use it for much more questionable luxury goods such as fine wines or antique cars.

THE RIGHT TO A DECENT MINIMUM OR ADEQUATE LEVEL OF HEALTH CARE

The force of these objections to the claim that there is an egalitarian right to health care helps to explain the popularity of the view that though there is a right to health care it is a limited one, a right to a decent minimum or adequate level of care. Such a position has several attractions (President's Commission, Vol. One 1983, 20). First, the notion that people have a right to a decent minimum (or adequate level), rather than to all health care that produces any net benefit, clearly acknowledges both that since not all health care is of equal importance allocational priorities must be set within health care and that resources must be allocated to goods other than health care as well. Second, it is also consonant with the intuitively plausible conviction that our obligations to the less fortunate, though fundamental enough to be expressed in the language of rights, are nonetheless *not unlimited*. Third, the decent minimum is a floor beneath which no one is to be allowed to fall, not a ceiling above which the better off are prohibited from purchasing services if they wish. Thus it avoids the troublesome interferences with individual liberty which an egalitarian right requires (President's Commission, Vol. One, 1983, 20).

The chief objection to this way of understanding the right to health care is that it is virtually contentless. The chief import of the claim that the right to health care is the right to a decent minimum or adequate level of care is negative: it only tells us that neither a right to all care that is of any net benefit nor to all technically possible care is appropriate. Beyond this cautionary function, little is conveyed unless some reasonable way of filling out the content is supplied.

Although it acknowledges the inadequacies of various ad hoc proposals for specifying the adequate level of care, The President's Commission offers little by way of a concrete alternative. At one point the report offers the apparently plausible suggestion that the fundamental idea behind the notion of an adequate level is the belief that everyone is to have access to ". . . enough care to achieve sufficient welfare, opportunity, information, and evidence of interpersonal concern to facilitate a reasonably full and satisfying life" (President's Commission, Vol. One 1983, 20). Unfortunately, this statement in effect takes back much of what was said about the obligation being a limited one, since there are some individuals who are so badly off that enormous amounts of resources could be spent in attempting to assure them of ". . . a reasonably full and satisfying life." Further, there may be considerable disagreement over what counts as a "reasonably full and satisfying life." This is simply the notion of "quality of life" that crops up elsewhere in medical ethics—often masking sharply conflicting values.

In an attempt to provide practical content to the notion of a decent minimum of care while avoiding an unlimited obligation that would raise the specter of the "black holes" problem, Alan Gibbard has proposed a seemingly simply but ingenious hypothetical choice procedure or thought experiment (Gibbard 1983, 153–178). To determine which health-care services should be included in the decent minimum, we are to think of a person as choosing among different lifetime health insurance policies, each of which represents a different mix of preventive and curative services, medical and nonmedical services, etc. Because different persons would choose different policies tailored to their own particular health-care needs if they could predict them, it is necessary to impose a veil of ignorance—a set of informational constraints—upon the choosers. Gibbard suggests that it would be necessary to think of a person as choosing among policies prior to his or her own conception, since from conception on our health prospects diverge. Granted this restriction, the rational choice of an insurance policy would be based on general statistical information about overall morbidity and mortality rates for one's society.

Before a determinate choice can be made, however, another parameter of the choice situation must be specified: the chooser must know his or her budget, what his or her total disposable wealth is. The choice of a particular health insurance policy will then depend not only upon one's estimate of the comparative health benefits of the different policies, but also upon how much one values the health benefits in question relative to benefits that could be obtained by using one's resources on goods and services other than health care.

The fundamental limitation on this strategy for specifying the ethically required decent minimum, of course, is not simply that it yields a determinate outcome if a fixed budget for the individual is assumed, but what that budget should be is itself an ethical question. Gibbard frankly acknowledges this when he describes his thought experiment as a way of giving content to the guaranteed decent minimum of health care once we know what the appropriate guaranteed income share is. In other words, until we know what individuals have a right to by way of the allocation of income, we cannot determine how health-care resources ought to be allocated. So it seems that we have merely substituted the problem of specifying one kind of decent minimum for another. Further, there is also a problem of circularity: whether something is a fair income share (or an adequate level of income) depends upon whether it would be sufficient for providing adequate levels of various important goods, including health care. Both of these objections point to the conclusion that the rational insurance chooser approach cannot settle the most fundamental ethical issues concerning the allocation of health-care resources and fails to provide a fully satisfying response to the objection that the notion of a right to a decent minimum or adequate level of care is too vague to be of much practical value (Baily 1986).[4]

Indeed, once the problem of vagueness is appreciated it may even become difficult to distinguish between the decent minimum view and the egalitarian view that its proponents reject. Those who believe that there is an egalitarian right to health care but who are not committed to egalitarianism across the board presumably hold that there is something special about health care that requires it to be distributed equally even if (some) other goods need not be. But if health care here means all forms of health care, then this is a most implausible position, since at best only some of the most important forms of health care could have this special status. Consequently, the claim that there is an egalitarian right to health care should be understood as meaning that everyone is to have equal access to some especially important subset of health-care services and resources. But until these are specified and until it is determined whether they exceed those included in a decent minimum, it will not be possible to distinguish between the egalitarian view and the decent minimum view. After all, the right to a decent minimum is an egalitarian right: Everyone is to have equal access to whatever it is that constitutes the decent minimum. Absent a clearer specification of what the decent minimum includes, it is possible to distinguish between it and the claim that there is an egalitarian right to health care only if the latter is taken in an unrestricted sense, as meaning that everyone is to have equal access to all beneficial forms of health care that anyone else is getting (assuming equal need).

BENEFICENCE RATHER THAN JUSTICE: OBLIGATIONS WITHOUT RIGHTS

Partly because of dissatisfaction with the foregoing attempts to settle major allocation questions by an appeal to principles specifying a right to health care and partly because of a growing perception that justice is not the only ethical value bearing on allocation, some recent works have begun to focus instead on principles of beneficence or charity. The President's Commission argues for a societal obligation to provide an "adequate level" (or "decent minimum") of care for all and that the ultimate responsibility and authority for seeing that this is achieved lies with the Federal government (President's Commission 1983, 3–6). The Commission ap-

---

[4]It would be a mistake, however, to conclude that the idea of an adequate level has no useful policy implications. See M. A. Baily. "Rationing Health Care: Defining the Adequate Level." In *What Price Health Care?* edited by G. Agich and C. Begeley, D. Reidel Publishing Co., forthcoming.

proach, like that advocated in an earlier article by this author, rejects a premise that has guided much of the ethical literature on allocation: the assumption that any policy for allocating health-care resources that involves nonvoluntary transfers of wealth from the better-off to the worse off is justifiable only if it can be shown to be based on a moral right to health care. Uncritical subscription to this assumption has led, quite naturally, to the belief that very little can be said about the ethical evaluation of the current pattern of health-care resource allocation in the absence of a convincing defense of the claim that there is such a moral right. This in turn would require a clear adjudication between rival theories of justice.

There may be an even more fundamental—and even less thoroughly examined—assumption that underlies the exclusively rights-based approach to allocation issues. This is the view that the government is morally justified in using coercion (in this case to enforce transfers of wealth) only for purposes of guaranteeing moral rights. This latter view is a very strong and usually inadequately defended assumption about the sole condition under which the use of state power is morally legitimate.

Implicit in the Commission's approach is the thesis that even if it is true that the need to guarantee rights is the strongest and most obvious moral justification for enforcing allocation policies, it is not the only justification. The Commission argues that, because of the special moral significance of health care (or, rather, of some forms of it), because health-care needs are often to a significant extent underserved, and because health-care needs are typically so unpredictable, costly, and unevenly distributed among people that it is implausible to expect everyone to be able to meet them using only their own resources, society has a moral obligation to provide an "adequate level" of care or set of health care services to those who cannot provide them for themselves. In effect, the Commission contends that this obligation is of such fundamental moral importance that it may be enforced, if necessary, whether or not there is a corresponding individual right to an adequate level of care.

In other words, I have attempted to flesh out this general line of argument in a more systematic and convincing way (Buchanan 1984a, 1985, 1987).[5] The basic premises employed are the following:

1. The provision of at least some of the more important forms of health care to the needy can be viewed as a collective goods, and strictly voluntary schemes for securing them may succumb to familiar obstacles to successful collective action—in particular, the free-rider problem and the assurance problem.
2. In some cases, enforcement of obligations to contribute is both necessary and sufficient for the successful provisions of collective goods, including important forms of health care for the needy.
3. The fact that enforcement is necessary and sufficient for achieving such a morally fundamental collective good as the provision of the most important

---

[5]The argument is drawn from Buchanan (1987), with the kind permission of the journal *Ethics*.

forms of health care to the needy is a strong prima facie justification for enforcement, independently of whether the individuals who will receive the good have an antecedent moral right to it.

Whether this strong prima facie justification is a decisive justification all things considered will depend, of course, upon a number of factors. Is this use of enforcement compatible with avoiding unacceptably dangerous concentrations of power in the government? Can a system of enforced contributions be achieved that fairly distributes the burden of providing for the needy among the better off and that avoids unpredictable, arbitrary, and excessively burdensome appropriations of individuals' wealth? Only if these questions can be answered affirmatively will the prima facie justification become a decisive justification, all things considered.

The attractiveness of this line of argument becomes clearer once premises 1 and 2 are explicated. Without an effective enforcement mechanism, strictly voluntary compliance with duties to aid the needy may founder due to the fact that a system of aid is a collective good. Even if rational individuals agree to a system of duties to contribute to the good, they may find it rational to defect from it, to be "free-riders," as long as compliance is voluntary. The situation has an incentive structure similar to that of a many-person Prisoners' Dilemma. Each individual may reason as follows. "Either enough others will contribute to the good in question, regardless of whether I do so, or they will not. Since my contribution is a cost to me, the rational thing for me to do is not to contribute, so long as I will be able to partake of the good regardless of whether I contributed."

It might be replied that in fact individuals will not behave thusly because their desire to maximize their own utility will be constrained by altruism. Now the extent to which individuals observe moral constraints on their individual utility-maximizing behavior is an empirical issue. But this much seems clear: since altruism is generally limited, the scope of duties to aid which we can expect people to fulfill voluntarily is probably considerably narrower than that of duties they would discharge if those duties were enforced.

The free-rider problem arises on the assumption that the good at which each individual aims is accurately described as "the provision of aid to the needy." If this is his goal, then as we have seen the individual may withhold his contribution if he believes that the needy will be provided for by others or that they will not, regardless of whether he contributes. And there are several different ways in which one may benefit from the attainment of this good without having contributed to it. Some may derive satisfaction or avoid discomfort simply by knowing that the needy are provided for. Others may view the provision of aid to the needy as instrumentally good: it makes for a more stable social structure, in which those who have wealth and power may enjoy them in greater security, and increases overall productivity by enabling more people to work. Indeed it is often said that the major social welfare programs initiated in western Europe in the late nineteenth century were motivated chiefly by the latter sorts of considerations rather than by a sense of justice or a direct concern for the well-being of the needy.

On the other hand, the free-rider problem will not block successful collective action if a sufficient number of people desire to provide for the needy, rather than simply desiring that the needy be provided for. If I regard the good to be attained as "a system of aid to the needy to which I contribute," then, of course, I cannot partake of that good without contributing to it.

Whether or not a sufficient number of people will be effectively motivated by the desire to be charitable to achieve a particular goal of collective charity (rather than simply by the desire that charity be done) is an empirical question whose answer will vary from case to case, depending upon the psychology of the individuals involved. But even if an individual does not himself wish to take a free ride on the contributions of others to a system of aid to the needy, he still may be unwilling to render aid to the needy unless he has assurance that others (with resources as great as or greater than his) will also render aid to those in need. He may be unwilling to contribute without assurance that others will do so for either or both of two distinct reasons: (1) He may conclude that it is better to expend his "beneficence budget" on an act of independent charity toward some particular person in need, rather than risk contributing to a collective charity in which the threshold of contributions needed for success is not reached; (2) his commitment to being charitable may be limited by a requirement of fairness or reciprocity. That persons who are strict individual utility-maximizers may fail to achieve systems of aid that are public goods is hardly surprising. What is striking is the more general conclusion that collective action to create and maintain systems of aid may falter even if some individuals are significantly altruistic.

Whether or not enforcement will be necessary to achieve goals of collective charity does not appear to admit of a general answer. Under certain rather strong conditions, strictly voluntary contributions may suffice. However, in the case of systems of aid that are collective goods, as with collective goods generally, there seem to be no strictly voluntary strategies which will work in all circumstances. If this is so, and if enforcement is justified in any such cases, then it is not the case that enforcement of a duty to contribute is justified only where there is an antecedent moral right to a share of the good in question, whether it be national defense or a system of health care for the needy.

The nonrights-based or enforced beneficence approach has four important advantages. First, it represents, in effect, a kind of end-run around the conceptual impasse created by the deadlock of rival theories of distributive justice in health care, because it provides an ethical basis for evaluating current allocations and for designing new allocation policies without having to adjudicate decisively among such theories. Indeed, the enforced beneficence arguments can be seen as providing moral support for establishing a legal right to health care in the absence of a clear justification for a moral right upon which to found the legal right.

Second, obligations of beneficence are traditionally understood to be limited by the proviso that rendering aid to the needy is not to be unduly burdensome to the benefactor. Consequently, the enforced beneficence approach avoids objections to which more demanding egalitarian conceptions of the right health care are vulnerable.

Third, the notion of enforced beneficence gains some plausibility from the widespread acceptance of the legitimacy of arguments for enforcement to secure more familiar collective goods, such as national defense. It is well-known that free-rider and/or assurance problems can block voluntary contribution to such goods and there is a rather broad agreement that enforced contribution is at least sometimes justifiable.

Fourth, the enforced beneficence approach can be seen as a step toward rectifying two unfortunate biases of much of contemporary ethical thinking, both within and outside medical ethics: a tendency to proceed as if morality were limited to justice and a propensity to concentrate exclusively on matters of individual, rather than collective, responsibility and action, thereby glossing over problems of social coordination.

On the other side of the ledger, there are two main difficulties with the enforced beneficence view. Perhaps the most important is that the obligation of beneficence in health care may be so vague that it, like the alleged right to a decent minimum, may not provide sufficient guidance for substantive policy decisions. In addition, a systematic, society-wide effort to specify and coordinate obligations to contribute may seem to run contrary to what many take to be a distinctive feature of those obligations of beneficence that do not have correlative rights. Such obligations, often called duties of charity, are traditionally thought to allow a broad sphere of discretion for the benefactor, who may choose either the form his aid will take or to whom it will be given, or both. If a coordinated, enforced system of contributions to the needy is to avoid this objection it must be designed in such a way as to allow a significant exercise of autonomy for benefactors, either within the system or outside it.

CONCLUSION

The foregoing critical survey has exposed a number of serious difficulties with each of the main strategies for making ethical evaluations of health-care resource allocation. None of these strategies has emerged as fully adequate or uniquely attractive. Such a result should prompt neither surprise nor pessimism. Systemic thinking about these difficult issues has barely begun. It is only in the past few years that economists, other policy analysts, and those who actually make policy, have begun to recognize that ethical issues are unavoidable and that they are not merely matters of taste, but can be reasoned about. Similarly, systematic ethical theorizing about matters of distributive justice is also a relatively recent phenomenon and the hard work of teasing out the concrete implications of such general theories for real-world allocation problems is in its infancy.

REFERENCES

Aaron, H., and R. Schwarz. *The Painful Prescription: Rationing Hospital Care.* Washington, D.C.: The Brookings Institution, 1984.

Baily, Mary Ann. "Rationing Health: Defining the Adequate Level." In *What Price Health?*, edited by George Agich and Charles Begeley. Dordrecht, Holland: D. Reidel, 1986.

Brock, D. W. "Recent Work in Utilitarianism." *Am Philosop Q* 10, no. 4 (1973): 8, 15.

Brock, D. W. "Ethical Issues in Recipient Selection for Organ Transplantation." In *Organ Substitution Technology: Ethical, Legal, and Public Policy Issues,* edited by D. R. Mathieu. Boulder, Colo.: Westview Press, 1988.

Buchanan, A. E. "Justice: A Philosophical Review." In *Justice and Health Care,* edited by E. E. Shelp. Dordrecht, Holland: D. Reidel, 1981.

———. "The Right to a 'Decent Minimum' of Health Care." *Philosophy and Public Affairs* 13, no. 1 (1984a).

———. "What's So Special About Rights?" *Social Philosophy and Policy* 2, iss. 1 (1984b): 63.

———. *Ethics, Efficiency, and the Market.* Totowa, N.J.: Rowman & Allanheld, 1985.

Buchanan, Allen. "Justice and Charity." *Ethics* 97, no. 3 (1987).

Childress, J. F. "Priorities in the Allocation of Health Care Resources." In *Contemporary Issues in Bioethics,* 2d ed., edited by T. L. Beauchamp and L. Walter. Belmont, Calif.: Wadsworth, 1982.

Cohen, G. A. "Robert Nozick and Wilt Chamberlain: How Patterns Preserve Liberty." In *Justice and Economic Distribution,* edited by J. Arthur and W. H. Shaw. Englewood Cliffs, N.J.: Prentice-Hall, 1978.

Daniels, N. *Just Health Care.* Cambridge, England: Cambridge University Press, 1985.

Dworkin, R. *Taking Rights Seriously.* Cambridge, Mass.: Harvard University Press, 1977.

Feinberg, J. "The Nature and Value of Rights." In *Rights,* edited by D. Lyons. Belmont, Calif.: Wadsworth, 1979.

Gibbard, A. "The Prospective Pareto Principle and Equity of Access to Health Care." President's Commission, *Securing Access to Health Care, Vol. Two, Appendices: Sociocultural and Philosophical Studies.* Washington, D.C.: Government Printing Office, 1983.

Gutman, A. "A Principle of Equal Access." President's Commission, *Securing Access to Health Care, Vol. Two: Appendices: Sociocultural and Philosophical Studies.* Washington, D.C.: Government Printing Office, 1983.

H.H.S. National Task Force on Organ Transplantation Report, 1986.

Mathieu, D. R., ed. *Organ Substitution Technology: Ethical, Legal, and Public Policy Issues.* Boulder, Colo.: Westview Press, 1988.

Menzel, P. T. *Medical Costs, Moral Choices.* New Haven, Conn.: Yale University Press, 1983.

Nozick, R. *Anarchy, State, and Utopia.* New York: Basic Books, 1974.

President's Commission. *Securing Access to Health Care, Vol. Two: Sociocultural and Philosophical Studies.* Washington, D.C.: Government Printing Office, 1983.

President's Commission for the Study of Ethical Problems in Medicine and Biomedical and Behavioral Research. *Securing Access to Health Care, Vol. One: Report,* 1983.

Rawls, J. *A Theory of Justice.* Cambridge, Mass.: Harvard University Press, 1971.

Report of the Task Force on Organ Transplantation. Washington, D.C.: U.S. Department of Health and Human Services, 1986.

Rescher, N. "The Allocation of Scarce Exotic Livesaving Therapy." In *Moral Problems in Medicine,* edited by S. Gorovitz et al. Englewood Cliffs, N.J.: Prentice-Hall, 1976.

Sartorius, R. E. *Individual Conduct and Social Norms.* Belmont, Calif.: Dickenson, 1975.

Veatch, R. M. *A Theory of Medical Ethics.* New York: Basic Books, 1981.

Weinstein, M., and W. Stason. "Foundations of Cost-Effectiveness Analysis for Health and Medical Practices." *N Engl J Med* 296 (1977): 716–721.

DISCUSSION QUESTIONS

1. What resources (time, energy, money, etc.) should be put into health care and into other social goods such as education, defense, eliminating poverty and homelessness, and improving the environment? Are professionals in health care appropriate persons for making these allocational decisions?

2. Within the area of health (once we have determined its budget), how much time, energy, money, etc., should we allocate for prevention and how much for rescue and crisis medicine? Are professionals within health care appropriate persons for making these decisions?

3. Within either preventive care of rescue medicine, who (if anyone) should receive resources such as vaccines or artificial hearts when we cannot meet everyone's needs?

4. Often because of their conditions the sickest and most needy patients are not the ones who would benefit the most from health-care interventions. For example, the worst-off heart patients may not benefit from a heart transplant as much as patients who are in somewhat better shape. Under ethical principles of utility and justice who should get the scarce resource?

5. If health care is to be allocated at least in part on the basis of need, do those people who have great need because of voluntary lifestyle choices they have made have high priority claims on scarce resources or have they waived their claim on these resources?

12

Death and Dying

Dan W. Brock

SUMMARY

Some of the most controversial moral issues and arguments in current medical ethics involve decisions about terminally ill patients and about what it means to be dead. The traditional criterion for determining death, i.e., the permanent cessation of heart and lung function, has largely been replaced by the contemporary criterion of cessation of brain function. Now some are maintaining that only the higher-brain must be destroyed for a person to be dead. The medical as well as judicial and conceptual changes which have occurred must be understood before we can know what it means for a person to be dead.

For those persons who are still alive we need an ethical framework for life support decisions. The authoritarian (paternalistic) model of the physician/patient relationship is contrasted in this chapter with the more patient-centered model aimed at promoting patients' well-being while respecting their self-determination. The role that quality-of-life considerations should play in life-sustaining treatment decisions is explored. Decisionmaking procedures for the incompetent patient are developed together with the moral principles that should guide these decisions so as to respect patients' wishes, or if they are not known, serve their best interests. Advance directives that can be used to state one's wishes about treatment and select a surrogate decisionmaker are explained.

The ethical framework presented for life-support decisions allows patients or their surrogates to weigh the benefits and burdens of treatment from the patient's perspective and to refuse any treatment. However, just because life itself is at stake some employ additional distinctions for these decisions. The chapter explores in some detail differences between withholding and withdrawing life support; killing and allowing to die; ordinary versus extraordinary treatment; whether foregoing life support constitutes suicide, active voluntary euthanasia, and pain relief that hastens death.

Finally, two issues are discussed that raise special policy concerns— decisions about critically ill newborns and life-sustaining nutrition and hydration.

In recent decades medicine has gained dramatic new abilities to prolong life. Patients with kidney failure can be placed on renal dialysis; patients who have suffered cardiac arrest can sometimes be revived with advanced life-support measures including drugs, electric shock, airway intubation and closed or open heart massage; patients with pulmonary disease can be assisted by mechanical ventilation on respirators; and patients unable to eat or drink can receive nourishment and fluids intravenously or with tube feedings. These are only some of the most dramatic and well-known additions to medicine's armamentarium for staving off death in the gravely ill. While these and other life-sustaining treatments often provide very great benefits to individual patients by restoring or prolonging functioning lives, they also have the capacity to prolong patients' lives beyond the point at which they desire continued life support or are reasonably thought to be benefitted by it. Thus, where once nature took its course and pneumonia was the "old man's friend," now increasingly someone must decide how long a life will be prolonged and when death will come. This chapter addresses some of the principal moral issues and arguments in current debates about life support. Below we address very briefly a related issue: the definition of death.

THE DEFINITION OF DEATH

The traditional criterion for determining death until recent years was the permanent ceasing to function of the heart and lungs. When a person stopped breathing and his or her heart stopped beating for more than a few minutes the loss of function was irreversible and the patient was declared dead. The loss of oxygen to the brain would quickly produce irreversible brain damage and loss of all cognitive function. However, the advent in recent years of new medical technology, and most importantly of respirators, has enabled modern medicine to continue artificially patients' heart and lung function after they would no longer function unassisted. As already noted, this can often save lives that previously would have been lost and sometimes permit the patient to recover a normal level of functioning. In some few other cases, however, heart and lung function can be restored or continued by these artificial means after brain function has been partially or completely destroyed, for example, from prolonged loss of oxygen or severe trauma to the brain. Such cases have forced a rethinking of the criteria for the determination of death (President's Commission 1981).

This rethinking has led to a widely acknowledged additional criterion for death, the complete and irreversible loss of all brain function, or so-called brain death. This allows a patient to be declared dead who has suffered complete and irreversible loss of brain function even if the patient's respiration and circulation are being continued by artificial means. There remains a single unitary concept of death, for example, "permanent cessation of the integrated functioning of the organism as a whole," or "irreversible loss of personhood" (Capron and Kass 1972, 102–104). What has been introduced is an additional criterion for when this condition of death obtains, namely the complete and irreversible loss of all brain function. Of course, once this additional criterion has been accepted, the practical question then is precisely which medical tests and procedures will establish this loss of brain function. This is a matter for medical determination given a particular level of medical knowledge and technology; it will change over time and will not be explored here (President's Commission 1981, Appendix F). However, we will consider the principal area of philosophical controversy between so-called whole brain and higher brain formulations in the new criteria for the determination of death.

The new definitions adopted by state courts and legislatures, as well as by various official bodies that have studied the matter such as the President's Commission, have adopted the whole brain formulation. In this formulation it is the loss of functioning of the whole brain, either as the integrating mechanism of the body's major organ systems or as the hallmark of life itself of the human organism, that is required for death. To quote from the President's Commission:

> When all brain processes cease, the patient loses two important sets of functions. One set encompasses the integrating and coordinating functions, carried out principally but not exclusively by the cerebellum and brainstem. The other set includes the psychological functions which make consciousness, thought, and feeling possible. These latter functions are located primarily but not exclusively in the cerebrum, especially the neocortex (President's Commission 1981, 38).

Thus, the whole brain formulation includes both the loss of integrating functions that make natural respiration and circulation possible as well as the functions that make consciousness, thought, and feeling possible. The higher brain formulations focus exclusively on the latter functions. In this view, it is consciousness, thought, and feeling that is necessary to personhood, and when they have been irreversibly lost the *person* has died or permanently ceased to exist (Green and Wikler 1980; Veatch 1975). Anyone dead by the whole brain formulation will obviously be dead as well by the higher brain formulation, but not vice versa. In particular, brain injury resulting from some stroke or trauma may permanently destroy all capacity for consciousness, thought, and feeling, but may allow respiration and circulation to continue either assisted or unassisted. This is essentially the condition of patients in so-called persistent vegetative states such as Karen Quinlan, who was able to breathe on her own for a number of years before she died.

There is not space to explore here deep philosophical questions about the nature of personhood and personal identity that divide whole and higher brain formulations. Some version of the higher brain formulation is probably supported by most accounts of personhood, but also at issue is whether the appropriate criterion is the death of a person, which would seem to be the issue of moral concern, or the death of a human being or organism. Since the determination of death is principally a legal determination, practical considerations of social and legal policy are also relevant. Use of the higher brain conception requires the willingness to declare as dead persons whose body's circulatory and respiratory functions remain intact; that is, those whose bodies are still breathing on their own. It would also require practical methods of discrimination of brain function that permit determinations of the permanent loss of higher brain function while some lower brain function persists, and to do so with the very high degree of certainty reasonably required for any declaration of death.

Since public and legal policy has for the present largely settled on the whole brain conception, we shall assume the perspective of that conception in the discussion that follows. It is to be emphasized that on that conception a patient such as Karen Quinlan who has suffered a permanent loss of consciousness and of all capacity for thought and feeling has *not* died. Such patients may, however, constitute a unique class of patients for decisions about foregoing life support because the permanent loss of all consciousness may imply the lack of any possible interest in continued life.

AN ETHICAL FRAMEWORK FOR LIFE-SUPPORT DECISIONS

Any account of morally appropriate procedures and content for life-support decisions presupposes a broader account of medical treatment decisionmaking generally, and of the physician/patient relationship. These broader issues are addressed more fully in the chapter on informed consent (Chapter 7). Here, we will set out only briefly the issues in a general account of treatment decisionmaking and the physician/patient relation to guide life-support decisions. It is all too easy to exaggerate the shift in actual practice regarding medical treatment decisionmaking that has taken place in recent decades, and to reduce discussions of models of physician/patient relations to caricatures. With that said, however, it is widely agreed that it was common historically to view the physician/patient relation as one in which the physician directed care and made decisions about treatment, while the patient's role was to comply with the "Doctor's orders." Patients were told only as much about their condition and treatment as was necessary to comply effectively with treatment.

This is sometimes called the authoritarian or paternalist model of the physician/patient relation. It reflects the medical training, knowledge, and experience possessed by the physician but lacked by the average patient, as well as the anxiety, fear, dependency and regression common in critically ill or dying patients. Moreover, if the end of medicine is seen as the preservation of the patient's health and life by the treatment of disease, it is not then surprising that physicians are viewed as possessing the necessary expertise to determine which treatment will best do so. With the dramatic increases in recent decades in medical knowledge and expertise, as well as the many new modes of treatment now possible, the case for the physician as primary treatment decisionmaker now would seem all the stronger. Yet the weight of argument and opinion has shifted substantially toward securing an enlarged, indeed principal, role in treatment decisionmaking for the patient (President's Commission 1982). Why has this happened? There are, of course, many historical reasons for this shift that we will not detail here, but there has also been a reconception of the ends of medicine and of the proper form of the physician/patient relation (Katz 1984; President's Commission 1982; Siegler 1981).

There are many ways of more precisely formulating this newer conception. One prominent version sees the goals of health-care decisionmaking as the promotion of the patients' well-being while respecting their self-determination (President's Commission 1982, Ch. 2). How is this different from promoting and preserving patients' health and life? What will best promote health and life is naturally thought to be an objective factual matter, an empirical question, and not a function of individual preference and value. So understood, what will best promote patients' health and preserve their lives is a factual matter about which the physician, not the patient, possesses expertise. Why then is a central role necessary for the patient in selecting the treatment best for the patient?

To conceive the endpoint of the health care process as the patient's well-being, instead of as health and life in general, is not to deny that physicians seek beneficially to affect patients' health and life. Rather, it is to stress that health and life extension are ultimately of value in the service of the broader overall well-being of the patient. They are of value in so far as they facilitate the patient's pursuit of his or her overall plan of life; the aims, goals and values important to the particular patient. In many instances the decision of which alternative treatment will best promote a patient's well-being, including the alternative of no treatment, cannot be objectively determined independent of that patient's own preferences and values.

In the case of life-support decisions, when the foregoing of life support is under serious consideration it is usually because 1) the patient is critically or terminally ill and likely to die soon no matter what is done, and 2) because the quality of the patient's life is seriously limited by the effects of disease, disability and sometimes the treatment itself. Whether treatment and continued life under such severely constrained conditions are better than no life at all must depend in significant part on how the particular patient views his or her life under those conditions. While the physician will be in the best position to predict the specific outcomes of different treatment alternatives and their effects for the patient, the patient will be in the best position to evaluate what importance should be given to any particular effect, such as the discomfort and restrictions on communication of intubation, or the restrictions on activities of dialysis. It is well established that different persons evaluate the importance of such burdens significantly differently—some will tolerate intubation or dialysis relatively well if it allows their lives to be prolonged, while others find that the limitations make life no longer worth living.

There is no single right answer to how such conditions should be valued; there are only the actual answers that real persons give for themselves. This is why many have urged that health care decisionmaking should be a process of shared decisionmaking between physician and patient (Katz 1984; President's Commission 1982; Siegler 1981). Each brings something to the decisionmaking process that the other lacks, and the communication is necessary to decisions that best serve the patient's well-being. The physician brings knowledge about the likely outcomes of alternative treatments; the patient brings knowledge of the personal aims, ends and values by which to evaluate those outcomes. Thus, even if treatment decisionmaking aims only best to serve the patient's well-being, shared decisionmaking, a process of conversation between the physician and patient, is necessary to identify the best alternative.

In this more recent view of health-care decisionmaking, the other value that should guide the process is the patient's self-determination or autonomy. Self-determination can be understood as the interest each person has in making important decisions that shape and affect one's life for oneself (Dworkin 1988). Self-determination reflects the everyday importance people give to having control over the course of their lives and thereby the level of responsibility they require to direct their lives. The claim of a right to self-determination is the claim of a right to define and revise one's desires and values in light of experience, and to pursue one's own conception of a good life. Involving patients in important treatment decisions, and leaving them free to refuse any proffered treatment, respects their self-determination. If the interest in self-determination is important in non-life-support cases that affect patients' lives in significant ways, then surely it is at least as important in decisions concerning whether treatment to sustain their lives will be employed or foregone, and thus when and under what conditions their lives will end. Valuing self-determination requires respecting both patients' own conception of their well-being (the subjective aspect of well-being noted above) as well as patients' interest in participating in the decisionmaking process about their care.

Both these values of patient well-being and self-determination support a process of shared decisionmaking between physician and patient in which the patient retains the right to refuse any offered treatment. Shared decisionmaking does not preclude, however, the important trust traditionally and commonly bestowed by patients on their physicians, even when patients ask their physicians to decide for them. There is a crucial moral difference, however, between patients transferring their right to decide to a trusted physician or family member and patients deferring to physicians because decisionmaking is considered to be physicians', not patients' business. The ultimate right of refusal of treatment rests with the patient because it is to or on the patient that treatment is done. It is the patient's body, and in turn the patient's life, that bears the principal effects of any treatment instituted.

The increased role for the patient in a process of shared decisionmaking has not, of course, gone unchallenged and unprotested (Kass 1985; Sider and Clements 1985). Some commentators have insisted that the proper goal of medicine is the objective (as opposed to subjective) promotion of health; for example, health defined in terms of species function. They argue that physicians are in the best position to determine what will best serve this goal and physicians should not be guided solely by the patient's preferences. Many physicians no doubt also share this resistance to any incursion on their traditionally dominant decisionmaking role. Nevertheless, the debates generally have not made clear to what extent, if any, these commentators would limit a competent patient's right to refuse any life-sustaining treatment. Disagreement probably more often concerns whether a physician must accede to a request, either from a competent patient or more likely from an incompetent patient's family, for life-sustaining treatment that the physician believes is inappropriate. All generally agree that no physician should be required or forced to provide treatment that he or she believes is not within the bounds of acceptable medical practice, but a substantive difference may remain about how these boundaries should in a particular case be defined and how responsive they should be to patient or family preferences.

The account of decisionmaking about life-sustaining treatment based on the values of patient self-determination and well-being empowers the competent patient, or the incompetent patient's surrogate, to weigh the benefits and burdens of alternative treatments, including the alternative of no treatment, according to the patient's own view of the relative value and importance of the various features of those alternatives (President's Commission 1983a). If the competent patient, or the incompetent patient's surrogate, judges that the overall benefits and burdens of the alternative employing life support are worse for the patient than the alternative of foregoing treatment with its expectation of death, that choice is to be respected. It essentially involves a judgment by the patient or surrogate that the expected duration and quality of the continued life possible for the patient is so bad that on balance it is worse than no further life at all.

It should be noted that in this view so-called quality of life considerations *do* quite properly and inevitably play a role in the assessment of alternatives and of their overall benefits and burdens. For most persons, whether the continued life made possible by a particular life-sustaining treatment is on balance a benefit to them will depend at least in part on the quality of that life. What is important to emphasize is that the assessment should be of the quality of life *to the patient* and whether its quality makes continued life on balance a benefit or burden to him or her. This view does not sanction giving weight to how the patient's continued life may affect the quality of other's lives, for example by making the patient a burden to others. Nor does it sanction any judgments that some peoples lives are not socially or economically worth sustaining because they are of low quality. The proper question is whether the patient's present and anticipated quality of life is sufficiently bad to make it, according to him or her, worse than no more life at all. This is a very narrowly constrained role for quality of life considerations that is fully compatible with respecting patient's self-determination and their own view of their well-being.

THE INCOMPETENT PATIENT

Our account of life-support decisionmaking thus far largely assumes that the patient is competent to make such decisions. Of course, this is often or even usually not the case when foregoing life-sustaining treatment is seriously at issue. The effects of illness and disease, as well as of treatments themselves, commonly compromise or eliminate patients' abilities to participate in decisionmaking. Someone else will then have to decide for them. This chapter is concerned with moral issues concerning life support and so we will not discuss in any detail the various legal and institutional practices and procedures that have been developed for decisionmaking for incompetent patients (President's Commission 1983a, Ch. 4, Appendices D, E, F). However, we will briefly discuss the moral principles that can guide decisionmaking for incompetent patients (Buchanan and Brock 1986).

Probably the most direct way for incompetent patients to participate in decisions about their care in a manner serving their well-being and self-determination is through use of advance directives. Advance directives, the best known of which are so-called Living Wills, enable persons while competent to specify their wishes about treatment should they later become incompetent. A majority of the states in the United States now have given these documents legally enforceable status. Nevertheless, advance directives are at best only a partial solution to the problem of decisionmaking for incompetent patients for several reasons. First, and probably most important, only a very small proportion of incompetent patients for whom such decisions must be made have ever given advance directives. This is likely to continue to be the case even with increased efforts to publicize advance directives and their value.

Second, to ensure the patient's competence when they are given, advance directives are usually made well in advance of the circumstances in which they are to be applied. Thus, they are inevitably framed in somewhat vague and general terms, and commonly make use of phrases like "if I am terminally ill and death is imminent, no further artificial or extraordinary means to prolong my life shall be employed," and so forth. While such instructions can provide others with general guidance as to the patient's wishes regarding life support, they inevitably leave much discretion to those who must interpret them in the patient's specific circumstances. At what point is death imminent? Are antibiotics extraordinary means? Even when advance directives have been given, others must unavoidably play a role in decisionmaking about life support for incompetent patients to interpret those directives. This has led many persons to conclude that so-called Durable Powers of Attorney, by which persons designate who is to make treatment decisions for them if they later become incompetent, are more helpful than Living Wills.

A third difficulty is that in order to guard against possible well-intentioned misuse or ill-intentioned abuse by others of advance directives the conditions bringing the directives into legal effect are often narrowly limited. For example, the condition that death be imminent on many natural interpretations restricts the directive so that it does not apply in many of the circumstances in which decisions about life support must be made. In any event, it is rarely the case that such directives are taken to court to enforce action in accordance with them. Instead, their function has been to serve in a more informal way as evidence of what the patient would have wanted in the circumstances.

In the absence of any advance directive, others must decide for the incompetent patient. The principle guiding such decisions most in accord with promoting the patient's well-being, as he or she conceives it, while also respecting his or her self-determination, is the principle of Substituted Judgment (Buchanan and Brock 1986; Capron 1982). This principle directs the surrogate decisionmaker to attempt to decide as the patient would have decided if he or she were competent. This essentially directs the surrogate to take account of any available information about the patient's preferences and values relevant to this decision, even if these preferences and values are different from most people's, in determining what the patient would have wanted.

In the absence of any information about what the particular patient would have wanted, for example because there are no available family or friends of the patient, it is generally accepted that the principle guiding decisions should be the Best Interest Principle. This principle directs the surrogate to decide about life support in a manner which best serves the patient's interests. Lacking any knowledge of this particular patient's wishes, such decisions will inevitably involve asking what most reasonable persons would want for themselves in the circumstances.

It is widely agreed that the surrogate decisionmaker who is to apply these principles should usually be the patient's closest family member. The presumption for the family member as surrogate is usually based on three reasons. First, in most instances the family member will know the patient best and so be in the best position to determine what the patient would have wanted. Second, in most cases the family member will care most about the patient's well-being and so be most concerned to represent it. Finally, the family in our society is commonly accorded a significant degree of decisionmaking authority and discretion in order to preserve the value of the family.

It should be emphasized that these considerations only establish a presumption for the family member as surrogate. They do not imply that the family member is always the appropriate decisionmaker, but only that in most cases a family member will be a better surrogate than anyone else who as a general practice might be turned to. When these reasons supporting the family member as surrogate do not hold in a particular case, for example because there is an evident conflict of interest between the patient and the family member or because the patient and family member have been estranged too many years, someone else should serve as surrogate. The physician may then have a positive obligation to ensure that the family member is removed as surrogate, through appeal to the courts if necessary.

There are a number of points of controversy concerning surrogate decision-making that we shall merely note here. One concerns the proper procedures and standards for determining whether the patient is incompetent to decide for him- or herself. In cases of questionable competence, this is a complicated matter that is dealt with in more detail in the chapter on informed consent. Very roughly, what is needed by a patient is adequate capacity to understand relevant information about alternatives and their consequences, together with the ability to apply one's own values to those alternatives and to select one as best (Buchanan and Brock 1986; Drane 1985). A second point of controversy is whether a surrogate should have the same range of discretion in choice that a competent patient would have. Third, in what cases and to what extent should it be required to involve others in the surrogate decisionmaking process? For example, when and how might institutional ethics committees within hospitals and other health-care delivery institutions become involved (Fost and Cranford, 1985; Rosner, 1985), and when is court review of decisions desirable? Despite these and other areas of controversy about surrogate decisionmaking for incompetent patients, however, the fundamental ethical framework discussed above for the competent patient that appeals to the values of patient well-being and self-determination can be extended to the incompetent patient as well.

SOME ADDITIONAL CONTROVERSIAL MORAL CONSTRAINTS ON FOREGOING LIFE SUPPORT

Many of the principal moral disputes about life-sustaining treatment do not focus on the broad issues discussed above of the proper role of the patient in health-care decisionmaking and of the proper form of the physician/patient relationship. Instead, these disputes are more specific to life-sustaining treatment, reflecting the important fact that death is the direct and expected result of foregoing such treatment, and have taken several forms. First, are there special constraints on what is morally permissible regarding life support because life and death is directly in the balance? For example, while it may be morally permissible not to start a particular life-sustaining treatment, is it also permissible to stop the treatment once it has begun? Would doing so be to kill the patient, not merely to allow him to die, and if so would it therefore be wrong? If life-sustaining treatment can be withdrawn with the expectation that death will result, is euthanasia permissible directly killing, for example, by a lethal injection, a terminally ill and suffering patient who voluntarily requests it?

These are only some of the special issues and distinctions that we shall consider below and that are important in the debates about moral limits on acceptable action concerning life-sustaining treatment because life and death are in question. Since the prohibition of the intentional killing of an innocent human being is one of our society's strongest moral and legal norms, it is hardly surprising that these issues should be difficult and controversial.

A second area of substantial recent concern is whether there are morally important differences between different kinds of treatment that would make foregoing some treatments impermissible in circumstances in which foregoing others would be permissible. For example, some persons believe food and water should never be withheld though treatments like mechanical ventilation and dialysis may be. Third, many persons find morally important differences between different kinds of patients, justifying either greater restrictions on withholding life support, or greater latitude in doing so. Examples of each sort include critically ill newborns and patients in a persistent vegatative state. In the remainder of this chapter, we shall work somewhat systematically through these moral issues in the care of the dying.

One issue that will not be addressed below is the economic costs of care of the dying. Whether these costs are excessive is controversial (Bayer et. al. 1983). The precise nature, basis and scope of a general social obligation to ensure access for all to an adequate level of health care, including life-sustaining care, is also controversial and complex (President's Commission 1983b). These issues are beyond the scope of this chapter, but are addressed in detail in the chapter on resource allocation (Chapter 11). However, since some 30 million Americans are substantially without access to health care, we will assume here that ability to pay should not be a general moral criterion limiting access to life-sustaining care.

Withholding and Withdrawing Life Support

One constraint that many persons accept on patient's rights to forego any life-sustaining treatment they judge to be excessively burdensome is that while it can be morally permissible not to start a particular life-sustaining treatment, it is not permissible to stop it once it has begun. Alternatively, even if such treatments can sometimes be stopped once begun, it is often held that it is a graver matter requiring weightier reasons to stop; stopping is at least sometimes not permissible in circumstances in which it would be permissible not to start. This accurately reflects much medical practice in which, for example, physicians who are prepared to honor patients' or their familys' requests for "Do Not Resuscitate" or "Do Not Intubate" orders nevertheless in similar circumstances will not stop respirators on which patients are dependent for life. Physicians commonly feel more responsible for a patient's death that results from stopping a respirator than from not starting one. But is there good reason to treat withdrawal of life-sustaining treatment as morally different and more serious than withholding such treatment? Consider the following case.

Case 1. A very gravely ill patient comes into a hospital emergency room from a nursing home and is sent up to the intensive care unit. The patient begins to develop respiratory failure that is likely to require intubation very soon. At that point the patient's family members and long-standing attending physician arrive at the ICU and inform the ICU staff that there had been extensive discussion about future care with the patient when he was unquestionably competent. Given his grave and terminal illness, as well as his state of debilitation, the patient had firmly rejected being placed on a respirator under any circumstances, and the family and physician produce the patient's Living Will to that effect. Most would hold that this patient should not be intubated and placed on a respirator against his will. Suppose now that the situation is exactly the same except that the attending physician and family are slightly delayed in traffic and arrive fifteen minutes later just after the patient has been intubated and placed on the respirator. Can this difference be of any moral importance? Could it possibly justify morally a refusal by the staff to remove the patient from the respirator? Do not the very same circumstances that justified not placing the patient on the respirator now justify taking him off it? Do not factors like the patient's condition, prognosis, and firmly expressed competent wishes morally determine what should be done, not whether we do not start, or fifteen minutes later stop, the respirator? Why should the stop/not start difference matter morally at all?

Cases such as this have led many to conclude that the difference between not starting and stopping, or withholding and withdrawing, life-sustaining treatment is not in itself of any moral importance (President's Commission 1983a; Rachels 1975; Steinbock 1980). Put differently, any set of circumstances that would morally justify not starting life-sustaining treatment would justify stopping it as well. If this conclusion is correct, then the fact noted above that persons feel more responsible for the patient's death when they stop life support, and are as a result more reluctant to stop than not to start, suggests that many people's natural reactions will here lead them to act in ways that are not morally defensible and that conflict with their own considered moral judgments. Consequently, this may be a place where physicians and others should be especially reflective about their behavior since their unreflective natural reactions may lead them morally astray. It is worth adding that in practice one often gains a reason to stop a treatment once it has been tried that one did not have earlier not to try it. Very often there is considerable uncertainty about how well a patient will do or what progress he or she will make with a particular form of life support such as mechanical respiration. The treatment will then usually be worth trying to see if it in fact has the hoped for positive effects. When it does not have the hoped for positive results, and so no longer holds out the reasonable but uncertain prospect of benefits to the patient, there is then a reason to stop the treatment that did not exist earlier not to start it.

Does it matter that many physicians and families are unwilling to stop treatments like respirators in circumstances in which they would be willing not to initiate them, even if there is no significant moral difference between the cases? There are at least two serious bad effects for patients of this reluctance to stop life support. The first and most obvious is patient overtreatment. Life-sustaining treatment will be continued beyond the point at which it is reasonable to believe that the patient either is benefitted by or still wants or would want the treatment. This is wasteful of what is commonly very costly care, but more important it fails to respect the patient's self-determination while often inflicting unnecessary emotional distress on patients, families and others.

The less obvious effect is at least as serious. A very common fear of patients, families, and physicians is that the patient will be "stuck on machines." To avoid this outcome, parties involved in decisionmaking may be reluctant to try life-sustaining treatment when its benefits are highly uncertain. This has the effect of denying life-sustaining treatment to some patients for whom it would have proved to be of genuine and substantial benefit and is indeed a serious harmful consequence of the reluctance to stop life support once it is in place. All parties should be much more willing than is now common to employ time-limited trials of therapies such as ventilator support, in which it is clearly understood that the trial, if unsuccessful, can be terminated, so as to allay this otherwise reasonable fear of patients and families of losing control of treatment and being stuck on machines.

It is worth adding that if the difference between stopping and not starting a life-sustaining treatment is thought to be of moral significance, it is then important how some common cases are to be classified. For example, with any therapy that involves multiple courses of treatment over time, such as dialysis or many medications, a decision to forego further treatment plausibly might be construed either as stopping the overall course of treatment or as not starting the next course of dialysis or dose of medication. That such cases might be plausibly interpreted either as stopping or not starting should give further pause about resting much moral importance on which is done.

Killing and Allowing to Die

The distinction between stopping and not starting a life-sustaining treatment corresponds in general to the distinction between acts and omissions leading to death. Ambiguities also abound about whether decisions to forego a life-sustaining treatment should be classified as an act or an omission. Does the postive decision make what happens an action, or the content of the decision not to start a treatment make it an omission? However these distinctions are more precisely drawn, if there is no moral importance to whether a life-sustaining treatment is stopped or not started, then it would seem to follow that it is not morally significant on this view whether it is an act or omission of the physician that leads to death. This implication has been explicitly accepted in some recent influential commentaries and court decisions (Barber and Nedjl 1983; Conroy 1985, Wanzer et. al. 1984). Yet the distinction between acts and omissions leading to death is also commonly understood to be the basis for the distinction between killing and allowing to die. Some have gone on to accept, or to explicitly argue, that killing is in itself no different morally than allowing to die, though of course many or most actual acts of killing are morally worse all things considered than most cases of allowing to die (Glover 1977; Steinbock 1980).

While this view has been increasingly widely accepted by philosophers and bioethicists, many health-care personnel, patients, and their families strongly resist it. For many, that killing is both wrong and also worse than allowing to die is a deeply and powerful held view. But the positive decision actively to turn off a life-sustaining treatment like a respirator seems to be an action, not an omission, leading to death, and so in this view is considered a killing, not a case of allowing to die. This line of reasoning uncovers a more general concern about whether all stopping of life support is killing and therefore morally wrong. In assessing this question it is important to be clear, first, about the meaning of the claim that killing is *in itself* no different morally than allowing to die. The claim is that the mere fact that one case is an instance of killing, another of allowing to die, does not make one any worse morally than the other, or make one justified or permissible but the other not. This is not to say that any particular instance of killing may not all things considered be morally worse than some instance of allowing to die. It is to say that if the killing is worse it will be because of its other properties such as the motives of the killer, whether the victim consented, and so forth, that differentiate it morally from the particular instance of allowing to die. Secondly, it is important to distinguish whether common instances of stopping life support should be understood as killing or as allowing to die from whether, if they are killings, they are for that reason morally wrong. Most commentators who have argued that stopping life-sustaining treatment is killing have insisted as well that it is not therefore wrong; some killing, including stopping life support, can be morally permissible and justified.

Are standard cases of stopping life-sustaining treatment killing or allowing to die (Brock 1986; Rachels 1975)? A physician who stops a respirator at the voluntary request of a clearly competent patient who is terminally ill and undergoing unrelievable suffering would commonly be understood by all involved as allowing the patient to die, with the patient's underlying disease the cause of death. If done with the consent of the patient, and with the intent of respecting his self-determination while promoting his well-being as he conceives it, it would be held by many to be morally justified. Let us agree that it can be morally justified, but is it allowing to die? Suppose the patient has a greedy nephew who stands to inherit his money and who has become impatient for the old man to die so that he will get the money. Thinking that his uncle is prepared to continue on the respirator indefinitely, he slips into the room, turns off the respirator, and his uncle dies. The nephew is found out, confronted, and replies, "I didn't kill him, I merely allowed him to die; his underlying disease caused his death." Surely this would be dismissed as specious nonsense. The nephew killed his uncle. However, it is plausible that he did exactly what the physician did in the other case. Both acted in a manner that caused the patient's death, expected it to do so, and might have performed the very same bodily movements in doing so. Of course, the physician acts with a different and proper motive, with the patient's consent, and in a professional role in which he is socially and legally authorized to carry out the patient's wishes concerning treatment. These differences in motive, consent and social role make what he does, but not what the nephew does, morally justified. That is not to say, however, that what he does, and whether he kills or allows to die, is any different from the nephew, only that his killing was justified while the nephew's was not. This general line of reasoning, then, accepts that standard cases of stopping life-sustaining treatment can sometimes be correctly understood as killing, but rejects any inference that they therefore must be wrong.

One explanation of why this account is resisted is that many physicians and others use the concept of killing as a normative concept to refer to unjustified actions causing death. In this view, killing may occur in medicine accidentally or negligently, but physicians do not knowingly and deliberately kill their patients. Yet, of course, physicians do stop life support in cases like the above and believe, quite rightly, that they can be justified in doing so. Thus, there is a powerful motive to understand what is done as allowing to die, not as killing. Common though this way of thinking may be, in this analysis it appears confused. It is a mistake to suppose that all killing must be unjustified, either morally or in the law. Killing in self-defense is an example outside of medicine, and stopping life support appears to be one within medicine.

There is another explanation of why standard cases of stopping life support are thought to be allowing to die and not killing. In the case of a terminally ill patient, a lethal disease process is already present. A life-sustaining treatment like a respirator may then be thought of as holding back or blocking the normal progress of the patient's disease. Removing that artificial intervention is then conceived of as standing aside and allowing the patient to die by letting the disease process proceed unimpeded to death. This may be a plausible explanation of why stopping life support is commonly understood to be allowing to die, but if it is to be any more than a metaphorical account, it must at the least explain why the nephew does not also allow to die. It is not clear how this is to be done consistent with the way killing and allowing to die are distinguished over a broad range of cases. It is worth adding that even understanding stopping life support as allowing to die along these lines, it remains possible still to argue that killing is in itself not morally different from allowing to die, though we shall not pursue that argument further here.

Is Foregoing Life Support Suicide?

Parallel to the concern that stopping life support is killing and therefore wrong is the concern that any foregoing of life support is suicide or assisted suicide and therefore wrong. Courts in particular try to distinguish foregoing life support from suicide, probably in significant part to insulate physicians, families and other health-care personnel from possible liability under laws prohibiting assisting in a suicide. The recent New Jersey Supreme Court decision in Conroy summarizes well the reasoning of many courts and others:

> . . . Declining life-sustaining medical treatments may not properly be viewed as an attempt to commit suicide. Refusing medical intervention merely allows the disease to take its natural course; if death were eventually to occur, it would be the result, primarily, of the underlying disease, and not the result of a self-inflicted injury. In addition, people who refuse life-sustaining medical treatment may not harbor a specific intent to die, rather, they may fervently wish to live, but to do so free of unwanted medical technology, surgery, or drugs, and without protracted suffering. . . . Recognizing the right of a terminally ill person to reject medical treatment respects that person's intent, not to die, but to suspend medical intervention at a point consonant with the "individual's view respecting a personally preferred manner of concluding life." The difference is between self-infliction or self-destruction and self-determination (Conroy 1985).

Although this way of distinguishing foregoing life support from suicide may seem plausible, it is at least problematic in some cases. The judgment of a person who competently decides to commit suicide is essentially that "my expected future life, under the best conditions possible for me, is so bad that I judge it to be worse than no further continued life at all." This seems to be in essence exactly the same judgment that some persons who decide to forego life-sustaining treatment make. The refusal of life-sustaining treatment is their means of ending their life; they intend to end their life because of its grim prospects. Their death now when they otherwise would not have died *is* self-inflicted, whether they take a lethal poison or disconnect a respirator. There need be, of course, no underlying lethal disease process present when a person commits suicide, whereas there must be when life-sustaining treatment is refused, but that is no reason to think that a person subject to a lethal disease process therefore could not commit suicide.

The Court's reasoning distinguishes some but not all cases of foregoing life-sustaining treatment from suicide, though it should be adequate to protect all instances from falling under legal statutes concerning suicide. Even if at least some instances of foregoing life-sustaining treatment are suicide that is no reason to conclude that they are morally wrong. The very same reasoning offered earlier in support of a competent patient's moral right to refuse any life-sustaining medical treatment will, of course, apply in these cases in which doing so may be suicide. The patient's self-determination and well-being support the moral permissibility of his or her declining any life-sustaining treatment, including any instance that might reasonably be construed as suicide. Cases of competent decisions to decline life-sustaining treatment that constitute suicide are commonly instances of rational and morally permissible suicide.

Ordinary and Extraordinary Treatment

A different way of distinguishing some foregoing of life support as impermissible is to hold that while extraordinary treatment can be permissibly foregone, ordinary treatment cannot be. This distinction has had special importance in cases of incompetent patients who are unable to decide about life support for themselves and so must have others decide for them. It is there often held that the surrogate decision-maker can decide to forego only extraordinary treatment for the patient. Many court decisions too have made reference to extraordinary treatment in endorsing the permissibility of foregoing life support, though often in passing and without any analysis of how ordinary and extraordinary treatment are to be distinguished.

There are two important questions regarding this distinction. First, what is the difference between treatments that the distinction is thought to mark? Second, is that difference of sufficient moral importance to mark a difference between the morally permissible and impermissible? With regard to the first question, it is clear that many different meanings have been intended. Among the differences that the distinction is thought to mark are: treatment that is usual, for example for a given condition, as opposed to unusual; treatment that employs high technology, artificial means as opposed to relatively simple means; treatment that is highly invasive as opposed to relatively noninvasive; treatment that is very costly as opposed to relatively inexpensive; treatment that is heroic in the sense of a long shot, last ditch attempt to keep the patient alive when other more ordinary means have failed.

Since there are so many interpretations of this distinction in use, confusion about what a particular user intends by it is inevitable unless its meaning is made explicit, as it usually is not. However, for any possible interpretation like those just mentioned, it is important to ask our second question: Why does this difference (for example, whether treatment employs high technology as opposed to relatively simple means) determine whether the treatment is morally justified, or whether foregoing it is morally permissible or impermissible. High-technology respirators or dialysis treatments sometimes promise benefits clearly outweighing any burdens of them so that a competent patient would choose them, while for another patient the life they continue may be of such limited duration and poor quality that the patient will competently choose to forego them. Why should it be at all morally important to whether the choice is justified that a treatment is common or unusual, employs high technology or is simple, is invasive or noninvasive, and so forth?

Instead, what is relevant is the overall balance of benefits and burdens of the treatment to the patient, according to the competent patient's own assessment, or the incompetent patient's surrogate's judgment of what the patient's assessment would have been if the patient were competent. Interpretations of the difference between ordinary and extraordinary treatment such as those noted above seem to appeal to differences that are not in themselves morally important, but instead are important only in so far as they affect the benefits and burdens of treatment to the patient.

It can be argued that all of these common and commonsense interpretations of the ordinary/extraordinary difference misunderstand it. The distinction probably originated within Roman Catholic moral theology where extraordinary treatment was understood, roughly, as treatment which was excessively burdensome for the patient (McCormack 1974). When treatment was judged by the patient (or by others acting as surrogates for an incompetent patient) to be excessively burdensome, then it was held that neither patient or surrogate were obliged to begin or continue it. But of course to determine whether a treatment is *excessively* burdensome it is necessary to weigh its burdens against whatever benefits it promises.

This interpretation of the ordinary/extraordinary difference simply appeals to the patient's assessment of the benefits and burdens of treatment and endorses the patient's right to refuse treatment he or she judges to be excessively burdensome. It thus can constitute no further moral constraint on a patient's right to refuse such treatment that it must be extraordinary and not ordinary. "Extraordinary treatment" is here only the label placed on treatment that has already and independently been assessed as excessively burdensome. The assessment of benefits and burdens, not any independent ordinary/extraordinary difference, is the criterion of whether any treatment is justified. "Ordinary" and "extraordinary" merely label the conclusions of that determination, but play no substantive role in making it. In this understanding, it is misleading to suppose that any list of treatments, some as ordinary, others as extraordinary, is possible which could help determine whether they should be employed with any particular patient. A treatment that is ordinary for one patient in particular circumstances can be extraordinary for another or for that same patient in different circumstances. While the ordinary/extraordinary distinction in this interpretation plays no positive or substantive role in an assessment whether to employ or to forego a treatment, its use does have one serious bad effect. The many possible and natural understandings of the ordinary/extraordinary distinction mean its use in decisionmaking about life support almost inevitably leads to confusion as different parties understand different things by it. It is for reasons of this sort that many recent commentators have concluded that, except within particular religious traditions where its meaning is clear, the distinction is unhelpful and best avoided in decisionmaking about life support (Conroy 1985; President's Commission 1983a).

Active Voluntary Euthanasia

If competent patients are morally entitled to refuse any life-sustaining treatment that they judge to be sufficiently burdensome, so as to make life no longer worth living with that treatment, are they also entitled in similar circumstances to have others, such as their physicians or family members, directly end their lives by administering a lethal injection or a poison? We have deliberately avoided until now using the term "euthanasia" because of its strong emotionally laden connotations, but it is this sort of active killing that is commonly understood as euthanasia. The very same values of patient well-being and self-determination that support a patient's right to refuse any life-sustaining treatment appear to support active voluntary euthanasia or direct killing in some circumstances as well. Does this show that if one accepts that foregoing life support is morally permissible, one must accept that this form of active voluntary euthanasia is permissible as well?

Some have argued that the case for active voluntary euthanasia can be strengthened further still by the argument from mercy (Rachels 1975). Consider the case of a terminally ill and imminently dying patient with a form of cancer that causes him very great and unrelievable suffering. With his competence not in question, the patient implores his physician to end his suffering by giving him a lethal poison. It seems cruelly perverse to hold that if a life-sustaining treatment were in place we should honor the patient's request to remove it and let him die, but that otherwise we cannot intervene and must leave him to suffer in pain until nature runs its course. How could any prohibition of voluntary euthanasia be morally justified if it prevents ending the excruciating suffering of great numbers of dying patients?

This argument from mercy for active voluntary euthanasia would be a powerful one indeed if its factual premises were true, but a crucial premise is false. There are not great numbers of patients undergoing severe suffering that can only be relieved by directly killing them. Modern methods of pain management enable physicians and nurses to control the pain of virtually all such patients without the use of lethal poisons, though often at the cost of so sedating the patient that interaction and communication with others is limited or no longer possible. The vast majority of cases in which such suffering is not relieved are due to wrongful failure to employ effective methods of available pain management, not to a prohibition of active voluntary euthanasia. Even if the unavoidable cost of a prohibition of active voluntary euthanasia is only exceedingly rarely the continuation of severe suffering, however, it does more commonly result in failure to respect the self-determination of patients who want their lives directly ended. This cost should not be lightly borne in a society such as our own that values self-determination highly in both its moral and legal traditions.

What reason is there to bear this cost by prohibiting active voluntary euthanasia? The most influential argument in support of maintaining this prohibition is the so-called "slippery slope" argument (Kamisar 1958). Even granting, so this argument goes, that there are a few cases in which such active killing might be justified, the consequences of socially and legally permitting it overall would nevertheless be bad. If we begin by permitting it in these few cases in which it is justified, we would inevitably end up permitting it in a great many other cases in which it would be wrong. It is the first step on the path to the Nazi policy of killing the old and weak and socially disfavored and must be firmly resisted. Since this path is slippery and steep, we must stay off it altogether.

What is to be made of this argument? If the factual claim is true that any relaxation of the prohibition of active euthanasia must inevitably lead to the Nazi's final solution, then all will agree that the prohibition must be firmly maintained. What is controversial, however, is whether this factual claim is true. We should have some reason or evidence for believing it, not the mere possibility that it might be true. Supporters of active voluntary euthanasia go on to urge that we have no serious reason to believe this claim. For example, we can and do make very clear and firm distinctions between voluntary and involuntary euthanasia; the values supporting the former in no way support the latter, and there is no significant reason to expect that permitting the former must inevitably lead to permitting the latter. This dispute is extremely difficult to resolve just because we possess very little evidence about the truth or falsity of the key factual claim in the argument. No one can reasonably deny the merest possibility that the claim might prove to be true, but on the other hand there is little persuasive evidence that in fact it is true.

There is at least some reasonable worry about possible abuse of an authorization of physicians or others to perform active voluntary euthanasia, even if it is not that it will lead to anything on the order of Nazism. Many frail and debilitated elderly who have become both financial and emotional burdens to others might be made increasingly vulnerable to having their lives wrongly ended by such an authorization. The magnitude of such risks is virtually impossible to estimate and, of course, depends on the exact form such authorizations take and the institutional safeguards built in against abuse. Besides such possible abuse, there are also the potential bad effects on the image of the medical profession, both the public's view and the profession's own view of itself. Public trust in the profession's commitment to fight with the patient against disease and death might be undermined if physicians also become "the angels of death." Physicians themselves might also find the role of euthanasiast in uneasy conflict with their role as medical caregivers to the sick and dying, even to an extent that it undermines their capacity to carry on effectively as caregivers to the dying.

The extent, if any, to which these bad effects would in fact occur from an authorization of active voluntary euthanasia is only speculative. Against these possible bad effects are the very real gains in self-determination and control over the process of dying that such an authorization would yield. Different persons can reasonably reach different conclusions about whether this tradeoff on balance argues in favor of or against permitting this form of euthanasia, but it would appear to be on this basis that the question ought to be decided.

Intended Versus Merely Foreseen Consequences

Some have seen a different issue at stake in active voluntary euthanasia. They argue that the intentional killing of innocent human beings is morally wrong, while actions from which a person's death is foreseen though not intended may sometimes be morally permissible (Fried 1978). This is the distinction embodied in the Roman Catholic Doctrine of Double Effect, sometimes also characterized as the difference between direct and indirect intention (Frey 1975). It is important not merely in its potential implications for active euthanasia but also for the issue of providing adequate relief of suffering to the dying. The following cases illustrate both implications. It sometimes happens that in the final stages of some terminal cancers adequate levels of medication (usually morphine) to control pain reach levels that risk depressing the patient's respiration and hastening his or her death. In such cases physicians often administer morphine at the patient's request with the intention or goal of relieving the patient's suffering, while foreseeing although not intending the patient's likely earlier death from respiratory depression. Virtually no physician, on the other hand, would give a lethal injection of strychnine at the patient's request to end the patient's suffering if morphine were unavailable or unavailing. Apart from what is legally permitted, is there an important moral difference between the two cases?

Many have thought that the difference lies in the physician's intentions. No fully adequate analysis exists of the concept of intention. Nevertheless, it does seem that the patient's earlier death is intended only in the morphine, not in the strychnine case. In each case, however, the physician's aim is to respond to the patient's request to end his suffering. The difference appears to be that in the strychnine case the means used to do so is to kill the patient; only through his death is the suffering ended. In the morphine case the administration of morphine is the means to the end of relieving the suffering while the earlier death is merely a foreseen side effect. The end sought is the same in each case, and the difference is that the death is the means to the end in one case and the foreseen consequence following the end in the other.

Can this difference be of sufficient moral importance to make the one morally permissible and the other prohibited? Many have argued that it cannot (Bennett 1981). In each case the physician's end or motive of relieving suffering at the request of the patient is the same. In each case it is causally impossible to end the patient's suffering without acting in a way that will cause his death. In each case both the patient and physician are prepared to end the suffering even at the cost of the patient's earlier death. The relief of suffering is judged to be of sufficient importance to justify acting in a way that leads to death. These seem to be the essential value judgments involved and they do not differ in the two cases. The difference in intention seems to be one of temporal structure—in one, the death precedes the end of relief of suffering, while in the other it temporally follows the end. It is hard to see why this difference in temporal structure should have much, or any, moral importance. It is tempting to reply that in the morphine case one would have given the morphine even if respiratory depression and death would not have followed, while the point of the strychnine was to cause death. However, if somehow strychnine would have relieved the suffering without causing death one would have still given it as well. In each case, in the circumstances that existed it was necessary to act in a way that the physician knew would lead to the patient's death in order to relieve his suffering.

There is a difference in the two cases in the certainty with which the earlier death will occur. It may never be certain that the dosage level of morphine is sufficient to cause death, and none would deny that this is a morally significant difference in the two cases. However, in some instances this difference in probability may be extremely small and so not support a great moral difference between the two cases. In any event, it is a difference in the risk of a bad outcome and not of intentions. Critics of this foreseen/intended distinction have argued that physicians are reasonably held equally morally responsible for all the foreseen consequences of their actions, whether or not intended, since all such consequences are under their control. In this perspective, in both cases it is a matter of weighing the relative benefits and burdens to the patient of relieving his suffering and shortening his life. If the patient judges that relief of suffering is paramount, the physician would be morally justified in acting in either the morphine or strychnine case. For the reason of public policy discussed above, it may be wise, nevertheless, not legally to authorize the performance of active voluntary euthanasia as in the strychnine case. It is important to emphasize that this would not be because the two cases are in themselves significantly different morally, but because of public policy concerns about the one and not the other. It is important to emphasize as well that the general right of the patient to decide about treatment does include the right to have adequate pain medication even if that may shorten his life. The relief of suffering is a longstanding, central, and fully legitimate aim of medicine.

SOME CASES OF SPECIAL POLICY CONCERN

Many of the issues addressed in this essay are of very great public and policy concern. We have sought above to cover the principal questions involved in the development of an overall ethical framework for decisions about life support. Of course, no such framework can be applied in any mechanical fashion to yield conclusions in particular cases. A framework is only that, and it must be applied with sensitivity and understanding to the unique features and details of any actual case. Nevertheless, the ethical framework should be applicable across the broad class of life-support cases. There are, however, two issues of special current concern that raise some questions not yet addressed: seriously ill newborns and life-sustaining nutrition and hydration.

Seriously Ill Newborns

Several cases of foregoing life support for seriously ill newborns have become front page news in recent years. Public and government attention was focused in this area a few years ago in the so-called "Baby Doe" case in Bloomington, Indiana, when an infant who suffered from Downs syndrome was allowed to die after its parents refused to permit surgery to repair its esophagus so that it could take nourishment. The federal government promulgated its "Baby Doe Rules," which went through extended negotiations and court challenges. These rules essentially require that all medically indicated treatment be provided to an infant unless the infant is irreversibly comatose, the treatment would merely prolong the dying of the infant and would be futile in terms of its survival, or the administration of the treatment would itself be virtually futile and inhumane. It is not yet clear how these proposed regulations will be interpreted or what their impact will be, but it is clear that their intent, both symbolic and for practice, was both to exclude the use of considerations about an infant's expected quality of life from decisions about its treatment and to seriously limit parents' and physicians' discretion in decisions to forego life support for such infants.

While the fundamental ethical framework developed above for life-support decisions generally applies to newborns, nevertheless, there are a few issues that are especially prominent with newborns (Singer and Kuhse 1986; Weir 1984). One is already implicitly noted in the proposed Baby Doe regulations. What role, if any, should the infant's expected quality of life play in decisions about treatment? As discussed earlier, a narrowly constrained role for quality-of-life considerations is inevitable if competent patients, or incompetent patients' surrogates, are to be free to decide whether a life-sustaining treatment and the life that it makes possible are on balance a benefit or excessively burdensome. Using this standard, the infant's prospects in relatively few cases will be so poor that it is reasonable to hold that continued life is clearly not in its interests. The clearest cases are probably when its life will be filled with substantial and unrelievable suffering and when the infant has suffered such severe brain damage as to preclude any significant social or environmental interaction. Other cases of very severe disabilities are more controversial and problematic, in part because of the wide variation in the weight adult patients give to such considerations and the fact that infants do not yet have preferences or values of their own.

A second issue is the relevance, if any, of the effects on others such as the parents of continued life support for the newborn. As a general matter our society rejects the involuntary sacrifice of one person's life for the benefit of others. The very high value we give to the protection of human life suggests that life-sustaining treatment for a seriously ill newborn should rarely if ever be foregone because of the burdens its continuing existence would place on others. Moral rights not to be killed are commonly understood to protect an individual from being killed, whatever the effects on others of the individual continuing to live. Nevertheless, it would be callously insensitive to deny the often overwhelming long-term burdens placed on the parents of these newborns, particulary in light of the often inadequate support services available to them. This issue reflects a fundamental difference between utilitarian moral conceptions, which weigh all the effects of a decision about treatment including the effects on others besides the patient, and moral rights conceptions, which exclude effects on others from consideration when a person's right to life is in question. As a practical matter, in most cases in which the parents judge the infant to be an excessive burden on them they have the alternative of giving it up for adoption.

A third issue concerns the moral status of infants. Should they be given the very same moral (and legal) protections as adults, particularly in light of common views on the moral permissibility of aborting fetuses. Birth seems a problematic point at which to draw a great moral difference in the moral permissibility of killing. Some commentators consider newborns closer morally to unborn fetuses than adults, or as somewhere between the two (Tooley 1983). Unborn fetuses, however, in this view are often considered replaceable and permissibly killed—for example, when found by amniocentesis to be defective—in order to try again for a normal pregnancy. This general issue concerns whether infanticide might be morally permissible in at least some circumstances in which killing an adult person would not be.

Finally, there is the policy issue of what review mechanisms, if any, are needed for parent's and physician's decisions to forego a life-sustaining treatment for a newborn. There are at least two important reasons to believe that conflicts of interest between seriously ill newborns and their parents may be more common than in most other cases of surrogate decisionmaking for incompetent patients.

First, the strong bonding that exists between parent and older child has not yet occurred with newborns, which can result in a weaker commitment of the parent to the infant's well-being. Second, the often enormous burdens of caring for the infant if life-sustaining treatment is continued will fall largely on the parents. Thus, serious conflicts of interest may be sufficiently likely in decisions to forego life-sustaining treatment of newborns to warrant some form of regular review, for example, by hospital ethics committees, so-called infant care review committees, or even the courts.

These are some of the issues of special importance in life-support decisions for newborns, but it bears emphasis that the fundamental ethical issues are not different from those with adults.

Life-Sustaining Nutrition and Hydration

The moral permissibility of a competent patient, or an incompetent patient's surrogate, deciding to forego treatments such as respirators or kidney dialysis has become fairly widely accepted by the public and health-care professionals, as well as in recent court decisions. More recently, concern has focused on the provision of artificial nutrition and hydration through the use of nasogastric tubes, intravenous lines, surgically inserted tubes, and so forth. Must nutrition and hydration, or food and water, always be continued or may it too permissibly be foregone (Lynn 1986)?

If nutrition and hydration are considered part of treatment, the same ethical framework discussed above for other kinds of life support can be applied to them. That framework calls for an assessment of the benefits and burdens to the patient of continuing nutrition and hydration as opposed to discontinuing it. For nearly all patients that assessment will favor continuing them, but in a few cases it need not do so (Lynn and Childress 1983). The process of providing nutrition and hydration can itself involve substantial ineliminable burdens for patients—for example, when patients' disease states makes taking in nutrition the cause of significant discomfort or when patients' dementia and resultant confusion requires physically restraining them to prevent their removing feeding tubes. In a very few other cases the quality of the life continued by nutrition and hydration may be substantially and unalterably burdensome to patients. Against possible burdens of continuing nutrition and hydration must be weighed the benefits and burdens of continuing it. For most patients, discontinuing nutrition and hydration would result in substantial subjective distress and likely not be in their interests even if death might otherwise be welcomed to them. Once again, however, for a few patients in the final stages of certain terminal diseases or in a persistent vegetative state in which all conscious experience is irretrievably lost, withholding nutrition and hydration and their resulting death by starvation or dehydration does not result in significant suffering. It bears repeating that the assessment of the benefits and burdens to a particular patient of continuing life-sustaining nutrition and hydration will in the vast majority of cases favor doing so, but there can be no assurance that this must always be so.

This conclusion has been challenged on several grounds: (1) human life is of infinite value and so deliberately shortening it can never be a benefit to the victim;

(2) a patient's choice to forego food and water is suicide and therefore wrong; and (3) life is a gift of God that we are not at liberty to destroy. We shall not pursue these objections in any detail here. The first two are really general challenges to foregoing any life support, not nutrition and hydration in particular, and so understood have already been addressed. The third appeals to religious views which could quite properly guide the choices of those individuals who share the particular religous faith, but should not form the basis for public policy in a pluralistic society.

A further concern about permitting the foregoing of nutrition and hydration centers on its symbolic effect together with worries about abuse (Siegler and Weisbard 1985). The provision of food and water is one of the very first acts of concern and support each person receives as he or she enters the world. Throughout life, feeding the hungry is properly invested with great moral importance, and starvation is associated with suffering and strong moral repugnance. This deep concern with not permitting suffering or death from starvation in general serves us well and, in this view, we should be extremely reluctant to do any thing that might weaken it. This is especially so since many of those who might be endangered by any weakening of the requirement to provide food and water are debilitated and vulnerable, unable to protect themselves and to assert their own interests. Permitting the withholding of food and water risks the deliberate killing of the vulnerable and burdensome on morally unacceptable grounds such as the economic costs of sustaining their lives. Moreover, many see any withholding of food and water as only a very small step from active voluntary or even unvoluntary euthanasia and oppose the former for fear that it will inevitably lead to the latter.

Like all "slippery slope" arguments based on a worry about potential abuse of a specific authorization, reasonable persons may disagree on several counts. Is it possible to discriminate clearly between cases in which withholding food and water is morally justified from those in which it is not? What procedures for making such decisions would provide the most effective safeguards against abuse? Given such procedures, how likely are abuses and are they sufficiently serious to outweigh the benefits of permitting withholding food and water that is excessively burdensome to the patient? Courts that have addressed the issue of withholding nutrition and hydration have been sensitive to the need for procedures with strong safeguards against abuse, but have nonetheless generally held that artificial measures for provision of nutrition and hydration are not in principle different than other treatments such as respirators that artificially provide oxygen to the patient (Barber and Nedjl 1983; Conroy 1985). All fall under a patient's general moral and legal right to decide about and to refuse any medical treatment.

CONCLUSION

We have sought in this chapter to address many of the most difficult and troubling ethical issues arising in decisions about life-sustaining treatment. Many of those issues are complex and no widespread agreement yet exists on them. We shall let the discussion of those issues in the body of the essay stand on its own and not attempt to summarize it here. There is, however, a central core of widespread agreement that is worth repeating and underlining. A competent patient, or an incompetent patient's surrogate, is ethically entitled to assess the benefits and burdens of any proffered treatment according to the patient's own aims and values and to accept or reject the treatment. The quite broad agreement on this seemingly simple principle should in no way be taken to imply, however, that the decisions themselves in concrete cases are simple or uncontroversial for those involved in them. There is much truth in the view that the particular circumstances and details of each case make it unique. No simple principles can be mechanically applied in a way that makes for easy choices. Decisions about life and death are inevitably and quite properly difficult and troubling and require sensitive, thoughtful and wise judgment from all involved.

REFERENCES

Barber and Nedjl v. Superior Court. 195 Cal. Rptr. 484 (Cal. App. 2 Dist.) 1983.

Bayer, R., et al. "The Care of the Terminally Ill: Morality and Economics." *N Eng J Med* 309 (15 Dec. 1983): 1490–1494.

Bennett, J. "Morality and Consequences." In *The Tanner Lectures in Human Value II*, edited by S. M. McMurrin. Salt Lake City: University of Utah Press, 1981.

Brock, D. W. "Foregoing Food and Water: Is It Killing?" In *Foregoing Life-Sustaining Food and Water*, edited by J. Lynn. Bloomington: Indiana University Press, 1986.

Buchanan, A., and Brock, D. "Deciding for Others." *The Milbank Quarterly* 64, Suppl. 2, (1986): 17–94.

Capron, A. M. "The Authority of Others to Decide About Biomedical Interventions with Incompetents." In *Who Speaks for the Child?* edited by W. Gaylin and R. Macklin. New York: Plenum Press, 1982.

Capron, A. M., and Kass, L. "A Statutory Definition of the Standards for Determining Human Death: An Appraisal and a Proposal." *U Penn Law Rev* 87 (1972): 102–104.

In re Conroy. 486 A.2d 1209 (N.J. 1985).

Drane, J. "The Many Faces of Competency." *Hastings Cent Rep* 15, no. 2 (April 1985): 17–21.

Dworkin, G. *The Theory and Practice of Autonomy.* Cambridge, Mass.: Cambridge University Press, 1988.

Fost, N., and Cranford, R. "Hospital Ethics Committees: Administrative Aspects." *JAMA* 253, no. 18 (10 May 1985): 2687–2692.

Frey, R. "Some Aspects to the Doctrine of Double Effect." *Can J Philos* (1985): 259–283.

Fried, C. *Right and Wrong.* Cambridge, Mass.: Harvard University Press, 1978.

Glover, J. *Causing Death and Saving Lives.* New York: Penguin Books, 1977.

Green, M., and Wikler, D. "Brain Death and Personal Identity." *Philosophy and Public Affairs* 9 (1980): 105–133.

Kamisar, Y. "Some Non-Religious Views Against Proposed Mercy Killing Legislation." *Minnesota Law Review* 42 (1958).

Kass, L. *Toward A More Natural Science: Biology and Human Affairs.* New York: Free Press, 1985.

Katz, J. *The Silent World of Doctor and Patient.* New York: Free Press, 1984.

Lynn, J., *Foregoing Life-Sustaining Food and Water.* Bloomington: University of Indiana Press, 1986.

Lynn, J., and Childress, J. "Must Patients Always Be Given Food and Water?" *Hastings Cent Rep* 13 (1983): 17–21.

McCormack, R. "To Save or Let Die: The Dilemma of Modern Medicine." *JAMA* 229 (1974): 172–176.

President's Commission for Ethical Problems in Medicine. *Defining Death.* Washington, D.C.: Government Printing Office, 1981.

————. *Making Health Care Decisions.* Washington, D.C.: Government Printing Office, 1982.

————. *Deciding to Forego Life-Sustaining Treatment.* Washington, D.C.: Government Printing Office, 1983a.

————. *Securing Access to Health Care.* Washington, D.C.: Government Printing Office, 1983b.

In re Quinlan. 70 N.J. 10, 355 A. 2d 647 (1976).

Rachels, J. "Active and Passive Euthanasia." *N Engl J Med* 292 (9 Jan. 1975): 78–80.

Rosner, F. "Hospital Medical Ethics Committees: A Review of Their Development." *JAMA* 253 (1985): 2693–2697.

Sider, R., and Clements, C. "The New Medical Ethics: A Second Opinion." *Arch Intern Med* 145, no. 12 (1985): 2169–2171.

Siegler, M. "Searching for Moral Certainty in Medicine: A Proposal for a New Model of the Doctor-Patient Encounter." *Bull NY Acad Med* 57 (1981).

Siegler, M., and Weisbard, A. "Against the Emerging Stream." *Arch Intern Med* 145 (1985): 129–131.

Singer, P., and Kuhse, H. *Should This Baby Live?* New York: Oxford University Press, 1986.

Steinbock, B., ed. *Killing and Letting Die.* Englewood Cliffs, N.J.: Prentice-Hall, 1980.

Tooley, M. *Abortion and Infanticide.* Oxford, England: Oxford University Press, 1983.

Veatch, R. "The Whole-Brain Oriented Concept of Death: An Out-Moded Philosophical Formulation." *J Thanatology* 13 (1975).

Wanzer, S. et al. "The Physicians' Responsibility Toward Hopelessly Ill Patients." *N Engl J Med* 310, no. 15 (12 April 1984): 955–959.

Weir, R. *Selective Non-Treatment of Handicapped Newborns.* New York: Oxford University Press, 1984.

DISCUSSION QUESTIONS

1. What criteria for death should be used for anencephalics or patients in a persistent vegetative state? Are they dead based on whole brain concepts of death? On higher brain concepts of death?

2. When, if ever, should life be prolonged on competent patients against their wishes? Why?

3. Is there any morally significant difference between starting a treatment such as a ventilator and stopping one once it has been started? Should physicians have an obligation to "withdraw" treatment when patients or surrogates withdraw their consent to it? Should they have to "pull the plug?"

4. In what cases and to what extent should it be required to involve others, i.e., institutional review boards, ethics committees, the courts, in the surrogate decisionmaking process?

5. What are the the medical and moral differences, if any, between killing and allowing to die, withholding and withdrawing treatment, euthanasia and suicide?

GLOSSARY OF TERMS

A priori   derived from self-evident proposition

Anencephalic   literally the condition of having no encephalon or brain (normally applied to infants with no cerebrum)

Anorexia nervosa   an eating disorder characterized by persistent, health-threatening loss of appetite

Antinomianism   the position that ethical action is determined independent of law or rules; cf. situationalism, rules of practice, legalism

Autonomy   the governing of one's self according to one's own system of morals and beliefs

Beneficence   the state of doing or producing good; cf. nonmaleficence

Best Interest Standard   judgment based on an idea of what would be most beneficial to a patient; cf. substituted judgment

Ceteris paribus   other things being equal; if all other conditions are the same

Chemotherapy   a form of treatment that consists in the use of chemicals to control disease

Consequentialism   the normative theory that the rightness or wrongness of actions is determined by anticipated or known consequences, cf. deontologism

Covenant   a solemn agreement between two or more parties

De facto   in reality, actual; cf. de jure

De jure   by right, by law; cf. de facto

Deontologism   a theory according to which actions are judged right or wrong based upon inherent right-making characteristics or principles rather than on their consequences

Double Effect, the Doctrine of   the theory that an evil effect is morally acceptable provided a proportional good effect will accrue, evil is not intended, the evil effect is not the means to the good, and the action is not intrinsically evil

Dyspepsia   indigestion

Egalitarian   a social philosophy that advocates human equality

Euthanasia   the merciful hastening of death, often limited to willful and merciful actions to kill of one who is injured or terminally ill

Fatuity   something foolish

Fidelity   the state of being faithful

Germ line   the cells which constitute gametes or reproductive cells

Gesisah   the state of being that immediately precedes death and during which, according to the Jewish faith, one ought not to intervene to interfere with the dying process

Histocompatible   the condition in which tissues will not react to produce a rejection during transplantation

Human Immunodeficiency-Virus (HIV)   a retrovirus responsible for acquired immune deficiency syndrome (AIDS)

Hypochondriasis   morbid concern about one's health

Immunodeficiency   the state of sub-standard expression of the immune system

Immunosuppression	that state of inhibiting the expression of the immune system
Intubation	the insertion of a tube into an organ
Legalism	the position that ethical action consists in strict conformity to law or rules; cf. antinomianism, rules of practice, situationalism
Macroallocation	the distribution of resources on a large scale
Maternal Serum Alpha-Fetoprotein	a protein secreted during gestation used to predict fetal abnormalities such as spina bifida
Metaethics	the branch of ethics having to do with the meaning and justification of ethical terms and norms
Metaphysical	the principles underlying a particular subject or system of beliefs
Microallocation	distribution of resources on a small scale
Nontherapeutic	something which does not serve the purposes of benefitting an individual patient
Nonmaleficence	the state of not doing harm or evil; cf. beneficence
Normative	the branch of ethics having to do with standards of right or wrong; cf. metaethics
Normativism	the doctrine that moral standards or norms determine the rightness or wrongness of actions
Null hypothesis	in scientific research, the hypothesis that there exists no difference in the effect of two or more treatments
Parentalism	the system of action in which one person treats another the way a parent treats a child, striving to promote the other's good even against the other's wishes; cf. autonomy, paternalism
Pareto Optimality	the system of distribution whereby pairs of individuals are permitted to make exchanges until no pairs are willing to make further exchanges thus leaving all parties as well off as possible without violating the interests of any party
Pareto Improvement	additions to aggregate good brought about by exchanges between pairs of individuals in which each believes his or her welfare increases
Paternalism	the system of action in which one person treats another the way a father treats a child striving to promote the other's good even against the other's wishes; cf. parentalism
Persistent vegetative state	a state of brain pathology in which the brain stem is intact but there is no content to consciousness; characterized by a state of profound dementia which is associated with a loss of awareness and ability to interact with the environment
Prima facie	all things being the same
Pythagorean	of or relating to the theories and beliefs of the Greek philosopher, Pythagorus
Randomized Clinical Trial (RCT)	A scientific research design in which treatment varies for two or more groups selected at random
Renal Dialysis	treatment by the use of an artificial kidney machine
Rules of Practice	the position that rules govern practices such that actions are normally judged by rules; cf. antinomianism, situationalism, legalism
Schizophrenia	a psychotic disorder characterized by personality disintegration and distortion in the perception of reality
Secular Ethics	theories of what is good and bad, or right or wrong, based on criteria other than religious doctrine

Seropositivity	the state of positive results of a study of antigen-antibody reactions in vitro
Situationalism	the position that ethical action must be judged in each situation guided by, but not directly determined by, rules; cf. antinomianism, rules of practice, situationalism
Somatic	all cells other than germ line cells
Substituted judgment standard	the standard of judgment based on an estimation of what an individual would have chosen
Surrogate	someone serving as a substitute decisionmaker
Taxonomy	a system of classification
Teleological	explaining phenomena by their design, purpose, or final causes
Therapeutic	relating to therapy
Therapy	the provision of remedies in the treatment of disorders or illnesses
Utilitarian	the view that an action is deemed morally acceptable because it produces the greatest balance of good over evil taking into account all individuals affected
Utility	the state of being useful or producing good
Vertigo	dizziness; confusion
Virtue	a persistent trait of good character

INDEX

neonatal screening, 213
prenatal diagnosis, 213–214
Gert, B., 59–60, 68, 180, 260, 265
Gibbard, A., 320
Gilligan, C., 45
Glover, J., 225, 342
Golden Rule, 32–33
Goldman, Emma, 99
Gomer, R., 137
Gordon, L., 98, 99
Graber, G. C., 86
Grady, D., 150
Graebner, W., 86
Green, M., 248, 332
Greene, B., 155–156
Gregory, John, 9
Griswold v. Connecticut, 96, 100–101
Grossman, M., 269
Gury, J., 99
Gutman, A., 318
Guttmacher, S., 37

Halevi, Yehuda, 14
Hammer, R. E., 221
Haney, R., 98
Harm principle, limitation of freedom, 275–276
Harris, G. W., 116
Harris, J., 245
Harris, L., 179
Harrison, M., 159, 241
Harris v. McRae, 117–118
Hauerwas, S., 219
Health care
"adequate" care, 247
in American society, 51–52
market model for, 246
"rights" approach to, 248
right to, 306, 321
beneficence over justice position, 323–325
decent minimum level of care position, 319–321
egalitarian approach, 318–319
equality of opportunity based theory, 314–317
features of "right," 307
justice based theory, 312–314
libertarian approach, 310–312
President's Commission approach (1983), 319–320, 321–322
utilitarian approach, 308–310

Health care resources
meaning of, 293
See also Allocation of health-care resources.
Health and disease
and American society, 51–53
and medical domain, 53–54
normativist view, 60–61
relationship between, 54–55
statistical approach, 57
value-free aspects, 56–57
Health and Human Services, Department of
institutional assurance system, human research, 146–148
policy for protection of human research subjects, Appendix 2, 165–172
Helmholz, R., 97
Heyd, D., 271
Heymann, R., 101
Hippocratic Oath, 7–9, 141
on abortion, 111
Christian version, 9
content of, 8
criticisms of, 9
origins of, 7, 8
Hock, R. A., 220
Hoffmeister, B., 239
Holder, A. R., 278, 280
Hollender, M. H., 69
Hough, D., 86
Human experimentation
American regulations, 129–131
bioethical principles and
beneficence, 140–142
justice, 142–145
respect for competent persons, 137–139
respect for incompetent persons, 139–140
concentration camps, 129, 131, 137, 143, 145–146
definitional aspects
benefits to others, 135
human subject, 167
interaction, 167
minimal risk, 167
practice, 132, 133–134, 135
private information, 167
research, 132–133, 135, 167
therapeutic vs. nontherapeutic research, 134–135